Self Assessment and Review of

PLASTIC SURGERY

Rajiv Agarwal

MBBS MS (Gen Surg) DNB (Gen Surg) MCh (Plast Surg) DNB (Plast Surg)
Recipient of Indian National Science Academy 'Young Scientist' National award
Professor,
Department of Plastic Surgery,
King George's Medical University, Lucknow, UP, India

Ramesh Chandra

MS (Gen Surg) MS (Plast Surg) FRCS (Eng)
Recipient of Dr BC Roy National Award
Past President—Association of Plastic Surgeons of India
Former Professor and Head, Department of Plastic Surgery,
Former Principal and Dean,
King George's Medical College, Lucknow, UP, India

Forewords by

Kenneth E Salyer, USA
Marita Eisenmann-Klein, Germany
K Mathangi Ramakrishnan, India

JAYPEE BROTHERS MEDICAL PUBLISHERS (P) LTD

New Delhi • Panama City • London • Dhaka • Kathmandu

Jaypee Brothers Medical Publishers (P) Ltd

Headquarters
Jaypee Brothers Medical Publishers (P) Ltd
4838/24, Ansari Road, Daryaganj
New Delhi 110 002, India
Phone: +91-11-43574357
Fax: +91-11-43574314
Email: jaypee@jaypeebrothers.com

Overseas Offices
J.P. Medical Ltd
83, Victoria Street, London
SW1H 0HW (UK)
Phone: +44-2031708910
Fax: +02-03-0086180
Email: info@jpmedpub.com

Jaypee-Highlights Medical Publishers Inc.
City of Knowledge, Bld. 237, Clayton
Panama City, Panama
Phone: +507-301-0496
Fax: +507-301-0499
Email: cservice@jphmedical.com

Jaypee Brothers Medical Publishers (P) Ltd
17/1-B Babar Road, Block-B, Shaymali
Mohammadpur, Dhaka-1207
Bangladesh
Mobile: +08801912003485
Email: jaypeedhaka@gmail.com

Jaypee Brothers Medical Publishers (P) Ltd
Shorakhute, Kathmandu
Nepal
Phone: +00977-9841528578
Email: jaypee.nepal@gmail.com

Website: www.jaypeebrothers.com
Website: www.jaypeedigital.com

Inquiries for bulk sales may be solicited at: jaypee@jaypeebrothers.com

Self Assessment and Review of Plastic Surgery

First Edition: **2013, Reprint: 2026**

ISBN : 978-93-5090-317-9

Printed in India

TRIBUTES

I (RC) would like to pay my special tributes to my parents, Dr BR Agarwal and Mrs SD Agarwal for their support, guidance, all the love and care all through my life. I am indebted to my teachers for having shaped my career—Prof SC Mishra, Prof RV Singh, Prof A Charan, Prof RN Sharma, Prof PC Dubey, Prof NC Misra, Prof GP Agarwal from the department of surgery besides Prof BN Sinha and Prof MK Goel from the department of orthopaedics. I owe my special gratitude to Prof Bruce Bailey of Aylesbury for his guidance and support to me during my stay in UK and to Prof RN Sharma, my mentor for shaping my career in plastic surgery.

FOREWORD

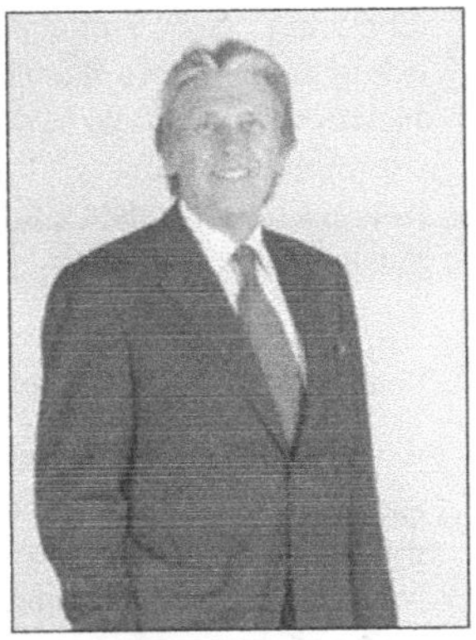

Rajiv Agarwal and Ramesh Chandra have produced a new 'Self Assessment and Review of Plastic Surgery' book for all students and scholars of plastic surgery interested in furthering their expertise in plastic surgery through studying and taking this multiple-choice examination. These authors published a book in 2002 which was favorably reviewed by the Journal of plastic and reconstructive surgery. Because of its high demand and the enthusiastic response for an updated expanded version these authors have compiled over 1000 multiple-choice questions in 8 categories of the specialty of plastic and reconstructive surgery. Its purpose is to provide for those interested in entrance examinations in plastic surgery and also exit examination or certification examinations in plastic surgery. Although there are a few other books available for study there is just one by the name of plastic surgery review published by WB Saunders Company. The authors felt there was a huge demand for a book of this nature in India and they feel that this broad-based multiple-choice question examination will be used by many others located throughout the globe interested in refining their knowledge and skill in taking multiple-choice examination in plastic surgery and broadening their knowledge base.

I was given a sample of questions from each of subspecialty sections and found these diverse and helpful. The design of answering the questions after a few questions with annotated references should provide a framework for detailed study of the various topics and questions which they have created. Although many of these questions seem straightforward and simple, they have provided answers which to some degree are all correct but there is one which is the answer for each question. Used properly students could achieve improvement in their knowledge while also practicing and learning the skill of multiple-choice examinations. This should serve as a useful additional tool for study by all those interested in plastic surgery examinations. The use of photographs is an added benefit in the examination process and is used today in various examinations for plastic surgery. I found the section of 51 questions on recent advances to be way too inadequate and short to cover the rapidly expanding recent knowledge base. I would encourage them to expand this section in there next edition to provide more updated expanded information.

Overall I find this to be a useful 'Self Assessment and Review of Plastic Surgery' book and think it should be in the hands of all students of plastic surgery.

Kenneth E Salyer MD
Founder and Chairman,
World Craniofacial Foundation,
Dallas Texas USA

FOREWORD

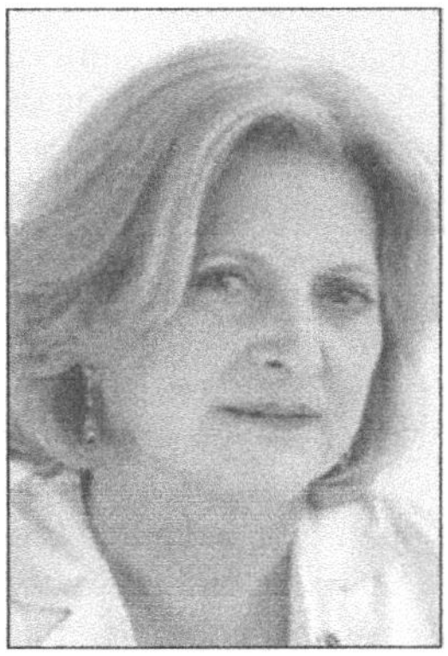

Choosing plastic surgery as a specialty means to commit yourself to treat all patients—babies, children, adults and seniors from head to toe. This is just one out of many fascinating aspects of our specialty. However, the variety of our beloved specialty becomes a big challenge, when it comes to preparing for an examination. Although trainees in plastic surgery experience much more exposure to our techniques than trainees in other fields, there are very few training centers which can provide adequate expertise in all the subspecialties.

While textbooks may give a basic insight, they cannot make the candidates feel well prepared for the challenge of an examination.

Therefore, with great joy, I recommend the new book of Professor Ramesh Chandra and Dr Rajiv Agarwal for trainees in plastic surgery. Studying questions and answers of previous examinations or, as in this case, fictive questions with profound explanations in their answers, is a very effective way to prepare for examinations. The insight, provided in this book, certainly will help the candidates to feel confident and well prepared for questions within all fields of plastic surgery, not only for those which they know from their daily work.

With the foundation of the IPRAS Trainees Association the International Confederation for Plastic Reconstructive and Aesthetic Surgery wants to create a forum for exchange and quality improvement in all aspects of plastic surgery training. Providing adequate tools for a successful examination is part of the program.

IPRAS thanks Prof Chandra and Dr Agarwal for contributing a tool to this ambitious project.

Marita Eisenmann-Klein
Prof hc Dr med Dr hc
President
International Confederation for
Plastic Reconstructive and Aesthetic Surgery

FOREWORD

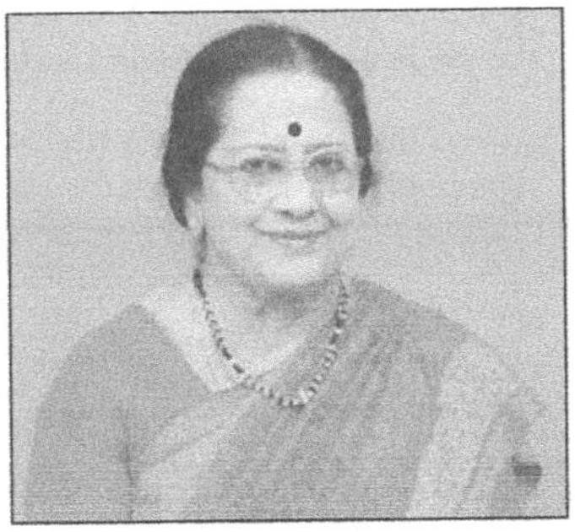

The concept of having a book on multiple choice questions "Self Assessment and Review of Plastic Surgery" in the super specialty of Plastic Surgery has been conceived by the former professor Dr Ramesh Chandra and his illustrious son Dr Rajiv Agarwal, the present professor is highly commendable. The current edition is the second book on the list. The editors have gone into great depth to formulate the questions, validate the important points and presented it in simple and explicit form to make the students understand.

In the group of super specialty plastic surgery assumes a very important place, particularly the topics on congenital malformations and reconstructions in head and neck. Inclusion of the recent and past developing surgical technique 'Robotics in Plastic Surgery' is highly appreciated. All the subdivisions have been dealt in a very concentrated manner.

This edition of the book must be in the armamentarium of every plastic surgeon who takes up postgraduation as well as seasoned teachers who need to get reaccredited to teach the students in an ongoing manner.

Prof **(Mrs) K Mathangi Ramakrishnan**

Chairperson, Childs Trust Medical Research foundation

Chief of Burns and Plastic Surgery Department

Kanchi Kamakoti Childs Trust Hospital

12–A, Nageswara Road,

Chennai–600 034. Tamil Nadu, India

Past President: National Academy of Burns

Past President: National Academy of Medical Sciences

Past President: Association of Plastic Surgeons of India

MESSAGE

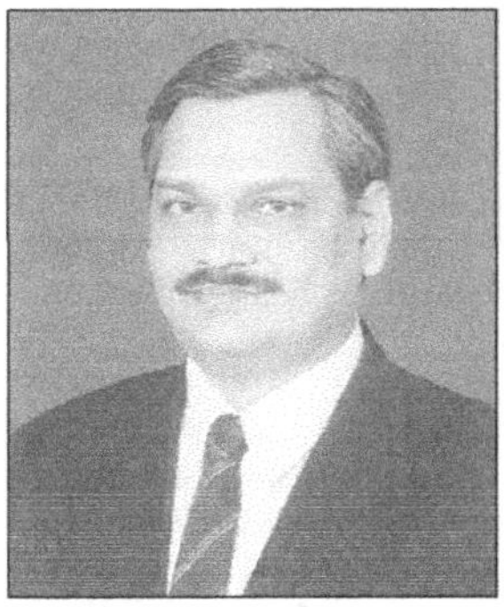

It is a pleasure to write a Message for the book on multiple choice questions in plastic surgery written by Dr Rajiv Agarwal and Dr Ramesh Chandra. They had earlier published a similar book in 2002.

This book "Self Assessment and Review of Plastic Surgery" is an updated version with the special feature that each question answer is referenced. An explanation for the answer has also been provided. It helps the person to understand the subject.

The book is comprehensive, covering all aspects of Plastic Surgery from history to the recent advances. The book will be an useful adjunct to both persons aspiring to enter the portals of Plastic Surgery and also for the already enrolled students.

I would strongly recommend this book as a teaching aid in Plastic Surgery.

A K Singh
Professor and Head,
Department of Plastic Surgery,
KG Medical University, Lucknow, UP, India
&
President
Association of Plastic Surgeons of India

PREFACE

Plastic Surgery is an amalgam of both science and art as these are the pillars of a successful plastic surgeon in achieving excellence, consistent results and harmony in performing this surgery. The classical textbooks and operative atlases help in understanding the core subject of plastic surgery while a book of this nature helps to train the reader in solving the multiple choice questions on the subject. The trend of giving such questions is on the rise over the last several years in examinations as these allow an in-depth assessment of the candidate which is totally objective precluding any bias which can hover on other methods of examination. Multiple choice questions in plastic surgery examination have become the norm for various entrance examinations, in-service examinations especially of the American boards and even passing out examination in plastic surgery in many national and international universities.

Currently very few books on multiple choice questions in plastic surgery exist in the market. These books often do not cover the vast expanse of the subject and leave many areas untouched. There was thus a genuine need among students, fellows, colleagues and established plastic and facial surgeons to develop a comprehensive text which is focussed on all the aspects of plastic surgery and which at the same time includes the key facts and knowledge of the subject which is relevant to the practice of plastic surgery. This book is an attempt to fill in this specific deficiency area and to provide the readers a comprehensive treatise of deft multiple choice questions which will not only test the knowledge of plastic surgery but will also assess the reader on his clinical skills and judgment based on the questions relating to clinical problems.

The subject matter of plastic surgery has been covered in a total of seven independent sections dealing with general principles, aesthetic surgery, head and neck, craniofacial and cleft, oncoplastic surgery, trunk and lower extremity and finally upper limb and hand surgery. This is followed by a section of multiple choice questions based on recent advances in plastic surgery. The questions have been based on various, notable publications in plastic surgery over the last ten years. The seven sections offer incisive questions based on the particular subject from the historical aspect to the intricacies of diagnosis and treatment. The last section on recent advances is an assortment of questions without any particular subject loyalty. This section will make the reader abreast with questions on the current advances in plastic surgery. To eliminate any type of ambiguity in the answer to the particular question item, each of the questions in this book has been supported by specific and complete references detailing the authors and the journal so that the reader can refer to these for more information on that particular question stem. All questions also have specific answers and explanations which will provide the reader a grasp of the particular point that has been raised and discussed in the subject stem. The answers, explanations and references follow at the end of each section so that the reader can turn the pages and review these at convenience while the answers also remain hidden from the eye at the time of reading the question item.

Plastic surgery is all about photographs and hence each section has also been augmented with succinct and unambiguous photograph based question items which would test the skill of the reader in clinical decision-making at the bedside.

Special care has been exercised in designing the question stems in this book. All the questions are single response correct type, meaning that only one answer is correct out of all the given options. Majority of the question items have a positive stem and the answers also have a positive response so that the candidates are not confused in attempting these questions. It has also been our endeavor to develop and design the answers in such a way that primarily on first look all of the options may appear to be correct. In fact most of the options or alternatives that are given after the question are correct to a certain degree but there is only one option which is 'most' correct. This type of designing of question items helps to maximally test the genuine candidate and especially helps in putting out those who rely on guess work while solving the questions. An attempt has also been made to give the options in such a way that no two options are contradictory to each other so that the candidate zeroes on these two options easily and decides between the two and leaves behind the rest. To further add value to the questions, we have made an attempt to avoid asking those questions whose answers end with numbers as these confuse the reader. It is submitted that while every attempt has been made to cross check the accuracy of the answers, in case of any ambiguity the reader is advised to refer to standard textbooks.

We hope that this work which has been based on our combined teaching experience of more than four decades in plastic surgery will prove useful and stimulating to the readers who will enrich their knowledge on the subject and will also help them in clearing the hurdle of examination in the discipline of not only plastic surgery but also allied specialities.

Rajiv Agarwal
drrajivagarwal@gmail.com

Ramesh Chandra
chandradoctorsclinic@gmail.com

ACKNOWLEDGMENTS

The authors are indebted to the following who have contributed in their own way to help reach this manuscript to its present standards.

Dr Abdul Halim, Former Professor and Head, Department of Anatomy and teacher of both the authors.

Dr SP Kharey, Former Director of Cancer Institute, Varanasi and Chief Medical Director, Railways and Professor Hospital Management for proof-reading and critical evaluation.

Prof Padam K Agarwal who has contributed immensely in the preparation of this book with her suggestions, ideas and proof-reading.

Dr AK Singh, Professor and Head, Department of Plastic Surgery, KG Medical University, Lucknow who has always supported in all our endeavors by his timely advise and guidance.

Colleagues in the department; Dr Vijay Kumar, Dr Brijesh Mishra and Dr Veerendra Prasad who have provided full support during this project. To all the residents of the department who have stimulated us to go for this new book namely Doctors Himanshu Saxena, Veena Kumari, Rimpi Jain, Saurabh Kr Gupta, Somshekhar G, Manish Jain, Rahul Kapoor, Prem Shanker, Shruti Patel and Varun Singla.

Dr Tulika Chandra, who has always supported and helped by taking over care of the children and other chores while the book was being prepared.

Dr Sanjeev Agarwal, FRCS (Orth) and Dr Jyoti Bansal, FRCR both consultants at the Cardiff University Hospital, UK who have been always at our side whenever we needed technical help and suggestions for this book.

Dr SC Mishra, Former Professor and Head ENT and Dr TC Goel, Former Professor of Surgery for encouragement and advise to produce such type of a book.

Our children, Devisha, Mallika, Rishabh, Suyash and Harshita who have undergone long periods of our absence and unavailability for them during the preparation of this book and have endeared and provided full moral support during the preparation of this book.

This book is dedicated to the senior colleagues in the Association of Plastic Surgeons of India and all over the world and the many students, fellows and residents who requested a book on this aspect to help them sail through the examinations in plastic surgery and other allied specialties.

Our thanks are due to Prof DK Gupta, Vice Chancellor, King George's Medical University, Lucknow for his blessings.

From the Publisher's Desk

We request all the readers to provide us their valuable suggestions/errors (if any) *at:*

jaypeemcqproduction@gmail.com

so as to help us in further improvement of this book in the subsequent edition.

CONTENTS

1

GENERAL PRINCIPLES

QUESTIONS

1. The earliest plastic surgery procedures for nose and earlobe reconstruction in the Before Christ era were performed in which of the following country?

A. Rome
B. France
C. India
D. United Kingdom

2. The famous text "Principalization of Plastic Surgery" elucidating knowing the ideal beautiful normal, to diagnose what is present, what is diseased, destroyed, displaced or distorted and what is in excess was authored by which of the following?

A. Harold D Gillies
B. D. Ralph Millard Jr
C. Thomas Kilner
D. Archibald McIndoe

3. The great ancient physician who wielded profound influence on the practice of medicine for 1500 years and made anatomic observations on the basis of animal experimentation was which of the following?

A. Michael Salmon
B. Carl Manchot
C. Galen
D. Sushruta

4. The earliest reference of plastic surgery procedures is described in which of the following?

A. Sushruta Samhita
B. De Humani Corporis Fabrica
C. Novum Organum
D. Principles of Plastic Surgery

5. The first successful human skin graft for covering the stump of an amputated thumb with skin from the amputated part was performed by which of the following?

A. Reverdin
B. Thiersch
C. Cooper
D. Ollier

6. Which one of the following study is considered as having the highest level of evidence in measuring outcomes after plastic surgery?

A. Case report with objective documentation
B. Prospective and retrospective cohort studies
C. Randomised controlled trial
D. Expert opinion

7. Which one of the following plastic surgeon won the noble prize for his work?

A. Harold Gillies
B. T.P Kilner
C. Paul Tessier
D. Joseph Murray

8. A malformation is defined as a morphologic defect of an organ, a part of an organ or a larger area of the body resulting from intrinsically abnormal development. Which of the following is a malformation?

A. Amniotic band syndrome
B. Cleft palate
C. Potter sequence
D. Ring constriction of finger

9. Which one of the following syndromes is associated with gynaecomastia?

A. Turner syndrome
B. Klinefelter's syndrome
C. Down syndrome
D. Apert's syndrome

10. Molecular genetic testing allows accurate diagnosis of syndromes for which a variety of clinical differential diagnoses may lead to confusion. Which of the following syndromes can be diagnosed by detection of Pro250Arg FGFR3 mutation?

A. Crouzon syndrome
B. Apert syndrome
C. Pfeiffer syndrome
D. Muenke syndrome

11. Which one of the following has been found to be genetically responsible for causing the common craniosynostosis syndromes like Apert's, Crouzon's and Pfeiffer syndrome?

A. Fibroblast growth factor receptor (FGFR)
B. Small nuclear riboprotein N gene (SNRPN)
C. UBE3A gene
D. Chromosome 22q11 microdeletion

12. The fibroblast growth factor receptors (FGFRs) are typically single trans-membrane proteins that have extracellular immunoglobulin like structural motifs. These motifs are linked by transmembrane region to the intracellular component. The number of extracellular domains in a typical FGFR is which of the following?

A. One
B. Two
C. Three
D. Four

13. The 9q22-31 gene is associated with a syndrome characterised by palmar pits, bifid ribs, keratocysts of the jaw and characteristic coarse facies. The syndrome is which one of the following?

A. Crouzon's syndrome
B. Apert's syndrome
C. Pfeiffer syndrome
D. Gorlin syndrome

14. Plastic surgery is effective and useful to patients as it has the power to change the body image. Which one of the following best describes the term body image?

A. It refers to image of the body as seen in the mirror or on photography.
B. It refers to the anthropometric dimensions of the body and its comparison with the established parameters.
C. It refers to the mind body relationship with subjective perception of the body and the psychological effects of what a person looks like.
D. It refers to the physical appearance of the body with description of various deformities existing in the body after mapping using whole body imaging.

15. The physician-patient relationship plays an important role in the outcome of plastic surgery. Both the surgeon and patient develop a relationship based upon the mutual interaction and response to such interactive reactions. Which one of the following phenomenon describes the patient's feelings towards the surgeon?

A. Reaction
B. Counterreaction
C. Transference
D. Countertransference

16. The physician-patient relationship plays an important role in the outcome of plastic surgery. Both the surgeon and patient develop a relationship based upon the mutual interaction and response to such interactive reactions. Which one of the following phenomenon describes the physician's emotional reaction in response to patient's feelings?

A. Reaction
B. Counterreaction
C. Transference
D. Countertransference

17. An overly grateful patient who idealizes the surgeon and professes undying love and admiration in addition to having persistent requests for seeking attention can be classified as which one of the following?

A. Paranoid personality disorder
B. Histrionic personality
C. Dependent clinger
D. Narcissistic personality

18. A patient having an excessive need for admiration, an exaggerated sense of self importance and grandiose notions of their beauty and power is best classified as which of the following?

A. Paranoid personality disorder
B. Histrionic personality
C. Dependent clinger
D. Narcissistic personality

19. A patient who is excessively emotional, lively, flirtatious and dramatic with exhibition of attention seeking behaviour so that the spotlight is always on them is best classified as which one of the following?

A. Paranoid personality disorder
B. Histrionic personality
C. Dependent clinger
D. Narcissistic personality

20. A patient who perceives herself to be ugly despite having a normal appearance and performs repetitive compulsive behaviour such as excessive grooming or skin picking is considered to be suffering from which one of the following?

A. Body dysmorphic disorder
B. Avoidant personality disorder
C. Conversion disorder
D. Trichotillomania

21. The modern medical ethical principle of the moral obligation to protect patients from harm and injustice as also embodied in the Hippocratic oath is which one of the following?

A. Beneficence
B. Nonmaleficence
C. Primum non nocere
D. Casuistry

22. Informed consent is an essential part of plastic surgery practice. The patient should be fully informed of the treatment's risks and consequences. All the following are constituents of a valid informed consent except which one of the following?

A. The diagnosis or suspected diagnosis of the deformity
B. Nature and purpose of the proposed treatment
C. Costs involved in delivering such treatment
D. Reasonable available alternatives

23. The first clinical photograph, a daguerreotype (first commercially successful photographic process) of a leg fracture and also the first preoperative and postoperative photographs in plastic and reconstructive surgery were taken by which one of the following?

A. Gurdon Buck
B. George Eastman
C. Harold Gillies
D. McIndoe

24. The focal length of a lens refers to the distance from the posterior element of the lens to the film plane when an object at "infinity" is in focus. A standard lens is one that produces minimal distortion at infinity. Lens with a focal length shorter than a standard lens is which one of the following?

A. Narrow angle
B. Wide angle
C. Telephoto
D. Macro

25. Depth of field is an important consideration in facial photography. It refers to the distance in front of and behind the focal plane of the film that appears to be in focus. Which one of the following camera setting is desirable for optimum clinical facial photography?

A. Increased aperture and minimum depth of field
B. Decreased aperture with maximum depth of field
C. Longer focal lengths with maximum shutter speed
D. Using automatic camera

26. The position of the flash in plastic surgery photography is important for quality of photograph. Which one of the following correctly describes the flash position for the above photograph showing a left lateral view of the face with a shadow outline on one side?

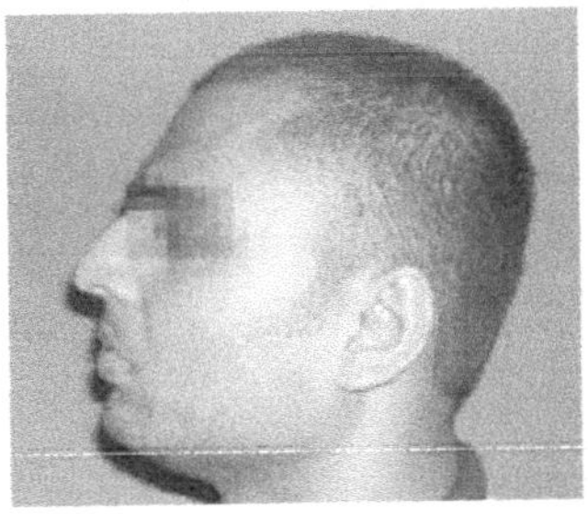

A. Flash mounted on top of the camera
B. Flash mounted on right side of camera
C. Flash mounted on left side of camera
D. Camera turned for vertical photograph with ring flash

27. Lateral view of the face of a young woman taken with standard positioning, lighting and background. Which one of the following lens, distance and camera setting is likely to give this result?

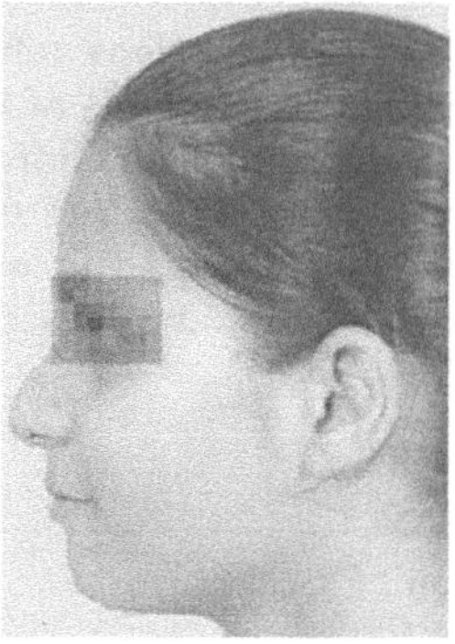

A. 50 mm lens with single flash
B. 50 mm lens with ring flash
C. 100 mm macrolens with servant flash
D. 100 mm macrolens with single flash

28. Which one of the following is the advantage of film photography over digital photography?

A. Ease of presentation
B. Cost
C. Stability of records
D. Ease of storage

29. Propofol as an induction agent for General Anaesthesia has the following features except which one of the following?

A. Short acting
B. Less chances of nausea and vomiting
C. Produces fall of B.P.
D. Produces broncho-constriction

30. Use of Ketamine produces the following effects except which of the following?

A. Dissociative anaesthesia i.e. a disconnected and painfree state with nystagmus.
B. Tachycardia
C. Rise in B.P.
D. Bronchodilatation
E. Patient likely to aspirate
F. Patient unlikely to aspirate

31. Halothane produces the following effects but can produce which one of the following complication?

A. Relaxes bronchial smooth muscles
B. Decreases blood pressure
C. Pulse rate/Heart rate is usually maintained
D. Cardiac arrythmias E. Hepatic necrosis

32. The local anaesthetic produces its anaesthetic effect by doing which one of the following?

A. Block the nerve
B. Prevent passage of sodium
C. Prevent passage of potassium
D. Prevent passage of calcium

33. Regional anaesthesia to the external nose can be achieved by blocking the following nerves except?

A. Infraorbital nerve
B. Infratrochlear nerve
C. External nasal nerve
D. Supraorbital nerve

34. Which one of the following techniques is the most favoured procedure for regional anaesthesia to the superior extremity?

A. Brachial block
B. Axillary block
C. Interscalene block
D. Intra-arterial block

35. Hand surgery can be done under regional block anaesthesia by blocking the three nerves as follows excepting which one of the following?

A. Median nerve lateral to the brachial artery at the elbow
B. Median nerve medial to the brachial artery at the elbow
C. Ulnar nerve in its groove behind the medial epicondyle
D. Radial nerve in front of the lateral epicondyle

36. Regional anaesthesia to the thigh for harvesting skin grafts can be achieved by blocking which of the following nerve?

A. Lateral femoral cutaneous nerve of thigh
B. Femoral nerve in the femoral triangle
C. Obturator nerve in the obturator canal
D. All of the above

37. Regional anaesthesia to the foot can be achieved by blocking all of the following nerves except which one of the following?

A. Posterior tibial nerve
B. Sural nerve
C. Anterior tibial nerve
D. Anterior interosseous nerve

38. Wound healing triggers release of various types of cells into the wound for achieving specific objectives. Which one of the following is the last cell to appear in a wound?

A. Lymphocytes B. Macrophages
C. Monocytes D. Platelets

39. Granulation tissue plays an important role in wound healing. All of the following cell types are associated with granulation tissue except which one of the following?

A. Neutrophils
B. Fibroblasts
C. Macrophages
D. Endothelial cells

40. Which one of the following characteristic would differentiate a keloid from a hypertrophic scar?

A. Excessive scarring
B. Scarring beyond the original scar
C. Scarring within the original scar
D. Tendency to recur

41. Keloids are preferably treated by all of the following procedures except which one of the following?

A. Surgical excision
B. Intralesion steroids
C. Pressure garments
D. Silicone sheet

42. The word 'scar' is derived from which one of the following?

A. Latin Literature
B. Greek Literature
C. English Literature
D. French Literature

43. Reorientation of scars can be achieved by Z–plasty. A 60° Z–plasty would increase the length of the two end points of a scar by which one of the following?

A. 50%
B. 60%
C. 70%
D. More than 70%

44. The Limberg flap is a type of which one of the following flap?

A. Rotation flap
B. Transposition flap
C. Interpolation flap
D. Free flap

45. Which one of the following flap requires a secondary flap from the lax surrounding skin to close the secondary flap defect?

A. Rotation flap
B. Transposition flap
C. Interpolation flap
D. Bilobed flap

46. Which one of the following suture technique is preferable for insetting the areola in breast reduction surgery to minimise suture marks?

A. Skin staples
B. Half buried horizontal mattress suture
C. Continuous over and over suture
D. Horizontal mattress suture

47. An acute wound is defined as the one that has occurred within which one of the following timelines?

A. Within past 3-4 days
B. Within past 3-4 weeks
C. Within past 3-4 months
D. Within past 3-4 years

48. Immunoglobins are antibodies and are of five types as mentioned below. Which one of the following is found on the surface of the lymphocytes?

A. IgM
B. IgA
C. IgG
D. IgE
E. IgD

49. Partial thickness skin grafting is indicated in all of the following conditions except which one of the following?

A. Large wounds
B. Hair restoration
C. Vitiligo
D. Nipple – Areola reconstruction

50. The donor sites for full thickness skin grafts include all of the following except:

A. Postauricular region
B. Cubital fossa
C. Groin (inguinal region)
D. Popliteal region

51. Full thickness skin grafts can be used in all of the following situations except which one of the following?

A. Defects of the lower eyelid
B. Defects on the nose/face
C. Reconstruction of the eyebrows
D. Large wounds

52. Defects on the palmar surface of the hand should preferably be covered by which one of the following?

A. Partial thickness skin graft from thigh
B. Partial thickness skin graft from arm
C. Graft from the sole/hypothenar eminence
D. Full thickness skin graft

53. Which one of the following sensation is the first to appear in the skin grafted area?

A. Pain
B. Touch
C. Temperature
D. Tactile discrimination

54. The cutaneous circulation of the human body was first studied by which one of the following scientist?

A. Manchot, C
B. Spalteholz, W
C. Salmon, M
D. Schafer, K

55. The term "Angiosome" is derived from which one of the following literature?

A. Greek
B. French
C. English
D. Latin

56. Muscles have been classified into four categories on the basis of their nerve supply. Latissimus dorsi belongs to which one of the following categories?

A. Type I with single nerve entering the muscle
B. Type II with the single nerve which branches before it enters the muscle
C. Type III with multiple branches from the same trunk which enter the muscle
D. Type IV with multiple branches from different nerve trunks entering the muscle

57. Which one of the following muscles will suffer ischaemia most due to rise in compartment pressure of the forearm in Volkmann's ischaemia?

A. Flexor digitorum sublimis
B. Flexor digitorum profundus
C. Supinator
D. Extensor digitorum longus

58. All of the following are 'indirect cutaneous vessels' which arise from the source arteries and penetrate the deep tissues before piercing the outer layer of the deep fascia to supply the skin except which one of the following?

A. Internal thoracic artery
B. Intercostal artery
C. Deep inferior epigastric musculocutaneous perforator
D. Radial artery

59. The external nose is supplied by which of the following?

A. External carotid artery
B. Internal carotid artery
C. Both of the above
D. None of the above

60. All of the following statements about choke vessels are true except which one of the following?

A. They serve as a connection between adjacent cutaneous arteries
B. They are plentiful in the integument and are important in regulating the blood flow to the intact skin
C. The calibre of the choke vessels is comparable to that of the true anastomotic vessels
D. The choke vessels dilate in response to flap delay

61. The most universally accepted system of muscle flap blood supply which elucidates that every muscle, in part or as a whole has a potential for use as a muscle flap was developed by which one of the following?

A. McGregor and Jackson
B. Bakamjian
C. Mathes and Nahai
D. Ponten

62. Muscles have been classified into five types based on the pattern of their arterial supply. Latissimus dorsi has which of the following vascular pattern?

A. Type I – Single vascular pedicle
B. Type II – Dominant vascular pedicle and minor pedicles
C. Type III – Two dominant vascular pedicles
D. Type IV – Many segmental vascular pedicles
E. Type V – One dominant and many segmental pedicles

63. Which one of the following muscle has type III blood supply containing two dominant vascular pedicles each of which can support the entire muscle?

A. Rectus femoris
B. Trapezius
C. Orbicularis oris
D. Tibialis anterior

64. Which one of the following muscles has type IV pattern of blood supply?

A. Extensor digitorum longus
B. Abductor hallucis
C. Temporalis
D. Vastus medialis

65. Which one of the following muscle has type I blood supply?

A. Tensor fascia lata
B. Sternocleidomastoid
C. Triceps
D. Peroneus brevis

66. A muscle flap which is elevated on its secondary pedicles requiring division of its dominant pedicle is designated as which one of the following?

A. Secondary flap
B. Reverse flap
C. Delayed flap
D. Ponten flap

67. Which one of the following muscle can be transferred to restore loss of function of the biceps muscle?

A. Latissimus dorsi
B. Pectoralis major
C. Teres major
D. Triceps

68. The pectoralis major musculocutaneous flap can be used for the reconstruction of the following defects except which one of the following?

A. Reconstruction of the pharynx
B. Reconstruction of the oesophagus
C. Reconstruction of the mandibular defects
D. Reconstruction of the nose

69. The latissimus dorsi musculocutaneous flap can be used for the reconstruction of following defects except which one of the following?

A. Reconstruction of shoulder
B. Restoration of flexion of the elbow
C. Reconstruction of breast
D. Reconstruction of the face, cheek and lips

70. The rectus abdominis is a Type III musculocutaneous flap. A transverse rectus abdominis musculocutaneous flap based on the superior epigastric artery consisting of lower abdominal skin and fat for breast reconstruction was popularised by which of the following ?

A. Mathes
B. Hartrampf
C. Elliot
D. Diner

71. The TRAM (transverse rectus abdominis musculocutaneous) flap has revolutionised breast reconstruction. All of the following can be considered advantages and indications of the free TRAM flap over pedicled TRAM except which one of the following?

A. Reduced abdominal dissection and muscle sacrifice
B. History of heavy cigarette use (>10 pack/years smoking)
C. Higher incidence of flap failure
D. Avoidance of disturbance of medial inframammary fold

72. The sacral pressure sore can be managed by the gluteus maximus muscle flap in all of the following ways except as which one of the following?

A. Superiorly based flap
B. Inferiorly based flap
C. Partial gluteus maximus flap
D. Free flap

73. Which one of the following statement best describes the "Law of equilibrium" described by Michel Salmon in relation to the cutaneous arteries?

A. The number of cutaneous vessels and anatomical territories is fixed in the human body to maintain the equilibrium.
B. The size of different cutaneous vessels in an anatomical territory is fixed to maintain the equilibrium.
C. The anatomical territories of adjacent arteries bear an inverse relationship to each other yet combine to supply the same region.
D. The anatomical territories of adjacent arteries bear an inverse relationship with the venous drainage to ensure effective drainage of the angiosome.

74. Which one of the following methods is considered the 'gold standard' for monitoring of a free flap?

A. Clinical examination
B. Ultraviolet lamp
C. Surface doppler
D. Implantable doppler

75. The word 'microscope' has been derived from which one of the following languages?

A. English
B. French
C. Greek
D. German

76. Sliding bar in double clamps used in microsurgery was developed by which one of the following?

A. Jacobson
B. O' Brien
C. Acland
D. Tamai

77. Which one of the following methods of microanastomosis is used when the size of the vessel ends is not equal?

A. End to end anastomosis
B. End to side anastomosis
C. Use of double approximating microvascular clamps
D. Adventitial stripping

78. An instrument system for fast and safe microvascular anastomosis with patency rates comparable to handsewn arterial anastomosis was developed by which of the following?

A. Ostrup
B. Acland
C. Carrel
D. Buncke

79. Which one of the following is the most favourable anticoagulation agent in common use?

A. Heparin
B. Aspirin
C. Dextran
D. Papaverine

80. Who first introduced the operating microscope which was initially used for otolaryngologic surgery?

A. Jacobson
B. Nylen
C. Acland
D. Zacharias and Hans Janseen

81. Who introduced the technique of first placing triangulating sutures to ensure equal traction on the blood vessels at the time of microvascular anastomosis?

A. Carrel
B. Nylen
C. Acland
D. Zacharias and Hans Janseen

82. Tissue expansion is a reliable method of providing additional skin in addition to providing optimum skin texture and colour match. The local changes produced by tissue expansion include which one of the following except?

A. Epidermal thickening
B. Thinning of dermis
C. Formation of fibrous capsule
D. Local muscle show hypertrophy

83. Which one of the following is credited with the first use of an expansile implant comprising of a latex balloon to enlarge periauricular skin for a traumatic ear deformity?

A. Eric Austad
B. Radovan
C. Neumann
D. Putti

84. Alloderm (acellular allogeneic dermis) which is composed of acellular dermis and extracellular matrix is obtained from which one of the following?

A. Sheep skin
B. Human skin
C. Pig skin
D. Cadaveric skin

85. Which one of the following scientists first used free fat autografts ?

A. Coleman
B. Leaf and Zarem
C. Neuberg
D. Romberg

86. Harvesting of fat prior to injection requires centrifugation. Which one of the following layers is used for injection ?

A. Upper layer
B. Middle layer
C. Basal layer
D. Middle and basal layer

87. Soft tissue fillers can lead to embolic complications as a result of entry of filler material into one of the arteries. All of the following are helpful in preventing this outcome except which of the following?

A. Use of fine cannulas to avoid the vessels
B. Use of vasoconstriction by epinephrine
C. Injection of 0.1 mL of filler per pass
D. Meticulous technique

88. Which one of the following is the preferred site for harvesting large free fascial grafts?

A. Temporoparietal fascia
B. Scarpa's fascia
C. Tensor fascia lata
D. Plantar fascia
E. Transversalis fascia

89. There are eight pulleys which hold the flexor tendons in contact with bones. Which of the following is a key pulley which prevents bow stringing of the flexor tendons?

A. A1 pulley
B. A2 pulley
C. Palmar aponeurosis pulley
D. C1 pulley
E. C2 pulley

90. Which one of the following core suture techniques comes closest to the ideal suture for flexor tendon repair in terms of being relatively easy to perform, stronger than the other repairs and places the knot outside the laceration site?

A. Modified Kessler suture
B. Cruciate four strand repair
C. Modified Kessler suture
D. Interlock suture
E. Kessler-Tajima suture

91. Which one of the following donor sites would provide the longest tendon graft?

A. Palmaris longus
B. Plantaris
C. Extensor digitorum longus
D. Exensor indicis proprius
E. Flexor digitorum superficialis

92. Which one of the following is the first change that occurs in a denervated muscle?

A. Atrophy
B. Fasciculation
C. Reinnervation
D. Fibrillation
E. Regeneration

93. Which one of the following muscles is responsible for 'smiling'?

A. Levator labii superioris
B. Levator labii superioris alaequae nasi
C. Zygomaticus minor
D. Zygomaticus major

94. The cartilages in the human body are mainly of three types. Which one of these cartilage is present in the external ear and larynx?

A. Hyaline cartilage
B. Elastic cartilage
C. Fibrocartilage
D. 50% hyaline and 50% elastic cartilage

95. The most prevalent technique for cartilage storage is which one of the following?

A. Refrigeration
B. Cryopreservation
C. Lyophilisation (Freeze-drying)
D. Irradiation
E. Merthiolate

96. The hyaline cartilage is present in all of the following locations except which one of the following?

A. Joints
B. Rib cage
C. Trachea
D. Intervertebral disc

97. Elastic cartilage is present in all of the following locations except which one of the following?

A. External ear
B. Corniculate cartilage of larynx
C. Apices of arytenoids
D. Epiglottis
E. Nasal septum

98. The white fibro cartilage is present in all of the following locations except which one of the following?

A. Intervertebral discs
B. Articular discs
C. Glenoidal labrum (shoulder joint)
D. Acetabulum labrum (hip joint)
E. Temporomandibular joint
F. Nasal septum

99. Which one of the following connective tissues is responsible for providing support and protects the axon from elongation injury?

A. Endoneurium
B. Perineurium
C. Epineurium
D. Mesoneurium

100. Which one of the following types of nerve injury is associated with an advancing Tinel's sign?

A. Neuropraxia
B. Axonotmesis
C. Neurotmesis
D. Neuroma in continuity

101. Which one of the following objective tests of sensory nerve injury uses an amino acid containing Ninhydrin?

A. Electrodiagnostic test
B. Moberg's test
C. O'Rain's wrinkle test
D. Nerve conduction velocity

102. Which one of the following site has the lowest normal value for two-point discrimination?

A. Chest
B. Fingertip
C. Back
D. Pulp of the great toe

103. Which one of the following nerves can provide the longest donor nerve graft material?

A. Sural nerve
B. Superficial radial sensory nerve
C. Lateral femoral cutaneous nerve
D. Great auricular nerve

104. Which one of the following nerves shows the best results of motor recovery after microsurgical repair?

A. Median nerve
B. Ulnar nerve
C. Radial nerve
D. Peroneal nerve
E. Tibial nerve repair

105. Which one of the following implants used in plastic surgery is made from titanium?

A. Nasal implants for augmentation
B. Chin implants
C. Ear implants
D. Breast implants
E. Mini-plates

106. The Food and Drug Administration (FDA) has classified medical devices into three classes depending upon the degree of complexity, invasiveness and other criteria. Which of the following medical device falls in Class 1 category?

A. Intravenous cannula
B. Pacemaker
C. Breast implant
D. Tongue blade
E. External midface distractor

107. The Food and Drug Administration (FDA) has classified medical devices into three classes depending upon the degree of complexity, invasiveness and other criteria. Which one of the following medical device falls in Class 2 category?

A. Intravenous cannula
B. Pacemaker
C. Breast implant
D. Tongue blade
E. Mayo's scissors

108. The Food and Drug Administration (FDA) has classified medical devices into three classes depending upon the degree of complexity, invasiveness and other criteria. Which one of the following medical device falls in Class 3 category?

A. Intravenous cannula
B. Pacemaker
C. Surgical marker
D. ECG multipara monitor
E. Mayo's scissors

109. Braiding of a suture material increases the break strength of the suture while making it more susceptible to infection. Which one of the following absorbable suture is braided ?

A. Chromic catgut
B. PDS (Poly-p-dioxanone)
C. Vicryl
D. Monocryl
E. Maxon

110. Braiding of a suture material increases the break strength of the suture while making it more susceptible to infection. Which one of the following non-absorbable suture is braided?

A. Silk
B. Stainless steel
C. Prolene
D. Gore-Tex
E. Ethilon

111. Which one of the following material comes in the form of polymer granules at time of surgery and requires to be mixed with a liquid to generate a mouldable compound which can be contoured and tailored to fit the surgical defect?

A. MEDPOR
B. PMMA (Polymethyl methacrylate)
C. Dacron (Polyethylene terephthalate)
D. Gore-Tex
E. Proplast

112. Which one of the following absorbable suture material has the fastest absorption?

A. Chromic catgut
B. PDS
C. Vicryl
D. Monocryl
E. Maxon

113. Nylon is a commonly used suture in plastic surgery for skin closure. It is rapidly encapsulated and maintains tensile strength for a long time. It is made up of which one of the following?

A. Polyester
B. Polyethylene
C. Polyamide
D. Polypropylene
E. Polytetrafluoroethylene (PTFE)

114. Prolene (Polypropylene) is considered inert and also maintains tensile strength for several years. It also has characteristics of long term stability and long lasting strength with minimal tissue reaction. The filament of prolene is which one of the following?

A. Braided
B. Twisted
C. Sheathed
D. Monofilament
E. Antibiotic coated

115. The word 'prosthesis' is derived from the noun 'prostithenai' and has a mythological importance in the Trojan War. It is derived from which one of the following languages?

A. English
B. French
C. German
D. Greek
E. Latin

116. Which one of the following is commonly used for colour matching for construction of a facial prostheses?

A. Clinical examination
B. Digital photography
C. Munsell colour system
D. Segall colour coding system
E. Computer digitisation

117. Which one of the following methods provides the most secure method of fixation of a nose prostheses?

A. Adhesives
B. Eyeglasses
C. Tissue undercuts around defect
D. Osseointegration

118. What is the minimum length of a finger or thumb stump for retention of a digital prostheses?

A. 0-5 cm
B. 1.5 cm
C. 2.5 cm
D. 3.5 cm
E. 4.5 cm

119. What is the minimum length of the proximal forearm for fitting an upper extremity prostheses ?

A. 5-10 cm
B. 10-15 cm
C. 15-20 cm
D. 20-25 cm
E. More than 30 cm

120. The myoelectric prosthesis is the current state of the art for prosthetic rehabilitation of the upper limb. The battery operated myoelectric prostheses capable of allowing many types of movements including pronation, supination and finger movements is activated by impulses from which one of the following source?

A. External power
B. Myoelectric impulses through cable system running across opposite shoulder
C. Myoelectric impulses from contraction of stump muscles
D. Do not require impulses for muscle movements
E. Brain generates myoelectric impulse for various movements

121. Toxic epidermal necrolysis is characterised by detachment of the epidermis from the dermis leading to extensive loss of the skin. It is associated with which one of the following syndrome?

A. Sjogren's syndrome
B. Stevens-Johnson syndrome
C. Sudden infant death syndrome
D. Stein-Leventhal syndrome
E. Sheehan's syndrome

122. Epidermolysis bullosa is a condition characterised by which one of the following?

A. Blisters
B. Cysts
C. Necrotising vasculitis
D. Folliculitis

123. The total body surface area (TBSA) is the best predictor in burn survival. In which one of the following regions, the value of TBSA actually decreases from birth to adulthood?

A. Right thigh
B. Right leg
C. Left thigh
D. Left leg
E. Head

124. The total body surface area (TBSA) is the best predictor in burn survival. In which of the following regions the value of TBSA does not change with the age of the patient?

A. Head
B. Left thigh
C. Right thigh
D. Leg
E. Foot

125. The amount of fluid replacement in a case of burns during the first eight hours should be which one of the following?

A. Half of the total requirement.
B. One third of the total requirement.
C. One fourth of the total requirement.
D. Three fourths of the total requirement

126. The urine output in an adult case of burns receiving fluid replacement should be maintained at a rate of which one of the following?

A. 1 c.c. per minute
B. 2 c.c. per minute
C. 3 c.c. per minute
D. 4 c.c. per minute
E. 5 c.c. per minute

127. Colloids are commonly used for restoration of intravascular volume and oncotic pressure in burns. Which one of the following resuscitation formulae advocates the use of colloids on Day 1?

A. Brooke
B. Modified Brooke
C. Parkland
D. Monafo

128. The amount of fluid (Ringer's lactate) to be given as per Parkland's formula in a case of 40% burn in an adult of 80 kg in the first 24 hours is which one of the following?

A. $80 \times 40 \times 4 = 12{,}800$ mL
B. $80 \times 40 \times 2 = 6{,}400$ mL
C. $80 \times 40 \times 1.5 = 4{,}800$ mL
D. $80 \times 40 \times 1 = 3{,}200$ mL

129. How much of Ringer's lactate is given to a case of burns on the second day according to the Parkland's formula?

A. 0.25 mL / kg / % burn
B. 0.50 mL / kg / % burn
C. 1 mL / kg / % burn
D. None

130. Biologic dressings are commonly used in burns as they are relatively abundant and inexpensive. Which one of the following biological dressing is derived from bovine collagen and shark chondroitin sulphate matrix ?

A. Porcine skin
B. Cadaveric skin
C. Integra
D. Transcyte
E. Alloderm

131. Biologic dressings are commonly used in burns as they are relatively abundant and inexpensive. Which one of the following biological dressing is derived from human fibroblast in collagen matrix?

A. Porcine skin
B. Cadaveric skin
C. Integra
D. Transcyte
E. Alloderm

132. Biologic dressings are commonly used in burns as they are relatively abundant and inexpensive. Which of the following biological dressing is composed of acellular human dermis?

A. Porcine skin
B. Cadaveric skin
C. Integra
D. Transcyte
E. Alloderm

133. The unit of radiation commonly used is gray (Gy). It is not the energy that leaves the machine but the energy that is absorbed by the tissue. It is equivalent to which of the following?

A. 1 Rad
B. 50 Rads
C. 100 Rads
D. 1000 Rads
E. 10,000 Rads

134. Hypothermia is a decrease in the core body temperature below which one of the following?

A. 35^{0}C
B. 33^{0}C
C. 31^{0}C
D. 29^{0}C
E. 27^{0}C

135. Severe exposure to cold may lead to a fatal outcome due to which one of the following changes?

A. Cardiac
B. Respiratory
C. Renal
D. Cerebral

136. Which one of these frost bite injuries is associated with haemorrhagic blisters?

A. 1st degree injury
B. 2nd degree injury
C. 3rd degree injury
D. 4th degree injury

137. All of the following are characteristic pathophysiologic changes in frost bite except which of the following?

A. Ice crystal formation
B. Denaturing of lipid-protein complexes
C. Tissue hypoxia
D. Alkalosis
E. Release of free oxygen radicals

138. Rewarming in a case of frost bite is best done by which one of the following?

A. Blankets
B. Central heating
C. Radiators/convectors
D. Submersion in hot water at 40^0 C.

139. Which of the following types of blisters would you consider for debridement in a case of frost bite?

A. Blisters with clear fluid
B. Blister with haemorrhagic fluid
C. Both of the above
D. None of the above

140. Acute mountain sickness occurs at an elevation above which one of the following?

A. 3000 feet
B. 5000 feet
C. 7000 feet
D. 9000 feet
E. 11,000 feet

141. Which one of the following medical complications is associated with high altitude climbing above 9000 feet?

A. Myocardial infarction
B. Pulmonary oedema
C. Bronchial asthma
D. Cyanosis
E. Hypertension

142. Debridement is the process of removal of which of the following?

A. Necrotic tissue
B. Slough
C. Bacteria/pus
D. Foreign material
E. All of the above

143. The dead muscle has all of the following features except which one of the following?

A. Dull in colour
B. Swollen
C. Friable
D. Contracts when grasped with forceps
E. Grainy on palpation

144. Paprika sign is characterised by punctate bleeding from which one of the following?

A. Donor area of thigh
B. Cut edge of the skin
C. Cut edge of the bone
D. Cut edge of muscle
E. Cut edge of tendon

145. Film dressings are those that allow exchange of oxygen, carbon dioxide and water vapour. Which one of the following dressing is not a film dressing?

A. Bioocclusive
B. Opsite
C. Tegasorb
D. Tegaderm
E. Polyskin

146. The word 'endoscope' is derived from which one of the following language?

A. English
B. Greek
C. Latin
D. German
E. French

147. The concept of optical cavity is important in endoscopic plastic surgery. Optical cavity allows the endoscope to be separated from the tissues being viewed, improves incoming light and also makes room for instrument movement. Which of the following types of optical cavity is used for endoscopic harvest of omentum?

A. Type 1 optical cavity
B. Type 2 optical cavity
C. Type 3 optical cavity
D. Type 4 optical cavity
E. All of the above

148. The concept of optical cavity is important in endoscopic plastic surgery. Optical cavity allows the endoscope to be separated from the tissues being viewed, improves incoming light and also makes room for instrument movement. Which of the following types of optical cavity is used for endoscopic latissimus dorsi based cardiac augmentation?

A. Type 1 optical cavity
B. Type 2 optical cavity
C. Type 3 optical cavity
D. Type 4 optical cavity
E. All of the above

149. The concept of optical cavity is important in endoscopic plastic surgery. Optical cavity allows the endoscope to be separated from the tissues being viewed, improves incoming light and also makes room for instrument movement. Which of the following types of optical cavity is used for endoscopic carpal tunnel release?

A. Type 1 optical cavity
B. Type 2 optical cavity
C. Type 3 optical cavity
D. Type 4 optical cavity
E. All of the above

150. The concept of optical cavity is important in endoscopic plastic surgery. Optical cavity allows the endoscope to be separated from the tissues being viewed, improves incoming light and also makes room for instrument movement. Which of the following types of optical cavity is used for endoscopic harvest of rectus abdominis?

A. Type 1 optical cavity
B. Type 2 optical cavity
C. Type 3 optical cavity
D. Type 4 optical cavity
E. All of the above

151. Which one of the following is the preferred modality for imaging of foetal anomalies?

A. Two dimensional ultrasonography
B. Three dimensional ultrasonography
C. Four dimensional ultrasonography
D. Magnetic resonance imaging

152. AFP is a protein made in the liver of the developing foetus. Which one of the following condition is associated with abnormally low AFP levels?

A. Down syndrome
B. Twins
C. Preterm delivery
D. Intrauterine growth retardation
E. Ectopia vesicae

153. Dexon is a synthetic absorbable suture made from which one of the following?

A. Polylactic acid
B. Polyglycolic acid
C. Polyhydroxy acid
D. Polyanhydride
E. Polyamino acid

154. Which one of the following commercially available skin substitutes is composed of porcine collagen?

A. Epicel
B. Alloderm
C. Integra
D. Biobrane
E. Apligraf

155. Which one of the following is considered the father of fetal surgery?

A. Sushruta
B. Lister
C. Liley
D. Gillies
E. Joseph

156. Congenital high airway obstruction syndrome (CHAOS) can be diagnosed by prenatal ultrasound examination. Which of the following is the most common cause of this syndrome?

A. Laryngeal atresia
B. Tracheal atresia
C. Buccopharyngeal membrane
D. All of the above

157. Foetal surgical intervention involves access inside the uterus. Which one of the following options best describes the standard intrauterine access for foetal surgery?

A. Uterine incision by a knife
B. Uterine incision by diathermy
C. Operative stapler
D. Ultrasonic knife

158. The term 'robot' is derived from which one of the following language?

A. Greek Word
B. German Word
C. French Word
D. Czech Word
E. Chinese Word

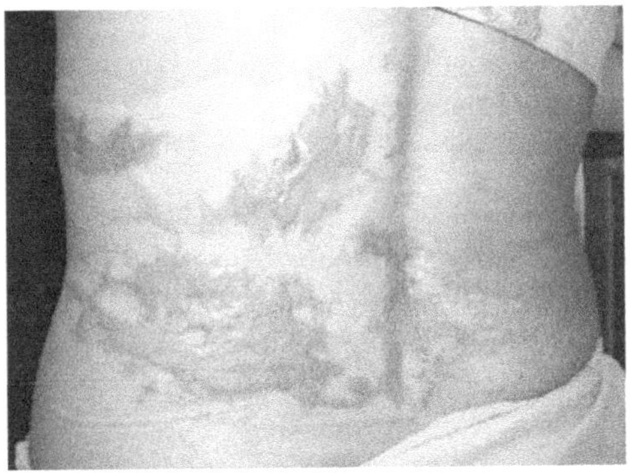

159. A 32-year-old woman presents with scarring on the back after sustaining thermal burns six months back. Which one of the following is the most critical consideration in planning further treatment?

A. Age of the patient
B. Anatomic location
C. Histologic findings
D. Severity of injury
E. Natural history

ANSWERS, EXPLANATIONS AND REFERENCES

1. The correct response is C.

Plastic Surgery historically started from the initial surgical procedures for nasal and earlobe reconstruction in ancient India as has been recorded in the writings of Sushruta to the advancement flaps described by Celsus in Roman times. This was followed by the discovery of the skin graft and flaps.

Reference:

Flexner A. Medical Education in the United States and Canada: A Report to the Carnegie foundation for the Advancement of Teaching. The Carnegie Foundation, Bulletin No.4, 1910.

2. The correct response is B.

D. Ralph Millard Jr was a master surgeon who trained with Harold Gillies and wrote the famous text "Principalization of Plastic Surgery". He started from the initial surgical procedures for nasal and earlobe reconstruction in ancient India as has been recorded in the writings of Sushruta to the advancement flaps described by Celsus in Roman times. This was followed by the discovery of the skin graft and flaps.

Reference:

Millard RD. The plastic surgeon's creed. In Millard RD: Principalization of Plastic Surgery. Boston, Little Brown, 1986: 648.

3. The correct response is C.

It was Galen, the great Greek physician who made his anatomic observations based on animal experimentation, as use of human cadavers was difficult because of social and cultural boundaries. This also led to errors regarding the structure and function of internal organs and circulation. The work by others was based on human studies.

Reference:

Lyons AS, Petrucilli RJ. Medicine, An Illustrated History. New York, Harry N. Abrams, 1978.

4. The correct response is A.

The earliest reference to plastic surgery grafts and flaps was published in Sushrut Samhita. The Gentleman's magazine reported a letter sent to them by an Englishman who had seen a forehead flap being used for nasal reconstruction in India to help a soldier. The letter was published in Oct 1794.

The rest of the books have been published much later. De Humani Corporis Fabrica was written by Vesalius. Novum Organum was written by Francis Bacon and Principles of Plastic Surgery was written by Millard.

Reference:

1. *Cormack GC, Lamberty BGH. The arterial anatomy of skin flaps. Philadelphia, Churchill Livingstone, 1986: 3.*
2. *Bacon F. Novum Organum: Aphorisms concerning the interpretation of nature and the kingdom of man, 1620.*
3. *Millard RD. The plastic surgeon's creed. In Millard RD: Principalization of Plastic Surgery. Boston, Little Brown, 1986: 648.*

5. The correct response is C.

In 1817, it was Sir Astley Cooper who performed the first successful human skin graft. The partial thickness graft was first applied by Reverdin, followed by Ollier and Thiersch in 1874.

Reference:

Hauben DJ, Baruchin A, Mahler A. On the history of the free skin graft. Ann Plast Surg. Sep 1982; 9(3): 242-5.

6. The correct response is C.

The randomised controlled trial is considered to have the highest level of evidence for measuring outcomes. Expert opinion is the lowest level of evidence. Case control and cohort studies provide a medium range of level of evidence for measuring outcomes.

Reference:

Offer GJ, Perks AG. In search of evidence-based plastic surgery: the problems faced by the speciality [review]. Br J Plast Surg 2000; 53: 427-433.

7. **The correct response is D.**

It was Joseph Murray who performed the first successful renal transplant in identical twins in 1955, for which he was conferred the Noble prize. The other options are of leaders and icons of plastic surgery based on their individual contributions to the speciality.

Reference:

Watts G. Joseph Murray: innovative surgeon and pioneer of transplantation. The Lancet 2011; 377(9770): 987.

8. **The correct response is B.**

A malformation is defined as a morphologic defect of an organ, a part of an organ, or a larger area of the body resulting from intrinsically abnormal development. Cleft palate is representative of abnormal morphogenesis resulting in malformation.

Amniotic band syndrome and ring constriction are the examples of a disruption. Disruption is a morphologic defect of an organ, a part of an organ, or a larger area of the body resulting from a breakdown of or interference with originally normal development.

Reference:

Spranger JW, Benirschke K, Hall JG et al. Errors of morphogenesis: concepts and terms. J Pediatr 1982; 100, 160.

1

9. **The correct response is B.**

Klinefelter's syndrome (47, XXY) is associated with gynaecomastia. Turners syndrome is associated with webbing of the neck. Down's syndrome is associated with Mongoloid facies. Apert's syndrome is associated with deformities of the cranial vault.

Reference:

Tyler C, Edman JC. Down syndrome, Turner syndrome, and Klinefelter syndrome: primary care throughout the life span. Prim Care 2004; 31(3), 627-648.

10. **The correct response is D.**

The demonstration of the specific and easily detectable Pro250Arg FGFR3 mutation clarifies the diagnosis of Muenke syndrome. The rest of the syndromes are the result of mutation in FGFR2.

Reference:

Muenke M, Gripp KW, McDonald-McGinn DM et al. A unique point mutation in the fibroblast growth factor receptor 3 gene (FGFR3) defines a new craniosynostosis syndrome. Am J Hum Genet 1997; 60: 555.

11. **The correct response is A.**

Fibroblast growth factors (FGFR) are a large family of multifunctional growth factors that are involved in wide range of developmental processes. FGFR mutations are responsible for causing common craniosynostosis syndromes like Apert's, Crouzon's, Pfeiffer, Jackson-Weiss and others.

The small nuclear riboprotein N gene (SNRPN) is associated with Prader-Willi syndrome which is maternally imprinted. This syndrome is characterised by obesity, hypogonadism, short stature and learning difficulty. The UBE3A gene, which belongs to the ubiquitin family is associated with the Angelman syndrome. Chromosome 22q11 microdeletion is associated with patients with velopharyngeal insufficiency.

Reference:

1. *Wilkie AOM. Molecular genetics of craniosynostosis. In Lin K, Ogle RC, Jane J, eds: Craniofacial Surgery: Science and Surgical Technique. Philadelphia, WB Saunders, 2002, 46.*
2. *Mueller RF, Young ID. Emery's Elements of Medical Genetics, 11th ed. London, Churchill Livingstone , 2001.*

12. **The correct response is C.**

The fibroblast growth factor receptors (FGFRs) are typically single trans-membrane proteins that have three extracellular immunoglobulin like structural motifs. These motifs are linked by transmembrane region to the intracellular component, which is made up of a split tyrosine kinase domain.

Reference:

Wilkie AOM. Molecular genetics of craniosynostosis. In Lin K, Ogle RC, Jane J, eds: Craniofacial Surgery: Science and Surgical Technique. Philadelphia, WB Saunders, 2002, 43.

13. The correct response is D.

The putative Gorlin syndrome gene was mapped to 9q22-31. On the basis of the similarity of defects seen in the mutations of the Drosophila patched gene, mutations in the human equivalent of this gene were identified as the principal cause of this disorder.

Reference:

Gailani MR, Bale SJ, Lefell DJ et al. Developmental defects in Gorlin syndrome related to putative tumour suppressor gene on chromosome 9. Cell 1992; 69: 111.

14. The correct response is C.

The term body image actually describes a complex physical and psychological interaction. The physical features and attributes of the body are only one part of the body image, and the body image is defined as the mind body relationship, the subjective perception of the body as seen through the mind's eye and the psychological effects of what a person looks like.

Reference:

Fisher GT, Fisher JB, Stark RB. The body image. In Stark RB, ed: Aesthetic Plastic Surgery. Boston, Little, Brown, 1980:1-32.

15. The correct response is C

Patients commonly put a lot of emotions on the surgeon who does the surgery for correction of their problems. Henceforth patients develop special feelings for their surgeons that are similar to those associated with figures of authority from their past. Transference is defined as the patient's feelings towards the surgeon who may be viewed as a "saviour". Grandparent, uncle, or aunt and sibling transferences can occur. The physician's emotional reaction to the patient's transferential feelings is termed counterreaction. Counterreaction is a common or "normal"response to the patient's emotions whereas countertransference is the physician's reaction to the patient based not on the real circumstances but on issues in the physician's own life.

Reference:

Small SM. Psychological and psychiatric problems in aged and high-risk surgical patients. In Siegel JH, Chodorr PD, eds: The Aged and High Risk Surgical Patient: Medical, Surgical and Anaesthetic Management. Orlando, Fla, Grune and Stratton, 1976: 307-328.

16. The correct response is B.

Patients commonly put a lot of emotions on the surgeon who does the surgery for correction of their problems. Henceforth patients develop special feelings for their surgeons that are similar to those associated with figures of authority from their past. Transference is defined as the patient's feelings towards the surgeon who may be viewed as a "saviour". Grandparent, uncle, or aunt and sibling transferences can occur. The physician's emotional reaction to the patient's transferential feelings is termed counterreaction. Counterreaction is a common or "normal"response to the patient's emotions whereas countertransference is the physician's reaction to the patient based not on the real circumstances but on issues in the physician's own life.

Reference:

Small SM. Psychological and psychiatric problems in aged and high-risk surgical patients. In Siegel JH, Chodorr PD, eds: The Aged and High Risk Surgical Patient: Medical, Surgical and Anaesthetic Management. Orlando, Fla, Grune and Stratton, 1976: 307-328.

17. The correct response is C.

Dependent clingers range from having mild requests for seeking reassurance to having demanding requests for attention. The warning signs of dependent clinger is the overly grateful patient who idealizes the physician and professes undying love and admiration. The best management of such patient is to set firm limits related to their requests.

Paranoid patients have a pervasive mistrust and suspicion of others. These patients experience surgery as an "intrusion" and attack on their bodies. Under stress, paranoid individuals can develop brief psychotic episodes.

Histrionic patients tend to be excessively emotional and exhibit attention seeking behaviour. They are often lively, flirtatious and dramatic and continually seek to be the centre of attention. They are easily influenced by others and current fashion trends.

Narcissistic patients have an excessive need for admiration with exaggerated sense of self importance. They have a sense of entitlement and can be exploitative of others to achieve their own ends. Such patients are anxious about their surgery and may be distressed in the event of surgical complications.

Reference:

1. *Groves J. Taking care of the hateful patient. N Engl J Med 1978; 298: 883-887.*
2. *Diagnostic and Statistical Manual of Mental Disorders, 4th ed. Washington, DC, American Psychiatric Association, 1994: 669-773.*

18. The correct response is D.

Narcissistic patients have an excessive need for admiration with exaggerated sense of self importance. They have a sense of entitlement and can be exploitative of others to achieve their own ends. Such patients are anxious about their surgery and may be distressed in the event of surgical complications.

Dependent clingers range from having mild requests for seeking reassurance to having demanding requests for attention. The warning signs of dependent clinger is the overly grateful patient who idealizes the physician and professes undying love and admiration. The best management of such patient is to set firm limits related to their requests.

Paranoid patients have a pervasive mistrust and suspicion of others. These patients experience surgery as an "intrusion" and attack on their bodies. Under stress, paranoid individuals can develop brief psychotic episodes.

Histrionic patients tend to be excessively emotional and exhibit attention seeking behaviour. They are often lively, flirtatious and dramatic and continually seek to be the centre of attention. They are easily influenced by others and current fashion trends.

Reference:

1. *Groves J. Taking care of the hateful patient. N Engl J Med 1978; 298: 883-887.*
2. *Diagnostic and Statistical Manual of Mental Disorders, 4th ed. Washington, DC, American Psychiatric Association, 1994: 669-773.*

19. The correct response is B.

Histrionic patients tend to be excessively emotional and exhibit attention seeking behaviour. They are often lively, flirtatious and dramatic and continually seek to be the centre of attention. They are easily influenced by others and current fashion trends.

Narcissistic patients have an excessive need for admiration with exaggerated sense of self importance. They have a sense of entitlement and can be exploitative of others to achieve their own ends. Such patients are anxious about their surgery and may be distressed in the event of surgical complications.

Dependent clingers range from having mild requests for seeking reassurance to having demanding requests for attention. The warning signs of dependent clinger is the overly grateful patient who idealizes the physician and professes undying love and admiration. The best management of such patient is to set firm limits related to their requests.

Paranoid patients have a pervasive mistrust and suspicion of others. These patients experience surgery as an "intrusion" and attack on their bodies. Under stress, paranoid individuals can develop brief psychotic episodes.

Reference:

1. *Groves J. Taking care of the hateful patient. N Engl J Med 1978; 298: 883-887.*
2. *Diagnostic and Statistical Manual of Mental Disorders, 4th ed. Washington, DC, American Psychiatric Association, 1994: 669-773.*

20. The correct response is A.

Body dysmorphic disorder (BDD) is a psychiatric disorder in the spectrum of obsessive compulsive disorder in which a preoccupation with a slight or imagined defect in appearance makes the individual seek plastic surgery. The preoccupation causes clinically significant distress or impairment in social, occupational, or other important areas of functioning.

Individuals with Avoidant Personality Disorder or Social Phobia may worry about being embarrassed by real defects in appearance, but this concern is usually not prominent, persistent, distressing, time consuming, and impairing.

Some individuals with Body Dysmorphic Disorder remove body hair or pick their skin in an attempt to improve their appearance; these behaviours should be distinguished from hair pulling in Trichotillomania, which does not occur in response to appearance concerns, and from skin picking that may be associated with other mental disorders.

Reference:

1. *Philips KA. Body dysmorphic disorder: the distress of imagined ugliness. Am J Psychiatry. 1991; 148: 1138-1149;*
2. *Diagnostic and Statistical Manual of Mental Disorders, 4th ed. Washington, DC, American Psychiatric Association, 1994: 669-773.*

21. The correct response is B.

Nonmaleficence directs that patients be protected from harm and injustice and by implication that the surgeon should not injure a patient. The widely quoted maxim primum non nocere is not actually in the Hippocratic oath and its origins are totally not clear.

Beneficence is the moral obligation to act in the best interest of patients. Casuistry means simply "case based" and involves a search for clinical examples with which clinical problems can be compared.

Reference:

1. *Beauchamp TL, Walters L. Contemporary Issues in Bioethics, 5th ed. Belmont, Calif, Wadsworth, 1999;*
2. *Jonsen AR, Toulmin S. The abuse of Casuistry: A history of moral reasoning, Berkeley, Calif, University of California Press, 1988.*

22. The correct response is C.

Informed consent is an essential part of plastic surgery procedures. Discussion of costs however is not an essential part of a valid informed consent.

The patient needs to be fully informed of the treatment's risks and consequences and necessary recordings should be obtained. A valid informed consent has six components consisting of the diagnosis or suspected diagnosis; the nature of the procedure and its anticipated benefits; the risks, complications or side effects; the probability of success; reasonable available alternatives and possible consequences if advice is not followed.

Reference:

del Carmen MG and Joffe S. Informed Consent for Medical Treatment and Research: A Review. The oncologist 2005; 10(8), 636-641.

23. The correct response is A.

The introduction of the daguerreotype in 1839 represents the first widely available photographic process. This coincided with introduction of photography for clinical conditions. Gurdon Buck is credited with the first clinical photograph of a leg fracture. This was followed by extensive preoperative and postoperative photographs of his patients especially in the Civil War and cleft lip repair.

George Eastman later on invented the dry plate technique and introduced the Eastman Kodak company.

Reference:

Rogers BO. The first pre- and post-operative photographs of plastic and reconstructive surgery: contributions of Gurdon Buck (1807-1877). Aesthet Plast Surg 1991; 15, 19-33.

24. The correct response is B.

The focal length of a lens refers to the distance from the posterior element of the lens to the film plane when an object at "infinity" is in focus. A standard lens is one that produces minimal distortion at infinity. Lenses with a focal length shorter than a standard lens are considered wide angle, those with a longer focal length are considered telephoto.

Reference:

1. *Galdino GM, Vogel JE, Vander Kolk CA. Standardising digital photography: it's not all in the eye of the beholder. Plast Reconstr Surg 2001; 108: 1334-1344.*
2. *DiBernardo BE, Adams RL, Krause J et al. Photographic standards in plastic surgery. Plast Reconstr Surg 1998; 102: 559-568.*

25. The correct response is B.

Depth of field is an important consideration in facial photography. It refers to the distance in front of and behind the focal plane of the film that appears to be in focus. Depth of field increases with smaller apertures and shorter focal lengths. Using a medium telephoto for facial photography in automatic setting will reduce the depth of field. Hence it is recommended to override the automatic settings to aperture priority or manual mode with small aperture and larger depth of field.

Reference:

1. *Galdino GM, Vogel JE, Vander Kolk CA. Standardising digital photography: it's not all in the eye of the beholder. Plast Reconstr Surg 2001; 108: 1334-1344.*
2. *DiBernardo BE, Adams RL, Krause J et al. Photographic standards in plastic surgery. Plast Reconstr Surg 1998; 102: 559-568.*

26. The correct response is B.

The position of the flash is as important as the camera in plastic surgery photography. Ideally in any side or oblique view, the flash should be on the same side of the camera as the anterior part of the patient. If a shadow is visible on the left side of the patient then that means that the flash is positioned on the right side of the camera and vice versa. Ring flashes have been used to eliminate shadows but these tend to make contour appreciation difficult hence are not recommended for flash photography.

Reference:

1. *Galdino GM, Vogel JE, Vander Kolk CA. Standardising digital photography: it's not all in the eye of the beholder. Plast Reconstr Surg 2001; 108: 1334-1344.*
2. *DiBernardo BE, Adams RL, Krause J et al. Photographic standards in plastic surgery. Plast Reconstr Surg 1998; 102: 559-568.*

27. The correct response is C.

Ideally all aspects of the clinical photograph should be standardised to achieve consistent results. This includes the camera, focal length, position, background, lighting and exposure settings. A 50 mm lens is recommended for chest, torso and lower extremity. A 100 mm macro lens is used for face, hands and close-up photography. Single flash does not eliminate shadows and these are visible on the photographs on the opposite side. If flash is kept on the left side of the lens, the shadow appears on the right side of the patient and vice versa. Use of servant flashes and background flash is helpful in eliminating shadows in clinical photography.

Reference:

1. *Galdino GM, Vogel JE, Vander Kolk CA. Standardising digital photography: it's not all in the eye of the beholder. Plast Reconstr Surg 2001; 108: 1334-1344.*
2. *DiBernardo BE, Adams RL, Krause J et al. Photographic standards in plastic surgery. Plast Reconstr Surg 1998; 102: 559-568.*

28. The correct response is C.

The conventional film photography is now being replaced by the digital photography, however there are certain advantages existing for film photography. The film represents a stable record which cannot be manipulated or modified as opposed to digital records which can be manipulated and modified. However there are certain disadvantages to film photography which include the expense of buying and processing the film, secondly scanning the slides for presentations in large numbers may be cumbersome, thirdly the storage of slides or films can occupy great deal of space when compared to digital photographs which can be stored easily.

Reference:

1. *Galdino GM, Vogel JE, Vander Kolk CA. Standardising digital photography: it's not all in the eye of the beholder. Plast Reconstr Surg 2001; 108: 1334-1344.*
2. *DiBernardo BE, Adams RL, Krause J et al. Photographic standards in plastic surgery. Plast Reconstr Surg 1998; 102: 559-568.*

29. The correct response is D.

Propofol causes bronchodilatation due to direct muscle relaxant action.

Reference:

1. *Hall RI, Murphy JT, Landymore R et al. Myocardial metabolic changes during propofol anesthesia for cardiac surgery in patients with reduced ventricular function. Anesth Analg 1993; 77: 680.*
2. *Boyle WA, White PF and Rendig SV. Negative inotropic effects of propofol versus etmidate and thiopental on rabbit papillary muscle. Anesth Analg 1989;68: 535.*
3. *Pagel PS, Warltier DC. Negative inotropic effects of propofol as evaluated by the regional preload recruitable stroke work relationship in chronically instrumented dogs. Anesthesiology 1993;78:100.*
4. *Conti G, Dell'Urti D, Vilardi V, et al. Propofol induces bronchodilation in mechanically ventilated chronic obstructive pulmonary disease (COPD) patients. Acta Anesthesiology Scand 1993; 37: 105.*

30. The correct response is F.

Patients under ketamine anesthesia are able to maintain the airway and the swallowing reflex and hence are unlikely to aspirate. Laryngeal and Pharyngeal reflexes are also well maintained.

Reference:

1. *Stanley T. Blood pressure and pulse rate responses to ketamine during general anesthesia. Anesthesioogy 1973; 39:648.*
2. *Zsigmond EK, Kelsch RC, Kothary SP et al. Plasma norepinephrine concentration during anesthetic induction with ketamine. Rev Brasil Anest 1972; 22: 443.*

31. The correct response is E.

Halothane can produce hepatic necrosis, hence care is required during use of Halothane as an anesthetic agent.

Reference:

Knill RL. Gelb AW. Ventilatory responses to hypoxia and hypercapnia during halothane sedation and anesthesia in man. Anesthesiology 1978;49:244.

32. The correct response is B.

The local anaesthetics prevents passage of sodium and hence the conduction of the impulse.

Reference:

Mulroy MF. In White PF, ed: Ambulatory Anesthesia and Surgery. Philadelphia, WB Saunders, 1997;421.

33. The correct response is D.

The supra-orbital nerve need not be blocked. The ophthalmic nerve has three branches, lacrimal, frontal and nasociliary. The lacrimal supplies the lacrimal gland and the surrounding areas of the eye. Frontal nerve divides into supratrochlear and supraorbital branches. Supratrochlear supplies the lower part of the forehead near the midline i.e. glabellar region. Supra-orbital supplies the scalp up to the occipital region. The nasociliary nerve during its intraorbital course turns upwards and is then renamed as anterior ethmoidal nerve, which further on emerges from the nose as the external nasal nerve. Its long ciliary nerves emerge to supply the iris and cornea. Its internal nasal branches supply the nasal septum and the lateral wall of the nasal cavity. Infratrochlear nerve is given off the nasociliary nerve, to run along the medial wall of the orbit and then emerges out through the trochlea to supply the medial side of the eye and the side of the nose. The infraorbital nerve is a branch of the maxillary branch of the trigeminal and emerges out through the infraorbital foramen. It supplies innervation to the ala of the nose.

Reference:

1. *Mulroy MF. Local and regional anesthesia. In White PF, ed: Ambulatory Anesthesia and Surgery. Philadelphia, WB Saunders, 1997;420.*
2. *Mulroy MF. In White PF, ed: Ambulatory Anesthesia and Surgery. Philadelphia, WB Saunders, 1997;421.*

34. The correct response is A.

Brachial block is the most favoured procedure for administering regional anaesthesia to the superior extremity.

Reference:

Mulroy MF. Local and regional anesthesia. In White PF, ed: Ambulatory Anesthesia and Surgery. Philadelphia, WB Saunders, 1997;420.

35. The correct response is A.

The median nerve lies medial to the brachial artery at the level of the elbow joint. The other options specify correct locations for blocking the nerves.

Reference:

Mulroy MF. Local and regional anesthesia. In White PF, ed: Ambulatory Anesthesia and Surgery. Philadelphia, WB Saunders, 1997;420.

36. The correct response is D.

All the three nerves need to be blocked for achieving effective regional anesthesia to the thigh.

Reference:

Mulroy MF. Local and regional anesthesia. In White PF, ed: Ambulatory Anesthesia and Surgery. Philadelphia, WB Saunders, 1997;420.

37. The correct response is D.

Anterior interosseous nerve is a predominantly motor nerve of the upper extremity hence is not relevant for foot anaesthesia. The rest of the options are correct nerves for achieving anaesthesia of the foot.

Reference:
Mulroy MF. Local and regional anesthesia. In White PF, ed: Ambulatory Anesthesia and Surgery. Philadelphia, WB Saunders, 1997;420.

38. The correct response is A.

Platelets are the first to arrive in a wound followed by neutrophils. Monocytes and macrophages follow neutrophils into the wound and appear 48 to 72 hours after injury. The lymphocyte is the last cell to enter a wound and enters between 5 and 7 days after wounding.

Reference:
Singer AJ, Clark RAF. Mechanisms of disease: cutaneous wound healing. N Engl J Med 1999; 341(10): 738-746.

39. The correct response is A.

Granulation tissue is composed of three cell types that play critical and independent roles in granulation tissue formation: fibroblasts, macrophages and endothelial cells. These cells form extracellular matrix and new blood vessels.

Reference:
Singer AJ, Clark RAF. Mechanisms of disease: cutaneous wound healing. N Engl J Med 1999; 341(10): 738-746.

40. The correct response is B.

A keloid tends to grow beyond the original scar in any direction while the hypertrophic scar remains confined to the wound.

Reference:
Singer AJ, Clark RAF. Mechanisms of disease: cutaneous wound healing. N Engl J Med. 1999;341(10):738–746.

41. The correct response is A.

Surgical excision per se is avoided in the treatment of keloids as recurrence is common after surgical excision. The rest of the options are plausible treatment methodologies for the treatment of keloids.

Reference:
Singer AJ, Clark RAF. Mechanisms of disease: cutaneous wound healing. N Engl J Med. 1999;341(10):738–746.

42. The correct response is B.

The word is derived from the Greek word 'Eskhara' which means a scab. Scar is a mark left in the skin or internal organs by the healing of a wound.

Reference:
1. *Lee TY, Chin GS, Kim WJ, et al. Expression of transforming growth factors beta 1, 2 and 3 proteins in keloids. Ann Plast Surg 1999;43:179-184.*
2. *Brissett A E, Sherris DA. Scar contractures, hypertrophic scars and keloids. Facial Plast Surg 2001;17:263-272.*

43. The correct response is D.

The Z plasty principle is useful for increasing the length of skin in a desired direction. The gain in length depends on the angle of the Z plasty besides other factors. The gain in length increases as the angle of Z plasty increases. The gain in length is around 73% to 75% for a 60 degree Z plasty.

Reference:
Furnas DW, Fischer GW. The Z-plasty: biomechanics and mathematics. Br JPlast Surg. 1971;24:144.

44. The correct response is B.

The Limberg flap is a type of transposition flap. The success of the flap depends upon the looseness of adjacent skin and is useful in older age group patients.

Reference:
Borges AF. Elective Incisions and Scar Revision. Boston: Little, Brown; 1973.

45. The correct response is D.

The bilobed flap principle involves two flaps. The primary flap is transposed into the defect while a secondary flap from the surrounding lax skin is used to cover the defect left behind after the primary flap has been moved. The transposition, rotation and interpolation flaps may need a skin graft to close the defect from where the flap has been raised.

Reference:

Borges AF. Elective Incisions and Scar Revision. Boston: Little, Brown; 1973.

46. The correct response is B.

The half buried horizontal mattress suture leaves knots on one side of the suture line with no suture marks on the other side. This is thus preferable in the clinical situation of insetting the areola in breast reduction. The other suture techniques are likely to leave suture marks on both the sides of the incision line.

Reference:

Borges AF. Elective Incisions and Scar Revision. Boston: Little, Brown; 1973.

47. The correct response is B.

An acute wound is one that has occurred within the past 3 to 4 weeks. If the wound persists beyond 4 to 6 weeks it is considered a *chronic wound*, a term that also includes wounds that have been present for months or years.

Reference:

Goldman R. Growth factors and chronic wound healing: past, present, and future. Adv Skin Wound Care. 2004;17: 24–25.

48. The correct response is E.

The Immunoglobin "Ig D" is found on the surface of lymphocytes. The others have the following characteristics; IgM – responds to microbial antigens, IgA – is secreted in saliva, breast milk, IgG – responds to microbial antigens and IgE – binds with eosinophils.

Reference:

Lee WPA, Rubin JP. Transplant immunology and allotransplantation in plastic surgery. In Achauer B, ed: Plastic Surgery: Indications, Operations, Outcome. St. Louis, CV Mosby, 2000: 227–237.

49. The correct response is B.

The partial thickness skin grafts are not indicated for restoration of hair where hair transplants are required. The rest of the conditions benefit from partial thickness skin grafting.

Reference:

Mutallik S, Ginzburg A. Surgical management of stable vitiligo: a review with personal experience. Dermatol Surg 2000;25:302.

50. The correct response is D.

The full thickness grafts can be taken from any one of the above sites except the popliteal region which is unacceptable for harvesting this type of graft.

Reference:

Branham GH, Thomas JR. Skin grafts. Otolaryngol Clin North Am. Oct 1990; 23(5): 889–97.

51. The correct response is D.

The full thickness grafts are not feasible for use in large wounds as large amount of graft would require the donor surface to be resurfaced by split skin graft hence making this procedure less preferred.

Reference:

Branham GH, Thomas JR. Skin grafts. Otolaryngol Clin North Am. Oct 1990; 23(5): 889–97.

52. The correct response is C.

Grafts from the sole of the foot / hypothenar region would give the best colour match and hence are preferred for resurfacing palmar defects. Partial thickness skin grafts from the thigh or arm should not be used, because these grafts are likely to get hyperpigmented with or without scarring and the colour match with the palmar skin may also be a point of concern. Full thickness skin grafts are also not acceptable for use on the palmar surface of hand for the same reasons.

Reference:

Schenck RR, Cheema TA. Hypothenar skin grafts for fingertip reconstruction. J Hand Surg 9A: 750-3, 9A, 1984.

53. The correct response is A.

Pain sensation is the first one to appear in the skin grafted area. The other sensations would appear in the sequence as listed above in the order as touch, followed by temperature and tactile discrimination.

Reference:

Mannerfelt L. Evaluation of functional sensation of skin grafts in the hand area. Plast Reconstr Surg 30(4): 496-497, 30(4), 1962.

54. The correct response is A.

The study of the cutaneous vascular circulation was first done by Manchot 1889, a German Anatomist who also published a treatise on the subject. Spalteholz published his work on cadaveric circulation in 1893, while Salmon 1930 defined about 40 cutaneous territories. Schafer published his work on lower extremity circulation in 1975.

Reference:

1. *Manchot C. The Cutaneous Arteries of the Human Body. New York:Springer-Verlag, 1983.*
2. *Spalteholz W. Die vertheilung der blutgefasse in der haut. Arch Anat. 1893.*
3. *Salmon M. Arteries of the skin. In: Taylor GI, Tempest M, eds. London: Churchill-Livingstone; 1988.*

55. The correct response is A.

The word is derived from the Greek word 'Angeion' meaning vessel and 'Soma' meaning body.

Reference:

Taylor GI, Palmer JH. The vascular territories (angiosomes) of the body: experimental study and clinical applications. Br J Plast Surg. 1987 Mar; 40(2): 113-41.

56. The correct response is A.

The Latissimus dorsi belongs to Type I category with a single nerve entering the muscle.

Classification of Muscles based on their Nerve Supply

Type I	Type II	Type III	Type IV
Latissimus dorsi, Extensor indicis, Ext. pollicis longus	Deltoid, Trapezius,	Gluteus medius	Rectus abdominis
Abd. pollicis longus	Gluteus maximus,	Sartorius	Levator scapulare
Palmaris longus	Vastus lateralis,	Gastrocnemius	Internal oblique
Teres minor	Serratus anterior,	Soleus	Digastric
Ext. hallucis longus	Flex.carpi. ulnaris,	Tibialis anterior	Erector spinae
Plantaris	Biceps brachii	Tibialis posterior	
Popliteus	Brachialis	Triceps, Teres major,	
	Flexor pollicis longus	Subscapularis,	
	Flexor hallucis longus,	Ext. carp. ulnaris	
	Adductor longus	Ext. digi. longus	
	Adductor brevis	Flexor dig. sublimis	

Reference:

Mathes SJ, Nahai F. Classification of the vascular anatomy of muscles: experimental and clinical correlation. Plast Reconstr Surg. 1981; 67: 177.

57. The correct response is B.

The answer is flexor digitorum profundus. This is because the muscle is furthest away from the source of its blood supply. This is manifested by involvement of the middle and ring fingers tendons which arise from the centre of the muscle. Supinator is more proximal while the extensor digitorum longus belongs to the extensor compartment of the forearm.

Reference:

Mathes SJ, Nahai F. Classification of the vascular anatomy of muscles: experimental and clinical correlation. Plast Reconstr Surg. 1981; 67: 177.

58. The correct response is D.

Radial artery is not a indirect cutaneous vessel but a primary axis of the upper limb. The rest are indirect cutaneous vessels which arise from the source arteries and penetrate the deep tissues, usually muscle, vertically or obliquely before piercing the outer layer of the deep fascia.

Reference:

Taylor GI, Palmer JH. The vascular territories (angiosomes) of the body: experimental study and clinical applications. Br Plast Surg. 1987; 40: 113.

59. The correct response is C.

The nose is supplied by both the external and the internal carotid artery. The external carotid artery supplies the nose, through its facial, superior labial and lateral nasal branches. The internal carotid artery supplies the nose through the ophthalmic artery. Its external nasal branch supplies the dorsum of the nose.

Reference:

Jafek BW. Anatomy and physiology of the nose. In: Jafek BW, Stark AK, eds. ENT Secrets. Philadelphia, Pa: Hanley and Belfus; 1996:77-83.

60. The correct response is C.

The connection between adjacent cutaneous arteries is by either true anastomoses, without change in caliber, or by reduced-caliber choke anastomotic vessels. The latter are plentiful in the integument (skin and subcutaneous tissues) and may be important in regulating the blood flow to the intact skin. These choke vessels play an important role in skin-flap survival, where, like resistors in an electrical circuit, they provide an initial resistance to blood flow between the base and the tip of the flap. When a skin flap is delayed by the strategic division of cutaneous perforators along its length, these choke vessels dilate to the dimensions of true anastomoses, thus enhancing the circulation to the distal flap.

Reference:

1. *Dhar SC, Taylor, GI. The delay phenomenon: the story unfolds. Plast Reconstr Surg. 1999; 104(7): 2079–2091.*
2. *Morris SF, Taylor GI. The time sequence of the delay phenomenon: when is a surgical delay effective? An experimental study. Plast Reconstr Surg. 1995; 95(1):526.*
3. *Taylor GI, Minabe T. The angiosomes of the mammals and other vertebrates. Plast Reconstr Surg. 1992; 89: 181.*

61. The correct response is C.

Mathes and Nahai developed the universally accepted muscle flap blood supply classification in which five patterns of circulation to the muscle have been identified. Type I muscles are those who have a single vascular pedicle; type II are those who have a dominant vascular pedicle with minor vascular pedicles; type III are those who have two large vascular pedicles ; type IV are those who have a series of segmental pedicles and type V are those who have a dominant vascular pedicle and secondary segmental vascular pedicles.

Reference:

Mathes SJ, Nahai F. Classification of the vascular anatomy of muscles: experimental and clinical correlation. Plast Reconstr Surg. 1981; 67: 177.

62. The correct response is E.

Latissimus dorsi has type V blood supply in which the muscle receives a large vascular pedicle but also has secondary vascular pedicles which enter the muscle at its opposite end from the site of entry of the dominant vascular pedicle. These secondary pedicles have capability to support the muscle if the dominant vascular pedicle is divided. Other muscles with similar vascular pattern include internal oblique and pectoralis major.

Reference:

Mathes SJ, Nahai F. Classification of the vascular anatomy of muscles: experimental and clinical correlation. Plast Reconstr Surg. 1981; 67:177.

63. The correct response is C.

Out of the given options, orbicularis oris alone has type III blood supply. Rectus femoris and trapezius have type II vascular pattern while tibialis anterior has type IV pattern of blood supply.

Reference:

Mathes SJ, Nahai F. Classification of the vascular anatomy of muscles: experimental and clinical correlation. Plast Reconstr Surg. 1981; 67:177.

64. The correct response is A.

The extensor digitorum longus has type IV pattern of blood supply. All the above muscles of the leg have Type IV blood supply. Abductor hallucis and vastus medialis have type II pattern and temporalis has type III pattern of blood supply.

Reference:

Mathes SJ, Nahai F. Classification of the vascular anatomy of muscles: experimental and clinical correlation. Plast Reconstr Surg. 1981; 67:177.

65. The correct response is A.

The tensor fascia lata has type I blood supply. All the other muscles have type II blood supply according to the Mathes Nahai classification.

Reference:

Mathes SJ, Nahai F. Classification of the vascular anatomy of muscles: experimental and clinical correlation. Plast Reconstr Surg. 1981; 67:177.

66. The correct response is B.

A muscle flap that is elevated on its secondary pedicles requiring division of its dominant pedicle is designated as a reverse flap e.g pectoralis major flap when it is elevated based on the secondary vessels coming from the internal mammary circulation for resurfacing midline sternal defects.

Reference:

Mathes SJ, Nahai F. Classification of the vascular anatomy of muscles: experimental and clinical correlation. Plast Reconstr Surg. 1981; 67:177.

67. The correct response is A.

The latissimus dorsi muscle is commonly used as a standard choice for restoration of function of biceps muscle. The other options are not judicious options for biceps reconstruction, hence are not used clinically.

Reference:

Terzis JK, Sweet RC, Dykes RW, et al. Recovery of function in free muscle transplants using microneurovascular anastomoses. J Hand Surg. 1978; 3: 37.

68. The correct response is D.

The pectoralis major musculocutaneous flap is not a flap of choice for reconstruction of the defects of the nose due to limitations of length of pedicle for this site. The other options are valid indications for the use of this versatile flap.

Reference:

1. *Mathes SJ, Nahai F. Clinical Applications for Muscle and Musculocutaneous Flaps. St. Louis: CV Mosby, 1982.*
2. *McCraw JB, Dibbell DG, Carraway JH. Clinical definition of independent myocutaneous vascular territories. Plast Reconstr Surg. 1977; 60: 341.*

69. The correct response is D.

The latissimus dorsi flap is not suitable for reconstruction of the face, cheek and lips. The other options are valid indications for the use of this versatile flap.

Reference:

1. *Mathes SJ, Nahai F. Clinical Applications for Muscle and Musculocutaneous Flaps. St. Louis: CV Mosby, 1982.*
2. *McCraw JB, Dibbell DG, Carraway JH. Clinical definition of independent myocutaneous vascular territories. Plast Reconstr Surg. 1977; 60: 341.*

70. The correct response is B.

The transverse elliptical musculocutaneous flap based on the superior epigastric artery was popularised and described by Hartrampf for breast reconstruction. He theorized that the lower abdominal skin and fat could be transferred to the chest to create a breast mound based on the circulation of the rectus abdominis muscle. The successful outcome of this procedure opened the doors for a new technique for breast reconstruction.

Reference:

1. *Hartrampf CR, Scheflan M, Black P. Breast reconstruction with a transverse abdominal island flap. Plast Reconstr Surg. 1982;96:216.*
2. *Hartrampf CR Jr. The transverse abdominal island flap for breast reconstruction. A 7-year experience. Clin Plast Surg. 1988 Oct;15(4):703-16.*

71. The correct response is C.

Both the pedicled and free TRAM procedures may be indicated for patients desiring breast reconstruction. Patients in high-risk categories, such as those with a history of heavy cigarette use (>10 pack/years smoking) and those who are overweight or obese, are more suitable for free than for pedicle TRAM reconstruction. Advocates for the free TRAM cite its advantages of reduced abdominal dissection and muscle sacrifice, enhanced flap vascularity, ease of flap inset, and avoidance of disturbance of the medial inframammary fold. Requirement of microvascular skills and significantly higher risk of total flap failure are disadvantages of the free TRAM flap technique.

Reference:

1. *Grotting JC, Urist MM, Maddox WA, et al. Conventional TRAM flap versus free microsurgical TRAM flap for immediate breast reconstruction. Plast Reconstr Surg. 1989; 83: 828.*
2. *Elliott LF, Eskenazi L, Beegle PH, et al. Immediate TRAM flap breast reconstruction: 128 consecutive cases. Plast Reconstr Surg. 1993; 92:217.*
3. *Schusterman MA, Kroll SS, Weldon ME. Immediate breast reconstruction: why the free TRAM over the conventional TRAM? Plast Reconstr Surg. 1992; 90: 255.*

72. The correct response is D.

Gluteus maximus flaps can be used in any of the above ways for the treatment of sacral sores. The gluteal flap can be based superiorly or inferiorly, part or all of the muscle or both muscles may be used, it can be constructed of muscle or muscle and skin, and it may be rotated, advanced, or turned over. However use as free flap is not required as this is a regional muscle for this type of defect.

Reference:

Vasconez LO, Schneider WJ, Jurkiewicz MJ. Pressure sores. Curr Probl Surg. 1977;14:1.

73. The correct response is C.

The correct response is C. This concept was described by Debreuil-Chambardel and is referred to constantly by Michel Salmon in his description of the cutaneous arteries.

According to this concept "the anatomical territories of adjacent arteries bear an inverse relationship to each other yet combine to supply the same region." If one vessel is small, its partner is large to compensate, and vice versa. This is well illustrated in the variability in size between each of the parasternal perforators of the internal mammary artery and between the internal mammary perforators and the cutaneous perforator of the adjacent angiosome.

Reference:

Salmon M. Arteries of the skin. In: Taylor GI, Tempest M, eds. London: Churchill-Livingstone; 1988.

74. The correct response is A.

The gold standard for assessing viability of transferred tissue is clinical examination. A doppler ultrasonic probe is helpful for flap monitoring. Doppler monitoring is, however, subject to error, both false-positive and false-negative readings may occur and therefore this modality should always be used in conjunction with clinical evaluations.

Reference:

1. *Neligan PC. Monitoring techniques for the detection of flow failure in the postoperative period. Microsurgery. 1993; 14: 162.*
2. *Swartz WM, Izquierdo R,Miller MJ. Implantable venous Doppler microvascular monitoring laboratory investigation and clinical results. Plast Reconstr Surg. 1994; 3: 152.*

75. The correct response is C.

The word is derived from the Greek word 'micros' meaning small and 'skopein' meaning to view. It is an instrument which helps us to view small objects under magnification. Surgery done with the help of microscope is called microsurgery which refers to a set of surgical techniques performed beyond the limits of normal human eyesight.

Reference:

1. *Acland RD. Microsurgery: A Practice Manual. St. Louis: Mosby; 1980.*
2. *Buncke HJ. Microsurgery-retrospective. Clin Plast Surg. 1986; 13: 315.*

76. The correct response is D.

Tamai (1972) developed the sliding bar concept in double clamps used in microsurgery. This concept has virtually made the technique of microsurgery anastomosis simple to perform.

Reference:

1. *Acland RD. Microsurgery: A Practice Manual. St. Louis: Mosby; 1980.*
2. *Buncke HJ. Microsurgery-retrospective. Clin Plast Surg. 1986; 13: 315.*

77. The correct response is B.

End to side anastomosis is frequently done when the size of the vessel ends are not equal.

End to end anastomosis is done when the size of vessels is equal. Double approximating clamps are routinely used for performing anastomosis for ease of procedure. Adventitial stripping is also a standard microvascular technique used to prevent the intrusion of adventitial tissue into the lumen during the anastomosis.

Reference:

1. *Acland RD. Microsurgery: A Practice Manual. St. Louis: Mosby; 1980.*
2. *Buncke HJ. Microsurgery-retrospective. Clin Plast Surg. 1986; 13: 315.*

78. The correct response is A.

Nakayama introduced a vascular anastomotic coupling device, subsequently modified by Ostrup, consisting of polyethylene rings secured with steel pins. Use of such a device requires everted vessel walls and may not be possible with vessels that have a small diameter or atherosclerotic changes. Commercially available systems are available for vessels 1 to 4 mm in diameter. The patency rates achieved using anastomotic coupling devices are comparable to those using handsewn arterial anastomoses.

Reference:

Ostrup LT, Berggren A. The Unilink instrument system for fast and safe microvascular anastomosis. Ann Plast Surg. 1986; 17: 521.

79. The correct response is A.

Heparin is the most favoured anticoagulation agent. Dextran is used as a volume expander. It also inhibits platelet aggregation. Dextran use can lead to acute respiratory distress syndrome is some cases. Aspirin is used to prevent aggregation of platelets while papaverine is an antispasmodic agent which is used in dissection and anastomosis to reduce vasospasm.

Reference:

1. *Acland RD. Microsurgery: A Practice Manual. St. Louis: Mosby; 1980.*
2. *Buncke HJ. Microsurgery-retrospective. Clin Plast Surg. 1986; 13: 315.*

80. The correct response is B.

Nylen introduced the operating microscope for otolaryngologic surgery. The first compound microscope was invented by Zacharias and Hans Janseen in 1950. The term microvascular surgery was coined by Jacobson, who desired operating on small blood vessels under microscope magnification and demonstrated a 100% patency rate in vessels from 1.6 to 3.2 mm in diameter.

Reference:

Lee S, Frank DH, Choi SY. Historical review of small and microvascular vessel surgery. Ann Plast Surg. 1983;11:53.

81. The correct response is A.

The technique of first placing triangulating sutures to ensure equal traction on the blood vessels was first described by Carrel, who received the 1912 Nobel Prize in Medicine and Physiology for his work in this field.

Reference:

Lee S, Frank DH, Choi SY. Historical review of small and microvascular vessel surgery. Ann Plast Surg. 1983;11:53.

82. The correct response is D.

The local muscle shows atrophy and even disorganisation of myofibrils. Hypertrophy is not observed. The rest of the changes include epidermal thickening, thinning of dermis and formation of a fibrous capsule.

Reference:

Neumann CG. The expansion of an area of skin by progressive distention of a subcutaneous balloon. Plast Reconstr Surg. 1957;19:124.

83. The correct response is C.

Neumann is credited with the first use of an expansile implant to enlarge the periauricular skin for a traumatic ear deformity. Radovan reintroduced the concept of expansion when he inserted a contemporary device with an internally placed port. Eric Austad produced a self-inflating device for tissue expansion.

Reference:

1. *Austad ED, Rose GL. A self-inflating tissue expander. Plast Reconstr Surg. 1982;70:588.*
2. *Neumann CG. The expansion of an area of skin by progressive distention of a subcutaneous balloon. Plast Reconstr Surg. 1957;19:124.*

84. The correct response is D.

Alloderm is obtained from the cadaveric skin. It is acellular allogenic skin. The freeze dried sheets are rehydrated in isotonic saline for 5 minutes before they are used.

Reference:

Scalafani AP, Romo T, Jacono AA, et al: Evaluation of acellular dermal grafts in sheet (AlloDerm) and injectable (micronized Alloderm) forms for soft tissue augmentation. Arch. Fascial Plastic Surg 2000; 2:130-136.

85. The correct response is C.

Neuberg is credited with the use of first free fat autografts. He repaired a cosmetic defect around the orbit by fat transplantation. Leaf and Zarem brought attention to the technique of filling facial contours with dermal fat grafts.

Reference:

Lexer E. Free transplantation. Ann Surg 60:166, 1914. Jacono AA, et al: Evaluation of acellular dermal grafts in sheet (AlloDerm) and injectable (micronized Alloderm) forms for soft tissue augmentation. Arch. Fascial Plastic Surg 2000; 2:130-136.

86. The correct response is B.

The middle layer of the centrifuge is the usable layer for fat injection. This is transferred to appropriate Luer-Lok syringes for injection through blunt tipped cannulas.

Reference:

Coleman SR. The technique of periorbital lipoinfiltration. Oper Tech Plast Reconstr Surg. 1994; 1:120–126.

87. The correct response is A.

Coleman recommends that use of larger blunt cannulas, vasoconstriction by epinephrine, injection of 0.1 mL of filler per pass and a meticulous technique are some of the ways to prevent the embolic complications associated with soft tissue fillers.

Reference:

Coleman SR. Avoidance of arterial occlusion from injection of soft tissue fillers. Aesth Surg. 2002; 22: 555–557.

88. The correct response is C.

The tensor fascia lata is the single largest source and donor site for free fascial grafts. It may be used as a free graft, as a pedicled flap or as a vascularised free flap. The harvesting of a fascia lata graft may be performed at the lateral aspect of the thigh by an open approach for large grafts or by use of a stripper for long thin grafts.

Temporoparietal fascia grafts are also used clinically for numerous clinical situations but the amount of graft material is smaller when compared to fascia lata. The other options are not clinically used for harvesting fascial grafts commonly.

Reference:

1. *Nahai F, Hill HL, Coleman SR. Avoidance of arterial occlusion from injection of soft tissue fillers. Aesth Surg. 2002; 22: 555–557.*
2. *Crawford JS. Nature of fascia lata and its fate after implantation. Am J Ophthalmol 1969; 67: 900-907.*

89. The correct response is B.

The sturdy annular pulleys A2 and A4 are primarily responsible for preventing bowstringing of flexor tendons. The cruciate pulleys are thin and pliable and collapse to allow full digital flexion. The palmar aponeurosis pulley adds to the biomechanical efficiency of the sheath system.

Reference:

1. *Strickland JW. Development of flexor tendon surgery: twenty-five years of progress. J Hand Surg Am 2000; 25: 214-235.*
2. *Doyle JR, Blythe WF. Anatomy of the flexor tendon sheath and pulleys of the thumb. J Hand Surg Am 1977: 2: 149-151.*

90. The correct response is B.

Strickland comprehensively reviewed and determined that any locking or cruciate four strand core suture in combination with circumferential epitenon suture comes closest to ideal suture for flexor tendon repair. It is relatively easy to perform and places the knots outside the laceration site. The advantages of achieving greater tensile strength and decreased gap formation with multistrand repairs must be weighed against possible increase in bulk of the tendon, increased gliding resistance within the sheath, potential compromise of vascularity and increased operating time.

Reference:

1. *Strickland JW. Development of flexor tendon surgery: twenty-five years of progress. J Hand Surg Am 2000; 25: 214-235.*
2. *McLarney E, Hoffman H, Wolfe SW. Biomechanical analysis of the cruciate four-strand flexor tendon repair. J Hand Surg Am 1999; 24: 295-301.*
3. *Zhao C, Amadio PC, Momose IT et al. The effect of suture technique on adhesion formation after flexor tendon repair for partial lacerations in a canine model. J Trauma 2001; 51: 917-921.*

91. The correct response is B.

Plantaris offers the longest tendon as a donor graft, there is no functional loss after harvest and the tendon can also be braided if a thicker graft is required. However the disadvantages are that there is no test to determine its presence before surgery and it may be missing in 20% of cases. In case plantaris is not present on one side, only one in three will have a plantaris tendon on the other side.

Reference:

1. *Strickland JW. Development of flexor tendon surgery: twenty-five years of progress. J Hand Surg Am 2000; 25: 214-235.*
2. *Harvey FJ, Chu G, Harvey PM. Surgical availability of the plantaris tendon. J Hand Surg Am 1983; 8: 243-247.*

92. The correct response is B.

Fasciculation is the first change that occurs in a muscle when a motor nerve is cut. The irregular contractions are caused by release of acetylcholine from the degenerating distal axon. Several days after denervation, fibrillation begins characterised by spontaneous repetitive contractions that are due to enhanced sensitivity of the denervated muscle to acetylcholine. Atrophy of muscle begins after 3-4 months of denervation followed by gradual replacement with fat and connective tissue after 1-2 years.

Reference:

1. *Murphy R. Muscle. In Berne R, Levy M, eds: Physiology, 4th ed. St. Louis, Mosby, 1998; 267.*
2. *Owens N. The surgical treatment of facial paralysis, collective review. Plast Reconstr Surg 1951; 7: 61.*

93. The correct response is D.

The zygomaticus major is the muscle responsible for smiling. It is approximately 5 cm in length and it can contract by 1.5-2 cm during smiling. The zygomaticus minor helps in accentuating the nasolabial fold and thus it partially helps the zygomaticus major in producing the smile. The rest of the muscles are related to the animation of lip and nose.

Reference:

1. *Manktelow RT, Zuker RM. Muscle transplantation by fascicular territory. Plast Reconstr Surg 1984; 73: 751.*
2. *O'Brien B, Pederson W, Khazanchi R et al. Results of management of facial palsy with microvascular free-muscle transfer. Plast Reconstr Surg 1990; 86: 12.*

94. The correct response is B.

Ear and larynx are composed of elastic cartilage. Yellow elastic cartilage is present in the external ear cartilage and the epiglottis. The main function of the elastic cartilage is to provide support. Hyaline cartilage is present in joints, rib cage and trachea. Fibrocartilage is present in intervertebral disks and menisci.

Reference:

1. *Myers ER, Mow VC. Biomechanics of cartilage and its response to biomechanical stimuli. In Hall BK, ed: Cartilage: Structure, function and biochemistry. New York, Academic Press, 1983: 313-341.*
2. *Herberhold C. Reconstruction of the auricle with preserved homologous rib cartilage. Facial Plasti Surg 1988; 5: 431-433.*

95. The correct response is B.

Cryopreservation is the most prevalent technique for cartilage preservation. Some chondrocytes are able to survive freezing at -20°C. Multiple freeze-thaw cycles are necessary to completely eliminate viable chondrocytes. Refrigeration is the simplest form of cartilage preservation which can be achieved at 3°C to 5°C for as long as 7 days. Other reported means of preservation of cartilage are freeze drying, irradiation and merthiolate treatment. Lyophilization is effective for completely eliminating the cellular elements of cartilage grafts and permits long term storage of cartilage matrix. The use of merthiolate and irradiation can result in mineralization of the graft.

Reference:

1. *Malinin TI, Mnaymneh W, Lo HK et al. Cryopreservation of articular cartilage. Ultrastructural observations and long term results of experimental distal femoral transplantation. Clin Orthop 1994; 303: 18-32.*
2. *Bumann A, Kopp S, Eickbohm JE et al. Rehydration of lyophilised cartilage grafts sterilised by different methods. Int J Oral Maxillofac Surg 1989; 18: 370-372.*

96. The correct response is D.

Hyaline cartilage is present in joints, rib cage and trachea where the function is to dissipate the load. Fibrocartilage is present in intervertebral discs and menisci where the function is transfer of load.

Reference:

1. *Happey F. Studies of the structure of the human intervertebral disc in relation to its functional and aging processes. In Sokoloff L, ed The joints and synovial fluids, Vol 2. Academic Press, New York, 1980: 95-137.*
2. *Naylor A. The design and function of the human intervertebral discs. In Owen R, Goodfellow J, Bullough P, eds. Scientific foundations of Orthopaedics and Traumatology. London, Heinemann, 1980: 97-105.*

97. The correct response is E.

Elastic cartilage provides support function and is present in the ear and laryngeal cartilages. It is not present in the nasal septum.

Reference:

1. *Happey F. Studies of the structure of the human intervertebral disc in relation to its functional and aging processes. In Sokoloff L, ed The joints and synovial fluids, Vol 2. Academic Press, New York, 1980: 95-137.*
2. *Naylor A. The design and function of the human intervertebral discs. In Owen R, Goodfellow J, Bullough P, eds. Scientific foundations of Orthopaedics and Traumatology. London, Heinemann, 1980: 97-105.*

98. The correct response is F.

Fibrocartilage serves to provide the function of transfer of load, hence it is present in intervertebral discs and joints. It is not present in the nasal septum.

Reference:

1. *Happey F. Studies of the structure of the human intervertebral disc in relation to its functional and aging processes. In Sokoloff L, ed The joints and synovial fluids, Vol 2. Academic Press, New York, 1980: 95-137.*
2. *Naylor A. The design and function of the human intervertebral discs. In Owen R, Goodfellow J, Bullough P, eds. Scientific foundations of Orthopaedics and Traumatology. London, Heinemann, 1980: 97-105.*

99. The correct response is A.

Nerves are composed of three types of connective tissues; the endoneurium, the perineurium and the epineurium. The endoneurium is the supporting connective tissue that fills the fascicle and also provides protection of the axon from elongation injury. The perineurium is a thin sheath of connective tissue that surrounds each fascicle and functions to protect the fascicle and provide skeletal support. The epineurium is the layer that supports the nerve and is loosely attached to surrounding structures by the mesoneurium.

Reference:

1. *Sunderland S. Nerve and nerve injuries, 2nd ed, New York, Churchill Livingstone, 1978.*
2. *Mackinnon S, Dellon A. Surgery of the peripheral nerve. New York, Thieme, 1988.*

100. The correct response is B.

Axonotmesis is characterised by loss of axonal continuity with intact surrounding connective tissue sheath components. Regeneration therefore occurs from the intact proximal nerve and proceeds as limited by the axonal transport and regrowth of approximately 1 mm/day. It is not observed in other types of nerve injuries.

Reference:

1. *Sunderland S. A classification of peripheral nerve injuries producing loss of function. Brain 1951; 74: 491-516.*
2. *Seddon H. Three types of nerve injury. Brain 1943; 66: 237-288.*

101. The correct response is B.

Purely objective measures of sensory nerve injury help to compliment the clinical diagnosis of nerve injury. Of these the Moberg's Ninhydrin test is based on the principle that the denervated areas are devoid of sweat hence will not chemically react with Ninhydrin. The O'Rain's test is based on the observation that a denervated finger will not wrinkle when it is placed for a prolonged period in water.

Reference:

1. *Moberg E. Objective methods of determining functional value of sensibility in the hand. J Bone Joint Surg Br 1958; 40: 454-459.*
2. *O'Rain S. New and simple test of nerve function in the hand. Br Med J 1973; 3: 615-616.*

102. The correct response is B.

The innervation density is decreased in nerve lesions. This can be commonly tested by static and dynamic two-point discrimination. The normal values of these vary according to the location in the body. The fingertip has the lowest value of static 2PD as varying from 2-6 mm, while the great toe pulp has the value of around 8 mm. Chest and back have far greater values of two-point discrimination.

Reference:

1. *Szabo RM, Gelberman RH, Williamson RV et al. Vibratory sensory testing in acute peripheral nerve compression. J Hand Surg Am 1984; 9: 104-109.*
2. *Dellon AL. Sensibility testing. In Gelberman RH ed, Operative nerve repair and reconstruction. Philadelphia, JB Lippincott, 1991: 136-158.*

103. The correct response is A.

The sural nerve can give graft material of 30-40 cm long which is one of the commonest site for harvesting nerve grafts. The rest yield material of shorter length. Superficial radial sensory yields 10-15 cm long; lateral femoral cutaneous yields 2-8 cm and great auricular nerve yields 3-5 cm of nerve graft material.

Reference:

1. *Millesi H. Indications and technique for nerve grafting. In Gelberman RH ed, Operative nerve repair and reconstruction. Philadelphia, JB Lippincott, 1991: 525-543.*
2. *Nunley J. Donor nerves for grafting. In Gelberman RH ed, Operative nerve repair and reconstruction. Philadelphia, JB Lippincott, 1991: 545-552.*

104. The correct response is A.

Median nerve shows the best results of motor recovery following microneurosurgical repair amongst all the nerves. The return of function graded as M4 or M5 may be seen in 77% to 90 % of the repairs. The results of ulnar nerve and radial nerve are not upto this level. The nerves of lower extremity fare worse in terms of motor recovery when compared with upper extremity nerves. Peroneal nerve repair carries a poor outcome when compared to the tibial nerve.

Reference:

1. *Tupper JW, Crick JC, Matteck LR. Fascicular nerve repairs. A comparative study of epineurial and fascicular (perineurial) techniques. Orthop Clin North Am 1988; 19: 57-69.*
2. *Mailander P, Berger A, Schaller E et al. Results of primary nerve repair to the upper extremity. Microsurgery 1989; 10: 147-150.*

105. The correct response is E.

Mini-plates and screws are used for treatment of fractures using principles of skeletal fixation. Stainless steel and titanium are the principal metals currently available for biologic implantation. The other options given are of various types of implants which are primarily used for soft tissue augmentation purposes. Nasal implants and breast implants are commonly made of silicone.

Reference:

1. *Williams DF, Roaf R, eds: Implants in Surgery. Philadelphia, WB Saunders, 1973.*
2. *Lynch W: Implants: Reconstructing the human body. New York, Van Nostrand Reinhold, 1982: 1.*

106. The correct response is D.

Medical devices are categorised into one of three classes, depending upon degree of complexity, invasiveness and several other criteria. A Class 1 device exposes patients to little or no risk and these are devices which are not implanted into the body but have only temporary contact with the body e.g tongue blade. Class 2 device exposes patients to intermediate risk and is comprised of those devices which are implanted temporarily into the body. Class 3 devices are those which expose the patients to significant risk and are those that are designed for permanent implantation.

Reference:

Angell M. Science on Trial: The Clash of Medical Evidence and the Law in the Breast Implant Case. New York, WW Norton, 1997: 95.

107. The correct response is A.

Medical devices are categorised into one of three classes, depending upon degree of complexity, invasiveness and several other criteria. A Class 1 device exposes patients to little or no risk and these are devices which are not implanted into the body but have only temporary contact with the body e.g tongue blade. Class 2 device exposes patients to intermediate risk and is comprised of those devices which are implanted temporarily into the body e.g intravenous cannula. Class 3 devices are those which expose the patients to significant risk and are those that are designed for permanent implantation.

Reference:

Angell M. Science on Trial: The Clash of Medical Evidence and the Law in the Breast Implant Case. New York, WW Norton, 1997: 95.

108. The correct response is B.

Medical devices are categorised into one of three classes, depending upon degree of complexity, invasiveness and several other criteria. A Class 1 device exposes patients to little or no risk and these are devices which are not implanted into the body but have only temporary contact with the body e.g tongue blade. Class 2 device exposes patients to intermediate risk and is comprised of those devices which are implanted temporarily into the body e.g intravenous cannula. Class 3 devices are those which expose the patients to significant risk and are those that are designed for permanent implantation e.g pacemaker.

Reference:

Angell M. Science on Trial: The Clash of Medical Evidence and the Law in the Breast Implant Case. New York, WW Norton, 1997: 95.

109. The correct response is C.

Vicryl is a braided suture amongst these with absorption rate of 40-70 days and having the highest break strength. The rest all are monofilament absorbable sutures with comparatively lesser break strengths.

Reference:

1. *Casey D, Lewis OG. Absorbable and nonabsorbable sutures. In Von Recum AF, ed: Handbook of Biomaterials Evaluation: Scientific, Technical, and Clinical Testing of Implant Materials. New York, MacMillan, 1986: 86-94.*
2. *Reiter D. Methods and materials for wound closure. Otolaryngol Clin North Am 1995; 28: 1069.*

110. The correct response is A.

Silk is a braided suture. The rest are all monofilament nonabsorbable sutures.

Reference:

1. *Casey D, Lewis OG. Absorbable and nonabsorbable sutures. In Von Recum AF, ed: Handbook of Biomaterials Evaluation: Scientific, Technical, and Clinical Testing of Implant Materials. New York, MacMillan, 1986: 86-94.*
2. *Reiter D. Methods and materials for wound closure. Otolaryngol Clin North Am 1995; 28: 1069.*

111. The correct response is B.

Polymethyl methacrylate (PMMA) is a biocompatible, inert, rigid polymer. The liquid monomeric methyl methacrylate is combined with powdered methyl methacrylate polymer granules at the time of surgical application. The mixture assumes mouldable consistency and can be tailored to fit the defect. The other materials are stable implants and do not exist in liquid form.

Reference:

1. *Breitbart AS, Ablaza VJ. Implant materials, In Aston SJ, Beasley RW, Thorne CHM, eds: Grabb and Smith's Plastic Surgery, 5th ed. Philadelphia, Lippincott-Raven, 1997: 39-46.*
2. *Sevin KA, Saray A, Yormauk E. Exposure of high-density porous polyethylene (Medpor) used for contour restoration and treatment. Br J Oral Maxillofac Surg 2000; 38: 44.*

112. The correct response is C.

Vicryl has the fastest absorption rate of 40-70 days amongst the sutures listed. Catgut absorbs in ~90 days, PDS in 90 days - 6 months and monocryl and maxion absorb in 90-120 days.

Reference:

1. *Casey D, Lewis OG. Absorbable and nonabsorbable sutures. In Von Recum AF, ed: Handbook of Biomaterials Evaluation: Scientific, Technical, and Clinical Testing of Implant Materials. New York, MacMillan, 1986: 86-94.*
2. *Reiter D. Methods and materials for wound closure. Otolaryngol Clin North Am 1995; 28: 1069.*

113. The correct response is C.

Nylon is a polyamide and comes under various trade names as surgilon, ethilon, dermalon etc. It is available as a braided, monofilament or as a sheath. It has a break strength of 460-710 MPa and an elongation to break percentage ranging from 17-65.

Reference:

1. *Casey D, Lewis OG. Absorbable and nonabsorbable sutures. In Von Recum AF, ed: Handbook of Biomaterials Evaluation: Scientific, Technical, and Clinical Testing of Implant Materials. New York, MacMillan, 1986: 86-94.*
2. *Reiter D. Methods and materials for wound closure. Otolaryngol Clin North Am 1995; 28: 1069.*

114. The correct response is D.

Prolene has a monofilament structure and is able to resist infection better. Multifilament / braided sutures run higher risk of infection but are also susceptible to failure by shear forces. The monofilament suture however can be damaged and weakened by crushing forceps and other instruments.

Reference:

1. *Casey D, Lewis OG. Absorbable and nonabsorbable sutures. In Von Recum AF, ed: Handbook of Biomaterials Evaluation: Scientific, Technical, and Clinical Testing of Implant Materials. New York, MacMillan, 1986: 86-94.*
2. *Reiter D. Methods and materials for wound closure. Otolaryngol Clin North Am 1995; 28: 1069.*

115. The correct response is D.

The word is derived from a Greek noun; 'Prostithenai', which means the act of addition. It was first mentioned in the Greek mythology involving the tale of Trojan War. In this war, Apollo's oracle at Delphi prophesised that Troy could be seized only if the prosthesis of Pelops was brought back to Troy.

Reference:

Flaum E. The Encyclopaedia of Mythology, Gods, Heroes and Legends of the Greeks and the Romans. Philadelphia, Running Press Books Publishers, 1993.

116. The correct response is C.

The Munsell colour system is the most commonly used colour matching scheme for the construction of facial prostheses. It uses three parameters; hue, value and chroma for the determination of appropriate colour. The prosthetist uses a portable Munsell colour meter to match the prosthesis to the patient's skin characteristics.

Clinical examination and digital photography have limited application for colour matching and can be unreliable.

Reference:

Robert A. Intrinsic and extrinsic colouration of prosthesis. In McKinstry R, ed: Fundamentals of Facial Prosthesis Surgery. Arlington, Va, ABI Professional Publications, 1995: 161-168.

117. The correct response is D.

Osseointegration currently provides the most secure method of fixation of nose prostheses than do other methods. The implants are placed in the anterior floor of the nose to allow easy access. This method is also applicable for large midfacial defects where the implants may be placed in the maxillary tuberosity, frontal process of maxilla, midzygoma or the superior orbital rim. A period of 4-6 months is required for the process of osteointegration of the implants.

Reference:

1. *Tolman DE, Taylor PF. Bone-anchored craniofacial prosthesis study: irradiated patients. Int J Oral Maxillofac Implants 1996; 11: 612-619.*
2. *Jensen OT, Brownd C, Blacker J. Nasofacial prostheses supported by osseointegrated implants. Int J Oral Maxillofac Implants 1992; 7: 203-211.*

118. The correct response is B.

The minimum length of a finger remnant stump is 1.5 cm for retention of a prostheses. The remnant stump may occasionally require surgical revision to ensure reliable fixation.

Reference:

1. *Pillet J. Esthetic hand prostheses. J Hand Surg Am 1983; 8: 778-781.*
2. *Beasley RW, de Beze GM. Prosthetic substitution for finger-nails. Hand Clin 1990; 6: 105-110.*

119. The correct response is B.

The minimum length of a proximal forearm stump with good elbow function is 10-14 cm. Lengthening of the bone or soft tissue release may be required for patients with a short proximal forearm amputation before prosthesis fitting and construction.

Reference:

1. *Pillet J. Esthetic hand prostheses. J Hand Surg Am 1983; 8: 778-781.*
2. *Burkhalter WE, Mayfield F, Carmona LS. The upper extremity amputee. Early and immediate post-surgical prosthetic fitting. J Bone Joint Surg Am 1976; 58: 46-51.*

120. The correct response is C.

Battery powered myoelectric prostheses are activated by myoelectric impulses generated from contraction of stump muscles. These devices use cutaneous sensors to detect the action potentials of remnant stump muscles that are processed by a microcomputer and magnified to activate an electric motor inside the prosthesis.

Reference:

1. *Battye C, Nightingale A, Whillis J. Use of myoelectric currents in the operation of prostheses. J Bone Joint Surg Br 1955; 37: 506.*
2. *Kobrinsky A. Problems of pio-electric control in automatic and remote control. First International Congress of the International Federation of Automation Control, vol 2. Oxford, Butterworth, 1960.*

121. The correct response is B.

Stevens-Johnson syndrome (SJS) is the one that is closely associated with toxic epidermal necrolysis (TEN). Its features closely resemble that of TEN and currently SJS and TEN are considered to be variants of the same drug-induced process and probably exist on a spectrum with TEN being the more severe form of the same process. The other syndromes are unrelated to TEN.

Reference:

1. *Roujeau JC, Stern RS. Severe adverse cutaneous reactions to drugs. N Engl J Med 1994; 331: 1272-1285.*
2. *Craven NM. Management of toxic epidermal necrolysis. Hosp Med 2000; 61: 778-781.*

122. The correct response is A.

Epidermolysis bullosa is characterised by 'blisters' on fingers and other parts due to trauma. This is due to a fault in the binding system (anchoring) of the various layers of the skin. In the severe form, the blistering process is followed by repeated cyclic scarring and healing resulting in severe contractures and deformity requiring plastic surgery intervention.

Reference:

1. *Fine JD, Bauer EA, Briggaman RA et al. Revised clinical and laboratory criteria for subtypes of inherited epidermolysis bullosa. A consensus report by the Subcommittee on Diagnosis and Classification of the National Epidermolysis Bullosa Registry. J Am Acad Dermatol 1991; 24: 119-135.*
2. *Lin AN, Carter DM. Epidermolysis bullosa. Annu Rev Med 1993; 44: 189-199.*

123. The correct response is E.

The TBSA at birth for head is 19 while the same in adults is 7. For the rest of the areas the value of TBSA remains the same or increases.

Reference:

1. *Neuwalder JM, Sampson C, Breuing KH et al. A review of computer-aided body surface area determination: SAGE II and EPRI's 3D Burn Vision. J Burn Care Rehabil 2002; 23: 55-59.*
2. *Muller MJ, Pegg SP, Rule MR. Determinants of death following burn injury. Br J Surg 2001; 88: 583-587.*

124. The correct response is E.

The percentage area for the foot is designated as 3.5% and this does not change with age of the patient. For head the value is 19% at birth which is reduced to 7% in adults; for thigh the values are 5.5% at birth and change to 9.5% in adults. For leg the values at birth are 5% which change to 7% in adults.

Reference:

1. *Neuwalder JM, Sampson C, Breuing KH et al. A review of computer-aided body surface area determination: SAGE II and EPRI's 3D Burn Vision. J Burn Care Rehabil 2002; 23: 55-59.*
2. *Muller MJ, Pegg SP, Rule MR. Determinants of death following burn injury. Br J Surg 2001; 88: 583-587.*

125. The correct response is A.

Half of the total amount of fluid to be given is replaced during the first eight hours. Fluid replacement is based on the observation that fluid loss from the vascular space occurs at a constant rate during the first day after injury. The amount of replacement fluid is predicted from the extent of the burn and size of the patient.

Reference:

1. *Salisbury RE. Thermal burns. In McCarthy JM, ed: Plastic Surgery. Philadelphia, WB Saunders, 1990: 787-789.*
2. *Neuwalder JM, Sampson C, Breuing KH et al. A review of computer-aided body surface area determination: SAGE II and EPRI's 3D Burn Vision. J Burn Care Rehabil 2002; 23: 55-59.*

126. The correct response is A.

The urine output is a standard measure of an adequate clinical response to the fluid therapy in burns. Inadequate urine output calls for an increase in fluids. It should be maintained around 1 c.c. /minute i.e. 60 c.c.in an hour and 1440 c.c. in 24 hours.

Reference:

1. *Salisbury RE. Thermal burns. In McCarthy JM, ed: Plastic Surgery. Philadelphia, WB Saunders, 1990: 787-789.*
2. *Neuwalder JM, Sampson C, Breuing KH et al. A review of computer-aided body surface area determination: SAGE II and EPRI's 3D Burn Vision. J Burn Care Rehabil 2002; 23: 55-59.*

127. The correct response is A.

Brooke's formula advocates the use of colloids on Day 1 of burns in dose of 0.5 mL/kg/% burns. The rest of the formulae specify use of colloids after Day 1 in different doses.

Reference:

1. *Salisbury RE. Thermal burns. In McCarthy JM, ed: Plastic Surgery. Philadelphia, WB Saunders, 1990: 787-789.*
2. *Neuwalder JM, Sampson C, Breuing KH et al. A review of computer-aided body surface area determination: SAGE II and EPRI's 3D Burn Vision. J Burn Care Rehabil 2002; 23: 55-59.*

128. The correct response is A.

The Parkland's formula for crystalloids is Lactated Ringer's solution @ 4 mL/kg/% burn. Option B is correct for Modified Brooke's formula; option C is good for Brooke's formula and option D is good for Evans formula.

Reference:

1. *Salisbury RE. Thermal burns. In McCarthy JM, ed: Plastic Surgery. Philadelphia, WB Saunders, 1990: 787-789.*
2. *Neuwalder JM, Sampson C, Breuing KH et al. A review of computer-aided body surface area determination: SAGE II and EPRI's 3D Burn Vision. J Burn Care Rehabil 2002; 23: 55-59.*

129. The correct response is D.

Ringer's lactate is not given on the second day according to the Parkland's formula. Colloids are given instead as per the requirements to stabilise the blood pressure and have an adequate amount of urine output.

Reference:

1. *Salisbury RE. Thermal burns. In McCarthy JM, ed: Plastic Surgery. Philadelphia, WB Saunders, 1990: 787-789.*
2. *Neuwalder JM, Sampson C, Breuing KH et al. A review of computer-aided body surface area determination: SAGE II and EPRI's 3D Burn Vision. J Burn Care Rehabil 2002; 23: 55-59.*

130. The correct response is C.

Integra is derived from bovine collagen and shark chondroitin sulphate matrix; cadaveric skin is derived from split thickness human skin; transcyte is derived from human fibroblast in collagen matrix and alloderm is derived from acellular human dermis.

Reference:

1. *Salisbury RE. Thermal burns. In McCarthy JM, ed: Plastic Surgery. Philadelphia, WB Saunders, 1990: 787-789.*
2. *Luce EA. Burn care and management. Clin Plast Surg. 2000; 27: 1.*

131. The correct response is D.

Transcyte is derived from human fibroblast in collagen matrix. Integra is derived from bovine collagen and shark chondroitin sulphate matrix; cadaveric skin is derived from split thickness human skin and alloderm is derived from acellular human dermis.

Reference:

1. *Salisbury RE. Thermal burns. In McCarthy JM, ed: Plastic Surgery. Philadelphia, WB Saunders, 1990: 787-789.*
2. *Luce EA. Burn care and management. Clin Plast Surg. 2000; 27: 1.*

132. The correct response is E.

Alloderm is derived from acellular human dermis. Transcyte is derived from human fibroblast in collagen matrix. Integra is derived from bovine collagen and shark chondroitin sulphate matrix and cadaveric skin is derived from split thickness human skin.

Reference:

1. *Salisbury RE. Thermal burns. In McCarthy JM, ed: Plastic Surgery. Philadelphia, WB Saunders, 1990: 787-789.*
2. *Luce EA. Burn care and management. Clin Plast Surg. 2000;27:1.*

133. The correct response is C.

1 gray is equivalent to 100 Rads. The former unit of Rad is equal to 1c Gy (centigray).

Reference:

1. *Paterson R. A dosage system for gamma-ray therapy. Part 1. Br J Radiol 1934; 7: 592.*
2. *Fletcher GH. Basic principles of the combination of irradiation and surgery. Int J Radiat Oncol Biol Phys 1979;5: 2091.*

134. The correct response is A.

Hypothermia is defined as a decrease in the core body temperature below 35°C. The severity of hypothermia is further classified as mild (32.2°C - 35°C); moderate (28°C - 32.1°C) and severe (below 28°C).

Reference:

1. *Orr KD, Fainer DC. Cold injuries in Korea during the winter of 1950-1951. Medicine (Baltimore) 1952; 31: 177.*
2. *Whayne TF, DeBakey MF. Cold injury, Ground type. Washington, DC, Office of the Surgeon General, Department of the Army, 1958.*

135. The correct response is A.

Cardiac changes are responsible for fatal outcome in severe hypothermia. To begin with these changes produce tachycardia, increased cardiac output due to release of catecholamines, but later bradycardia sets in and blood flow to brain, heart, kidneys becomes less. Cardiac changes include development of a J- wave between QRS and ST segment, auricular fibrillation, ventricular fibrillation and death due to asystole.

Reference:

1. *Orr KD, Fainer DC. Cold injuries in Korea during the winter of 1950-1951. Medicine (Baltimore) 1952; 31: 177.*
2. *Whayne TF, DeBakey MF. Cold injury, Ground type. Washington, DC, Office of the Surgeon General, Department of the Army, 1958.*

136. The correct response is C.

Frostbite has been categorised into four degrees of injury. In the first degree injury there is erythema, numbness and oedema. In the second degree, which affects the upper dermis, there is blister formation. Third degree injury is deep dermal and results in development of haemorrhagic blisters. In the fourth degree injury there is tissue loss.

Reference:

1. *McCauley RL, Hing DN, Robson MC et al. Frostbite injuries: a rational approach based on the pathophysiology. J Trauma 1983; 23: 143.*
2. *Reamy BV. Frostbite: review and current concepts. J Am Board Fam Pract 1998; 11: 34.*

137. The correct response is D.

Alkalosis is not a feature of frostbite. Formation of ice crystals, irreversible denaturing of lipid-protein complexes, local tissue hypoxia, vasoconstriction, acidosis and release of cytokines, thromboxane A_2 etc are associated with frostbite.

Reference:

1. *McCauley RL, Hing DN, Robson MC et al. Frostbite injuries: a rational approach based on the pathophysiology. J Trauma 1983; 23: 143.*
2. *Reamy BV. Frostbite: review and current concepts. J Am Board Fam Pract 1998; 11: 34.*

138. The correct response is D.

Rapid rewarming is indicated in frostbite to decrease further tissue damage and prevent further release of secondary mediators. Immersion of the part in hot water at 40 degree C for 15-30 minutes is ideal to reverse the process and arrest further damage. This should be supported by local dressings, symptomatic treatment and antibiotics.

Reference:

1. *McCauley RL, Hing DN, Robson MC et al. Frostbite injuries: a rational approach based on the pathophysiology. J Trauma 1983; 23: 143.*
2. *Reamy BV. Frostbite: review and current concepts. J Am Board Fam Pract 1998; 11: 34.*

139. The correct response is A.

Blisters with clear fluid should be debrided because these contain high concentrations of inflammatory mediators. In patients where the fluid is haemorrhagic, blisters should not be debrided as these represent deep tissue injury and following debridement there is risk of desiccation of deeper structures due to uncovering.

Reference:

1. *McCauley RL, Hing DN, Robson MC et al. Frostbite injuries: a rational approach based on the pathophysiology. J Trauma 1983; 23: 143.*
2. *Reamy BV. Frostbite: review and current concepts. J Am Board Fam Pract 1998; 11: 34.*

140. The correct response is C.

Acute mountain sickness can occur at an elevation above 7000 feet and is characterised by nausea, insomnia, headache, palpitation and shortness of breath. This is not considered a serious illness.

Reference:

Larson EB, Roach RC, Schoene RB et al. Acute mountain sickness and acetazolamide. JAMA 1982; 248: 328.

141. The correct response is B

Pulmonary oedema is associated with high altitude climbing and occurs when the climber ascends beyond 7000 feet. It is characterised by acute shortness of breath, cough and cyanosis. Immediate decrease in elevation and administration of oxygen can alter the course of this potentially fatal illness.

Reference:

Larson EB, Roach RC, Schoene RB et al. Acute mountain sickness and acetazolamide. JAMA 1982; 248: 328.

142. The correct response is E.

Debridement is the removal of necrotic tissue, foreign material, and infecting bacteria from an acute or chronic wound. These tissues impede the body's attempt to heal by producing proteases, collagenases and elastases that obstruct wound healing.

Reference:

1. *Heimbachs DM, Engrav L. Surgical management of the Burn wound. New York, Raven Press, 1985.*
2. *Steed DL, Donohoe D, Webster MW et al. Effect of extensive debridement and treatment on the healing of diabetic foot ulcers. J Am Coll Surg 1996; 183: 61.*

143. The correct response is D.

The dead muscle has all the features listed except that it will not contract when grasped with forceps. Healthy muscle has a bright red appearance and bleeds on cutting.

Reference:

1. *Heimbachs DM, Engrav L. Surgical management of the Burn wound. New York, Raven Press, 1985.*
2. *Steed DL, Donohoe D, Webster MW et al. Effect of extensive debridement and treatment on the healing of diabetic foot ulcers. J Am Coll Surg 1996; 183: 61.*

144. The correct response is C.

Paprika sign is punctate bleeding from the cut edge of the bone during debridement. This signifies that healthy bone has been reached.

Reference:

1. *Heimbachs DM, Engrav L. Surgical management of the Burn wound. New York, Raven Press, 1985.*
2. *Steed DL, Donohoe D, Webster MW et al. Effect of extensive debridement and treatment on the healing of diabetic foot ulcers. J Am Coll Surg 1996; 183: 61.*

145. The correct response is C.

Tegasorb is a type of hydrocolloid dressing, the rest are types of film dressings. Film dressings are those that allow exchange of oxygen, carbon dioxide and water vapour. The exchange of water vapour prevents fluid buildup in low-secreting wounds. Hydrocolloid dressings consist of a water impermeable polyurethane film outer covering over a layer of hydrocolloid. They can absorb some fluid but are best on minimally exudative wounds.

Reference:

1. *Falanga V. Occlusive wound dressings. Why, when, which? Arch Dermatol 1988; 124: 872.*
2. *Alvarez OM, Hefton JM, Eaglstein WH. Healing wounds: occlusion or exposure. Infect Surg 1984; 3: 173.*

146. The correct response is B.

The term endoscope is derived from two Greek words, 'endon' meaning within and 'skopein' meaning to examine. An endoscope is therefore most simply described as a device for allowing the viewer to see within a space or a cavity.

Reference:

1. *Bostwick J, Eaves FF, Nahai F. Endoscopic Plastic Surgery. St. Louis, Quality Medical Publishing, 1995.*
2. *Gordon AG, Magos AL. The development of laparoscopic surgery. Baillieres Clin Obstet Gynaecol 1989; 3: 429-449.*

147. The correct response is A.

The endoscope needs to be placed in an optical cavity inside the body. The concept of optical cavity is important in endoscopic plastic surgery. Optical cavity allows the endoscope to be separated from the tissues being viewed, improves incoming light and also makes room for instrument movement. The optical cavities are classified on the basis of space, support, medium and pressure. Type 1 cavities are based on potential spaces that exist within the body e.g peritoneal cavity. Type 2 cavities are also potential spaces but rigid tissues themselves provide the support. e.g. thorax. Type 3 optical cavities are similar to type II but differ in that the space already exists and does not require development. e.g carpal tunnel release, nasoendoscopic procedures. Type 4 optical cavities are those that must be established through dissection followed by a need to maintain it mechanically. e.g endoscopic procedures of head and neck, breast, abdomen and extremities.

Reference:

1. *Miller MJ, Robb GL. Endoscopic technique for free flap harvesting. Clin Plast Surg 1995; 4: 755-773.*
2. *Karp NS, Bass LS, Kasabian AK et al. Balloon assisted endoscopic harvest of the latissimus dorsi muscle. Plast Reconstr Surg 1997; 100: 1161-1167.*
3. *Bostwick J, Eaves FF, Nahai F. Endoscopic Plastic Surgery. St. Louis, Quality Medical Publishing, 1995.*

148. The correct response is B.

The endoscope needs to be placed in an optical cavity inside the body. The concept of optical cavity is important in endoscopic plastic surgery. Optical cavity allows the endoscope to be separated from the tissues being viewed, improves incoming light and also makes room for instrument movement. The optical cavities are classified on the basis of space, support, medium and pressure. Type 1 cavities are based on potential spaces that exist within the body e.g peritoneal cavity. Type 2 cavities are also potential spaces but rigid tissues themselves provide the support. e.g. thorax. The type 2 optical cavity may be used in latissimus dorsi muscle cardiac augmentation. Type 3 optical cavities are similar to type II but differ in that the space already exists and does not require development. e.g carpal tunnel release, nasoendoscopic procedures. Type 4 optical cavities are those that must be established through dissection followed by a need to maintain it mechanically. e.g endoscopic procedures of head and neck, breast, abdomen and extremities.

Reference:

1. *Miller MJ, Robb GL. Endoscopic technique for free flap harvesting. Clin Plast Surg 1995; 4: 755-773.*
2. *Karp NS, Bass LS, Kasabian AK et al. Balloon assisted endoscopic harvest of the latissimus dorsi muscle. Plast Reconstr Surg 1997; 100: 1161-1167.*
3. *Bostwick J, Eaves FF, Nahai F. Endoscopic Plastic Surgery. St. Louis, Quality Medical Publishing, 1995.*

149. The correct response is C.

The endoscope needs to be placed in an optical cavity inside the body. The concept of optical cavity is important in endoscopic plastic surgery. Optical cavity allows the endoscope to be separated from the tissues being viewed, improves incoming light and also makes room for instrument movement. The optical cavities are classified on the basis of space, support, medium and pressure. Type 1 cavities are based on potential spaces that exist within the body e.g peritoneal cavity. Type 2 cavities are also potential spaces but rigid tissues themselves provide the support. e.g. thorax. The type 2 optical cavity may be used in latissimus dorsi muscle cardiac augmentation. Type 3 optical cavities are similar to type II but differ in that the space already exists and does not require development. e.g carpal tunnel release, nasoendoscopic procedures. Type 4 optical cavities are those that must be established through dissection followed by a need to maintain it mechanically. e.g endoscopic procedures of head and neck, breast, abdomen and extremities.

Reference:

1. *Miller MJ, Robb GL. Endoscopic technique for free flap harvesting. Clin Plast Surg 1995; 4: 755-773.*
2. *Karp NS, Bass LS, Kasabian AK et al. Balloon assisted endoscopic harvest of the latissimus dorsi muscle. Plast Reconstr Surg 1997; 100: 1161-1167.*
3. *Bostwick J, Eaves FF, Nahai F. Endoscopic Plastic Surgery. St. Louis, Quality Medical Publishing, 1995.*

150. The correct response is D.

The endoscope needs to be placed in an optical cavity inside the body. The concept of optical cavity is important in endoscopic plastic surgery. Optical cavity allows the endoscope to be separated from the tissues being viewed, improves incoming light and also makes room for instrument movement. The optical cavities are classified on the basis of space, support, medium and pressure. Type 1 cavities are based on potential spaces that exist within the body e.g peritoneal cavity. Type 2 cavities are also potential spaces but rigid tissues themselves provide the support. e.g. thorax. The type 2 optical cavity may be used in latissimus dorsi muscle cardiac augmentation. Type 3 optical cavities are similar to type II but differ in that the space already exists and does not require development. e.g carpal tunnel release, nasoendoscopic procedures. Type 4 optical cavities are those that must be established through dissection followed by a need to maintain it mechanically. e.g endoscopic procedures of head and neck, breast, abdomen and extremities. The harvest of rectus abdominis endoscopically is an example of a type 4 optical cavity.

Reference:

1. *Miller MJ, Robb GL. Endoscopic technique for free flap harvesting. Clin Plast Surg 1995; 4: 755-773.*
2. *Karp NS, Bass LS, Kasabian AK et al. Balloon assisted endoscopic harvest of the latissimus dorsi muscle. Plast Reconstr Surg 1997; 100: 1161-1167.*
3. *Bostwick J, Eaves FF, Nahai F. Endoscopic Plastic Surgery. St. Louis, Quality Medical Publishing, 1995.*

151. The correct response is D.

Magnetic resonance imaging currently is the preferred imaging modality for foetal anomalies as the soft tissue contrast, multiple planes for reconstruction and a large field of view allow unparalleled insight into the anomaly which is superior to ultrasonography. MRI is also being used for cases in which foetal complications have occurred with nonspecific ultrasound diagnoses.

Reference:

1. *Ohgiya Y, Gokan T, Hamamizu K et al. Fast MRI in obstetric diagnoses. J Comput Assist Tomogr 2001; 25: 190-200.*
2. *Levine D. Ultrasound versus magnetic resonance imaging in fetal evaluation. Top Magn Reson Imaging 2001; 12: 25-38.*

152. The correct response is A.

AFP is a protein made in the liver of the developing foetus. It circulates through the foetal blood stream and is excreted by the foetal kidney. Elevated levels of AFP are seen in open neural tube defects, twins, late pregnancy complications like preterm delivery, IUGR and haemorrhage. Down's syndrome, trisomy 18 etc are associated with low AFP levels.

Reference:

1. *Davidson RG. Policy on screening for maternal serum alphafetoprotein [editorial]. CMAJ 1987; 136: 1247.*
2. *Main DM, Mennuti MT. Neural tube defects: issues in prenatal diagnosis and counselling. Obstet Gynecol 1986; 67: 1-16.*

153. The correct response is B.

Dexon is made from polyglycolic acid (PGA) by polymerisation. It constitutes the most widely used polymers in tissue engineering. The other options are also used in tissue engineering and belong to the family of aliphatic polyesters.

Reference:

1. *Frazza EJ, Schmitt EE. A new absorbable suture. J Biomed Mater Res 1971; 5: 43-58.*
2. *Vacanti JP, Langer R. Tissue engineering: the design and fabrication of living replacement devices for surgical reconstruction and transplantation. Lancet 1999; 354 (suppl 1) : SI32-SI34.*

154. The correct response is D.

Biobrane is the one which is composed of silicone, nylon mesh, porcine collagen with or without human matrix proteins. Epicel is composed of cultured autologous human keratinocytes, alloderm is composed of acellular lyophilized human dermal matrix, integra is composed of bovine collagen with chondroitin sulphate matrix and apligraf is composed of human keratinocyte epidermis with a collagen lattice and human fibroblast dermis.

Reference:

1. *Lorenz C, Petracic A, Hohl HP et al. Early wound closure and early reconstruction. Experience with a dermal substitute in a child with 60 percent surface area burn. Burns 1997; 23: 505-508.*
2. *Boyce ST, Kagan RJ, Meyer NA et al. The 1999 clinical research award. Cultured skin substitutes combined with Integra Artificial skin to replace native skin autograft and allograft for the closure of excised full-thickness burns. J Burn Care Rehabil 1999; 20: 453-461.*

155. The correct response is C.

Sir William Liley is considered the father of fetal surgery for his treatment of fetal anaemia secondary to isoimmunisation-induced haemolysis by transuterine intraperitoneal transfusion of red blood cells. Sushruta is father of plastic surgery; Lister is considered the father of modern surgery; Gillies is father of modern plastic surgery and Joseph is father of rhinoplasty.

Reference:

Liley AW. Intrauterine transfusion of foetus in haemolytic disease. Br Med J 1963; 2: 1107.

156. The correct response is A.

Congenital high airway obstruction syndrome (CHAOS) is not an uncommon diagnosis and is being increasingly diagnosed with the help of ultrasound which shows characteristic findings. The lungs are large and echogenic with flattened diaphragms and dilated airways distal to the obstruction. Tracheal atresia does not produce CHAOS as it is associated with tracheo-esophageal fistula. The fistula acts as a conduit to vent the intrabronchial accumulation of excess foetal lung fluid.

Reference:

1. *Silver MM, Thurston WA, Patrick JE. Perinatal pulmonary hyperplasia due to laryngeal atresia. Hum Pathol 1988; 19: 110.*
2. *Hedrick MH, Longaker MT, Harrison MR. A fetal surgery primer for plastic surgeons. Plast Reconstr Surg 1998; 101: 1709.*

157. The correct response is C

The standard technique of intrauterine access in foetal surgery is by use of an operative stapler. This is used to cut and staple the uterus simultaneously as the uterus is vascular and a regular approach using knife or diathermy is not indicated. After the foetal portion of the procedure is complete, the foetus is returned to the womb and the amniotic fluid is reconstituted with isotonic electrolyte solution.

Reference:

1. Harrison MR, Adzick NS. The foetus as a patient: surgical considerations. Ann Surg 1991; 213: 279.
2. Hedrick MH, Longaker MT, Harrison MR. A fetal surgery primer for plastic surgeons. Plast Reconstr Surg 1998; 101: 1709.

158. The correct response is D.

The term 'robot' has been derived from a Czech word 'robota'. It refers to the free services done by peasants, like slaves doing their work for the Elites and Nobel's of the city. In similarity to this, slave robots now serve surgeons by replicating their hand movments during microsurgeries.

Reference:

1. Das H, Ohm T, Boswell C et al. Robot assisted microsurgery development at JPL. In Akay M, Marsh A, eds: Information technologies in Medicine, vol II. Rehabilitation and Treatment. New York, John Wiley and Sons, 2001: 85-99.
2. Merriam-Webster's Collegiate Dictionary, 10th ed. Springfield, Mas, Merriam-Webster, 1999.

159. The correct response is E.

This patient has a hypertrophic scar following thermal burns. Correct diagnosis of the abnormal scar will directly influence treatment options for this patient. Hypertrophic scars and keloid scars are clinically distinct entities with different treatment approaches. Hypertrophic scars can occur at any age and develop soon after the injury (within six to eight weeks). They can worsen up to six months but subside with time. The extent of scarring relates to the initial depth of injury. Hypertrophic scars can produce contractures, especially over joints however the boundaries of the original scar are maintained. Hypertrophic scars have a predilection to occur over the flexor surface of joints.

Keloid scars may develop months after the injury. They seldom regress and are not associated with contractures. They exceed the boundaries of the original wound. Keloid scars are commonly found on the deltoid, chest, and ear lobes. Pruritus is a common feature of keloid scars.

Reference:

1. *Niessen FB, Spauwen PH, Schalkwizk J, et al. On the nature of hypertrophic scars and keloids: a review. Plast Reconstr Surg. 1999; 104: 1435-1458.*
2. *Shahrad RR, Garner WL. Fibroproliferative scars. Clin Plast Surg. 2003; 30: 77-89.*
3. *Su CY, Alizadeh K, Boddie A, et al. The problem scar. Clin Plast Surg. 1998; 25: 451-465.*

2

AESTHETIC SURGERY

QUESTIONS

1. Which one of the following is the central point in the midline where the forehead skin joins the hairline?

A. Vertex
B. Nasion
C. Trichion
D. Gnathion
E. Menton

2. Soft tissue landmarks are used as anthropometric reference points. Which one of the following is the central point in between the eyebrows?

A. Vertex
B. Nasion
C. Trichion
D. Gnathion
E. Glabella

3. Which one of the following is the midline point of the junction of the frontonasal suture and the superior border of nasal bones?

A. Vertex
B. Nasion
C. Trichion
D. Gnathion
E. Glabella

4. Soft tissue landmarks are used as anthropometric reference points. Which one of the following is the most superior point of the external auditory meatus?

A. Porion
B. Nasion
C. Trichion
D. Gnathion
E. Glabella

5. Soft tissue landmarks are used as anthropometric reference points. Which one of the following is the palpable point of the lowest margin of the inferior orbital rim?

A. Porion
B. Nasion
C. Orbitale
D. Gnathion
E. Glabella

6. The Frankfort horizontal is an important radiological landmark of the face and is a line which joins which one of the following two points on the face?

A. Porion with subnasale
B. Nasion with orbitale
C. Gnathion with glabella
D. Orbitale with porion
E. Horizontal line in the middle of the face

7. Soft tissue landmarks are used as anthropometric reference points. Which one of the following is the most prominent point of the nasal tip?

A. Nasale
B. Pronasale
C. Supranasale
D. Subnasale
E. Glabella

8 Soft tissue landmarks are used as anthropometric reference points. The point where the columella joins the upper lip is called which one of the following?

A. Nasale
B. Pronasale
C. Supranasale
D. Subnasale
E. Glabella

9. Soft tissue landmarks are used as anthropometric reference points. The most inferior point on the chin is called which one of the following?

A. Porion
B. Nasion
C. Orbitale
D. Gnathion
E. Glabella

10. Soft tissue landmarks are used as anthropometric reference points. The most prominent point on the chin is called which one of the following?

A. Porion
B. Nasion
C. Pogonion
D. Gnathion
E. Glabella

11. Soft tissue landmarks are used as anthropometric reference points.The point where the upper lip touches the lower lip is called which one of the following?

A. Labiale
B. Sublabiale
C. Stomion
D. Menton
E. Gnathion

12. Modern anthropometry is based on the reference points on the face. The deepest point below the lower lip in the labiomental groove is called which one of the following?

A. Labiale
B. Sublabiale
C. Prolabiale
D. Menton
E. Gnathion

13. Soft tissue landmarks serve as useful anthropometric reference points. The point where the upper and lower eyelids join medially is called which one of the following?

A. Caruncle
B. Medial canthus
C. Canthion
D. Endocanthion
E. Limbus

14. Dividing the face into proportions is convenient for patient evaluation and analysis. The concepts using proportions have been based on neoclassical canons. The distance from trichion to nasion is equal to which of the following ?

A. Nasion to stomion
B. Nasion to subnasale
C. Nasion to pronasale
D. Stomion to gnathion
E. Porion to orbitale

15. Dividing the face into proportions is convenient for patient evaluation and analysis. The length of the nose is equal to which one other part of the face?

A. Chin
B. Ear
C. Interpupillary distance
D. Width of lip
E. Forehead

16. Dividing the face into proportions is convenient for patient evaluation and analysis. The distance between the medial canthi is equivalent to which one of the following ?

A. Width of mouth
B. Two thirds of width of mouth
C. One half of width of mouth
D. Width of ala
E. Width of root of nose

17. Dividing the face into proportions is convenient for patient evaluation and analysis. The width of the mouth is equal to which one of the following?

A. Width of ala
B. 1 ½ the width of ala
C. Two thirds of width of ala
D. Twice the width of ala
E. No correlation with width of ala

18. Which one of the following statements correctly describes an overbite?

A. Horizontal overlap of maxillary incisors over the mandibular incisors
B. Vertical overlap of mandibular incisors over the maxillary incisors

C. Horizontal overlap of mandibular incisors over the maxillary incisors
D. Vertical overlap of maxillary incisors over the mandibular incisors
E. None of the above

19. Cephalometry is the radiological study of which of the following?
A. Facial bones
B. Upper jaw
C. Lower jaw
D. Teeth
E. All of the above

20. Cephalometric analysis and planning is done with the help of cephalometric planes. These are based on standard cephalometric lines. All of the following are valid reference planes for cephalometric analysis except which one of the following?
A. Sella nasion (SN)
B. Frankfort horizontal (FH)
C. Maxillary plane (PP)
D. Occlusal plane (OP)
E. Sella menton (SM)

21. The angle SNA is an important parameter for analysis of the maxilla. Its normal range for men and women is which one of the following?
A. 78 ± 2 degrees
B. 80 ± 4 degrees
C. 82 ± 4 degrees
D. 84 ± 4 degrees
E. 88 ± 4 degrees

22. The angle SNB is an important parameter for analysis of the mandible. Its normal range for men and women is which one of the following?
A. 79 ± 4 degrees
B. 83 ± 4 degrees
C. 87 ± 4 degrees
D. 91 ± 4 degrees
E. 95 ± 4 degrees

23. The cranial base is an important measurement for analysis of craniofacial deformities. Which one of the following statement regarding cranial base is incorrect ?
A. It is the measurement from sella to subnasale
B. The average range for men is 83 ± 4 mm
C. The Frankfort horizontal makes an angle of approximately 5-9 degrees inferior to this plane
D. Length of cranial base can be increased by monobloc LeFort III advancement
E. Length of cranial base can be increased by monobloc LeFort III advancement with distraction

24. Which of the following patients could be a source of trouble and are not good candidates for surgery?
A. Showing rudeness in behaviour
B. Showering praise for the surgeon
C. Refuses to undress for the photograph
D. Indecisive
E. All of the above

25. Which of the following correctly describes the aesthetic brow position in respect of the medial end of the eyebrow? It is almost in the same vertical plane as which one of the following?
A. Medial canthus
B. Alar base
C. Philtrum
D. Angle of mouth
E. Nasal bone

26. The curve of the normal eyebrow has a convexity upwards which lies aesthetically in which one of the following configuration?
A. Above its centre
B. At junction of its medial one third and lateral two third
C. At junction of its medial two third and lateral one third
D. Medial to the midpupillary line
E. None of the above

27. Transverse lines on the forehead are due to which one of the following?
A. Contraction of the galea aponeurotica
B. Contraction of the frontalis
C. Contraction of the procerus
D. Contraction of the corrugator supercilii
E. Contraction of the depressor supercilii

28. Transverse skin lines above the root of the nose are due to which one of the following muscle?
A. Contraction of the galea aponeurotica
B. Contraction of the frontalis
C. Contraction of the procerus
D. Contraction of the corrugator supercilii
E. Contraction of the depressor supercilii

29. Vertical and oblique lines in the upper part of the nose are due to which one of the following muscle?
A. Procerus
B. Corrugator supercilli
C. Nasalis
D. Levator labii superioris alaequae nasi
E. Transverse nasalis

30. Which one of the following brow lift procedures would produce minimal scarring?

A. Suprabrow excision
B. Coronal browlift
C. Frontal browlift
D. Temporal browlift
E. Endoscopic brow lift

31. Botox is an exotoxin, produced by Clostridium botulinum. The complications of Botox therapy could be following except which one of the following?

A. Bruising
B. Ptosis
C. Diplopia
D. Fat atrophy
E. Depigmentation

32. Botox is an exotoxin, produced by Clostridium botulinum. The therapeutic and lethal doses of Botox are calculated and expressed by which one of the following?

A. millilitres (ml)
B. milligram / ml (mg/ml)
C. cubic centimetre (cc)
D. mouse units (MU)
E. joules per sq.cm (J/cm^2)

33. A beautiful eye irrespective of ethnicity is characterised by all of the following features except which one of the following?

A. Upper lid crease 9-12 mm above lid margin
B. Intercanthal axis tilt from medial to lateral
C. Upper lid covering the cornea by 2 mm
D. Vertical height of aperture should expose the full cornea
E. Lower lid (1- 1.5 mm) below the cornea

34. The orbital cone is made up of seven bones. Which one of these listed below is the smallest?

A. Zygomatic
B. Lacrimal
C. Ethmoid
D. Palatine
E. Sphenoid

35. The medial canthal ligament is attached to which one of the following bone?

A. Zygomatic
B. Lacrimal
C. Ethmoid
D. Palatine
E. Sphenoid

36. The lateral canthal ligament is attached to which one of the following bone?

A. Zygomatic
B. Lacrimal
C. Ethmoid
D. Palatine
E. Sphenoid

37. The lateral retinaculum is anchored on the lateral orbit and serves to maintain the integrity, position and function of the globe. It is composed of the following parts except which one of the following?

A. Lateral canthal tendon
B. Lateral part of levator aponeurosis
C. Lockwood's ligament
D. Whitnall's ligament
E. Muller's muscle

38. The four muscles which control the movement of the eyebrows are listed. Which of these pulls the eyebrow medially?

A. Frontalis
B. Procerus
C. Corrugator supercilii
D. Orbicularis oculi

39. The number of fat compartments in the upper eyelid is which one of the following?

A. Two
B. Three
C. Four
D. Five
E. Six

40. Muller's muscle originates on the deep surface of the levator near the point where the muscle becomes aponeurotic. It inserts into which one of the following?

A. Superior rectus
B. Superior tarsus
C. Medial rectus
D. Whitnall's tubercle
E. Lateral rectus

41. Which one of the following statements about frontalis muscle is correct?

A. Vertically placed
B. Horizontally placed
C. Directed downwards and medially
D. Directed upwards and laterally
E. Directed upwards and medially

42. A patient with true ptosis would have all the following characteristic features except:

A. Upper lid would cover more than 1.0 mm of cornea
B. Upper lid cannot be moved upwards to clear the cornea
C. Upper lid skin fold is almost non- existent
D. The upper eyelid skin hangs down to cover the lid margin

43. All of the following are advantages of anchor blepharoplasty except?

A. Requires greater surgical skill and expertise
B. Produces crisp lid folds
C. Minimal excision of eyelid skin
D. Provides easy access for adjustment of the levator aponeurosis

44. Which one of the following is the procedure of choice for treatment of epicanthal folds ?

A. Direct excision and closure
B. W plasty
C. V- W epicanthoplasty
D. Z plasty
E. W-V epicanthoplasty

45. Coronocanthopexy is a procedure designed for periorbital aesthetic rejuvenation. It consists of all of the following procedures except ?

A. Coronal brow lift
B. Lateral canthopexy
C. Mid-face lift
D. Upper blepharoplasty
E. Lower lid blepharoplasty

46. Ptosis affects individuals of all ages and can be due to all of the following causes except which one of the following?

A. Congenital
B. Traumatic
C. Involutional
D. Neoplastic
E. Spastic disease

47. The upper eyelid is lifted upwards by attachment of two muscles. Which one of these is involuntary in nature?

A. Levator palpebrae superioris
B. Muller's muscle
C. Superior rectus
D. Orbicularis oculi
E. Preseptal part of orbicularis oculi

48. Which one of the following muscle takes attachment on the upper border of the tarsal plate?

A. Levator palpebrae superioris
B. Muller's muscle
C. Superior rectus
D. Orbicularis oculi
E. Preseptal part of orbicularis oculi

49. Which one of the following statements about the insertion of levator palpebrae superioris on the tarsal plate is correct?

A. Insertion on the anterior surface of the tarsal plate
B. Insertion into the posterior surface of the tarsal plate
C. Insertion into the upper border of the tarsal plate
D. It is not inserted directly on the tarsal plate
E. It is inserted in only 20% of cases on the tarsal plate

50. Which one of the following procedures is indicated in patients with ptosis with no levator function?

A. Plication of LPS (Levator palpebrae superioris)
B. Shortening of LPS (Levator palpebrae superioris)
C. Advancement of LPS (Levator palpebrae superioris)
D. Frontalis sling procedure

51. The procedures used for correction of the lower eyelid ptosis include all of the following except:

A. Shortening
B. Stenting
C. Lateral canthoplasty
D. Static sling (Fascia lata)
E. Dynamic sling (Temporalis)

52. The nasojugal groove is an important consideration in treatment of periocular ageing. This groove occurs anatomically due to attachment of which one of the following to the orbital rim?

A. Orbicularis oculi
B. Arcus marginalis
C. Whitnall's ligament
D. Muller's muscle
E. Canthal ligament

53. The term SMAS bears relevance to facial aesthetic surgery. It is used for which of the following?

A. Subfacial musculoaponeurotic system
B. Superficial musculoaponeurotic system
C. Subcutaneous musculoaponeurotic system
D. Suprafacial musculoaponeurotic system
E. Subperiosteal musculoaponeurotic system

54. In facelift surgery, it is important to preserve the innervation of the facial muscles. The superficial group of muscles encountered in a face lift procedure get their nerve supply from which one of the following?

A. Superficial surface
B. Deep surface
C. Lateral to zygomaticus minor
D. Medial to zygomaticus minor
E. Superficial to SMAS layer

55. In facelift surgery, it is important to preserve the innervation of the facial muscles. The deep group of muscles encountered in a face lift procedure get their nerve supply from which one of the following?

A. Superficial surface
B. Deep surface
C. Lateral to zygomaticus minor
D. Medial to zygomaticus minor
E. Superficial to SMAS layer

56. Which one of the following nerve supplies the platysma muscle?

A. Cervical branches of facial nerve
B. Platysmal branches of cervical nerve
C. Platysmal nerve
D. Submental nerve
E. Marginal mandibular nerve

57. The platysma muscle takes origin from all of the following except:

A. Fascia covering the pectoralis major
B. Fascia covering the deltoid muscle
C. Fascia over the mastoid process
D. Occipital bone
E. Hyoid cartilage

58. The platysma muscle is inserted into which of the following?

A. Lower border of mandible
B. Lower part of face
C. Angle of the mouth
D. Lower lip (skin and subcutaneous tissues)
E. All of the above

59. Surgery of the face may lead to injury to vital structures including the parotid duct and the facial nerve. Which one of the following correctly describes the location of these structures in the face?

A. Superficial to the parotid-masseteric fascia
B. Deep to the parotid-masseteric fascia
C. They cross the midbelly of the sternocleidomastoid muscle 6.5 cm inferior to the external auditory canal
D. They cross the midbelly of the sternocleidomastoid muscle 6.5 cm anterior to the external auditory canal
E. None of the above

60. The temporal branch of the facial nerve is at risk of injury in the temporal region where an incision through the SMAS can produce a direct injury to the nerve. Which one of the following is not correct regarding the location of this structure?

A. It is likely to be injured on incising the temporal skin and subcutaneous tissue
B. It is likely to be injured on incising the temporal SMAS layer
C. It travels along a line connecting the base of the tragus to a point 1.5 cm above the eyebrow
D. Multiple branches of this nerve may be observed crossing the zygomatic arch
E. The nerve is located medial and inferior to the frontal branch of the superficial temporal artery

61. The facial artery and vein serve as landmarks for the marginal mandibular nerve. Which one of the following statement correctly describes the relationship of facial vessels with the marginal mandibular nerve?

A. The facial artery and vein lie superficial to the marginal mandibular nerve
B. The marginal mandibular nerve travels 1.5 cm all along the lower border of the mandible
C. It travels along a line connecting the base of the tragus to a point 1.5 cm above the eyebrow
D. The marginal mandibular nerve crosses the facial vessels at the anterior border of the masseter
E. The marginal mandibular nerve runs along with the facial vessels in the lower part of the face

62. The parotid duct after emerging from the gland terminates in the sulcus opposite the second maxillary molar. It crosses all the following structures in its path except which one of the following?

A. Buccal fat
B. Buccinator muscle
C. Buccal mucosa
D. Masseter
E. Zygomaticus minor

63. The retaining ligaments of the face hold the skin in position against the effects of gravity. The number of known ligaments are which one of the following?

A. Two
B. Three
C. Four
D. Five
E. Six

64. **The great auricular nerve provides sensation to the earlobe and the lateral portion of the cheek. It is commonly encountered while elevating the cervicofacial flap. What is the correct location of this nerve below the external auditory canal?**
   A. 2.5 cm
   B. 4.5 cm
   C. 6.5 cm
   D. 8.5 cm
   E. 10.5 cm

65. **Which is the sensory nerve most commonly injured in rhytidectomy?**
   A. Great auricular nerve
   B. Buccal branch of facial nerve
   C. Marginal mandibular nerve
   D. Infraorbital nerve
   E. Buccal nerve

66. **Which is the motor nerve most commonly injured in rhytidectomy?**
   A. Great auricular nerve
   B. Buccal branch of facial nerve
   C. Marginal mandibular nerve
   D. Infraorbital nerve
   E. Buccal nerve

67. **The frontal branch of the facial nerve may be injured in rhytidectomy. All of the following are the features of this injury except which one of the following?**
   A. Drop in the level of the eyebrow
   B. Inability to lift the eyebrow
   C. Loss of forehead wrinkles
   D. Ptosis
   E. Neuroma

68. **The anatomy of the zygoma is particularly important with relevance to the attachment of the temporal fascia for endoscopic brow lifts. The insertion of the intermediate temporal fascia and of the deep temporal fascia is directly onto the zygoma at which one of the following location?**
   A. Over the entire zygomatic arch
   B. In the central zygoma
   C. Through the zygomatic arch
   D. Under the zygomatic arch
   E. At the junction of the anterior and posterior thirds of the zygoma

69. **The term 'SOOF' in relation to midfacial aging refers to which one of the following?**
   A. Suborbicularis oculi fat
   B. Suborbicularis oris fat
   C. Supraorbicularis oris fascia
   D. Superficial orbicularis oris fat resection
   E. Suprafascial orbicularis oris fat transfer

70. **Modern techniques of fat injection have revolutionised surgical rejuvenation of the face. In patients with thin skin, which one of the following location is particularly unsuitable for fat injection ?**
   A. Nasolabial fold
   B. Upper lip
   C. Lower lip
   D. Infraorbital hollow
   E. Malar fat pad

71. **The deformity "crow's feet" is located at which one of the following region?**
   A. Feet of the crow
   B. Perioral region
   C. Perineal region
   D. Periorbicular region
   E. Periumbilical region

72. **Who amongst the following is credited with describing the continuous periauricular and hairline incision for face lift?**
   A. Rogers (1971)
   B. Barton (1985)
   C. Bames (1927)
   D. Skoog (1974)
   E. Mitz and Peyronie (1976)

73. **The dominant anatomic change of midfacial ageing is the gravitational descent of the malar fat pad. The term 'malar fat pad' was originally introduced in the surgical literature by which one of the following?**
   A. Skoog
   B. Rogers
   C. Bames
   D. Owsley
   E. Fagien

74. **The malar fat pad is triangular in shape with the base of the triangle along the paralabial nasolabial crease. Which one of the following muscle lies beneath the malar fat pad?**
   A. Orbicularis oris
   B. Orbicularis oculi
   C. Zygomaticus major
   D. Masseter
   E. Buccinator

75. The function of malar fat pad is which one of the following?
A. To provide insulation
B. To provide cushioning of the maxillary sinus
C. To provide protection to the eye
D. To provide attachment of muscles
E. All of the above

76. The midfacial ageing is characterized by a TRIAD comprising of infraorbital flattening, prominent nasolabial fold and which one of the following?
A. Eyelid bags
B. Xanthelasmas
C. Under eye hyperpigmentation
D. Lateral orbital wrinkles
E. Jowls

77. Which one of the following technique accomplishes complete mobilisation of all the facial soft tissue structures over the zygoma and maxilla?
A. Suspension suture
B. Subperiosteal midface lift
C. Midface alloplastic implant
D. SMAS plication and resection
E. Submalar implant

78. Perioral rhytids are due to which of the following?
A. Frequent perioral motion
B. Subcutaneous atrophy
C. Loss of skin elasticity
D. Accentuated by smoking
E. All of the above

79. The nasolabial fold is due to combined actions of all of the following muscles except which one of the following?
A. Levator labii superioris
B. Levator labii superioris alaequae nasi
C. Zygomaticus major
D. Risorius
E. Masseter

80. Which one of the following is the procedure of choice for treating an eighty year old man with significant skin excess in the neck?
A. Suction lipectomy
B. Lipectomy and platysmaplasty
C. Face lift using pre-auricular and post-auricular incisions
D. Direct neck lift
E. Neck implants

81. The corset platysmaplasty allows satisfactory rejuvenation of the neck. The shape of skin incision is which one of the following?
A. Horizontal arc shaped submental incision
B. Vertical 'T' shaped
C. 'Z' plasty
D. Two parallel horizontal incisions
E. 'W' shaped

82. Which one of the following gland requires consideration for treatment if found ptotic in neck rejuvenation?
A. Jugulodigastric lymph gland
B. Enlarged sublingual gland
C. Submandibular gland
D. Parotid gland
E. Branchial cyst

83. 'Jowls' occur in relation to which one of the following bone?
A. Maxilla
B. Mandible
C. Orbit
D. Nasal
E. Zygoma

84. The structures that lie superficial to the parotid gland are the following except which one of the following?
A. Skin and subcutaneous tissue
B. Superficial musculoaponeurotic fascia (SMAS)
C. Superficial parotid lymph glands
D. Superficial temporal artery and vein
E. Buccal nerve

85. The structures that lie on the surface of the sternocleidomastoid muscle are the following except which one of the following?
A. Skin and platysma
B. External jugular vein
C. Great auricular nerve/ Transverse cervical nerves
D. Parotid gland
E. Vagus nerve

86. Which of the following statement is correct regarding the marginal mandibular nerve?
A. It is a sensory nerve
B. It supplies the buccinator muscle after penetrating the deep cervical fascia near the inferior border of the mandible
C. It supplies the depressor labii inferioris muscle near the buccal space

D. It is vulnerable to injury before exiting the deep cervical fascia near the border of the mandible
E. It courses beneath the deep cervical fascia over the outer surface of the submandibular gland to reach the undersurface of the platysma where it arborizes to supply the entire platysma muscle.

87. Injury to a motor branch of the facial nerve is the most dreaded complication of a facelift surgery. Which one of the following surgical plane of facelift does not have any branches of the facial nerve?
A. Subcutaneous plane
B. Sub-SMAS plane
C. Composite facelift plane
D. Subperiosteal plane
E. None of the above

88. After a face lift procedure, if the patient is not able to have a 'full denture smile', it indicates injury to which of the following nerve?
A. Zygomatic nerve
B. Buccal nerve
C. Marginal mandibular nerve
D. Posterior auricular nerve
E. Frontal nerve

89. Which one of the following muscle is supplied by the marginal mandibular nerve?
A. Levator anguli oris
B. Mentalis
C. Zygomaticus major
D. Zygomaticus minor
E. Risorius

90. Dark brown skin falls in which type of Fitzpatrick classification?
A. Type I
B. Type II
C. Type III
D. Type IV
E. Type V

91. Lasers produce their effect through which one of the following?
A. Thermocoagulation
B. Photocoagulation
C. Photothermolysis
D. Vaporisation

92. 'Fluence' is a measure of which one of the following?
A. Laser wavelength
B. Laser type
C. Pulse duration
D. Laser energy
E. Laser skin damage

93. All of the following need special protection in patients undergoing laser surgery of the face except which one of the following?
A. Eyes
B. Teeth
C. Endotracheal tube
D. Nose

94. Which one of the following complications of laser therapy is likely to require a surgical intervention later on?
A. Edema
B. Erythema
C. Dermatitis
D. Milia
E. Hypertrophic scarring

95. Which one of following procedures should be used for resurfacing a capillary haemangioma?
A. Laser
B. Chemical peel
C. Dermabrasion
D. Skin grafting
E. Flap procedure

96. Vitamin A helps in rejuvenation of the skin by which of the following actions?
A. Stimulates exfoliation
B. Promotes collagen formation
C. Promotes vascularisation
D. Diminishes pigmentation
E. All of the above

97. The histological changes seen after Vitamin A therapy include all except which one of the following?
A. Increase in stratum corneum
B. Increase in stratum spongiosum
C. Increase in water retention in cells
D. Atrophy of the skin appendages
E. Improvement in dermal-epidermal junction

98. Alphatocopherol is the biologically active form of which one of the following Vitamin?
A. Vitamin A
B. Vitamin C
C. Vitamin B
D. Vitamin E
E. Vitamin K

99. Silicon is a commonly used implant for aesthetic facial augmentation. Chemically it is composed of which one of the following?

A. Polytetraflouroethylene
B. Polysiloxane
C. Polyethylene
D. Polypropylene
E. Acrylic

100. The relationship of the eye to the orbital rims determines the appearance of the upper third of the face. The eye is normally placed behind the overlying supraorbital ridge by which one of the following distance?

A. 5 mm
B. 10 mm
C. 15 mm
D. 20 mm
E. 25 mm

101. The advantages of the open rhinoplasty approach over the closed rhinoplasty are the following except which one of the following?

A. Complete anatomical exposure
B. Direct binocular view
C. Ease of architectural alterations in the bones and cartilages
D. Ease of obtaining cartilage grafts from the septum
E. Transcolumellar scarring

102. Which one of the following is a preferred source for cartilage grafts for use in rhinoplasty?

A. Nasal septum
B. Conchal cartilage
C. Rib cartilage
D. Articular cartilage
E. MEDPOR

103. The open approach for rhinoplasty by making an incision in the columella was first introduced by which one of the following?

A. Rethi
B. Goodman
C. Rohrich
D. Byrd
E. Daniel

104. Name the clinical condition for which an open rhinoplasty was done for the first time?

A. Hump Nose
B. Broad Nose
C. Long Nose
D. Short Nose
E. Cleft lip Nose

105. The columellar labial angle defines and determines the aesthetics of the nasal tip. Its normal value in women ranges from which one of the following?

A. 90 – 100°
B. 100 – 108°
C. 110 – 118°
D. 120 – 128°
E. 130 – 138°

106. All of the following can be considered important indications for open rhinoplasty approach except which one of the following?

A. When nasal tip surgery is required to be done
B. When cartilage grafts are to be used
C. When cleft lip nose deformity is required to be corrected
D. When spacer grafts are to be used to widen the upper lateral cartilage
E. Hump nose reduction

107. Which one of the following suture is likely to provide a better definition to the tip of nose?

A. Transdomal suture
B. Interdomal suture
C. Intercrural suture
D. Lateral crural suture
E. Columellar-septal suture

108. Which of the following structure can be responsible for producing the oversized and over projected tip of the nose?

A. Long septum
B. Long lateral crus
C. Long medial crus
D. Long middle crus
E. All of the above

109. Sir Harold Gillies laid out principles of Plastic Surgery in his book on "The Principles and Art of Plastic Surgery" in 1957. Which of the following is correct regarding these principles?

A. Diagnose before you treat
B. Put the parts in their normal positions and retain them there
C. Replace missing tissues in kind
D. Never do anything today which you can honourably put off till tomorrow
E. All of above

110. Provision of healthy nasal lining is essential for nose reconstruction. Which one of the following flap options for nasal lining is usually based on scarred tissues?

A. Contralateral septal flap
B. Ipsilateral septal flap
C. Bipedicle lining flap
D. Turnover flap
E. Nasolabial lining flap

111. The bilobed flap is suitable for nose reconstruction for defects in which one of the following zone?

A. Zone 1
B. Zone 2
C. Zone 3
D. Zone 4
E. Zone 5

112. Who among the following is credited with the first description of bilobed flap?

A. Millard
B. Converse
C. Esser
D. Zitelli
E. Tanzer

113. The nose is divided into separate zones based on texture, subcutaneous fat and sebaceous gland content. The nose tip falls majorly in which one of the following zone?

A. Zone 1
B. Zone 2
C. Zone 3
D. Zone 4
E. Zone 5

114. The nose is divided into separate zones based on texture, subcutaneous fat and sebaceous gland content. The sidewalls of the nose fall in which one of the following zone?

A. Zone 1
B. Zone 2
C. Zone 3
D. Zone 4
E. Zone 5

115. The nose is divided into separate zones based on texture, subcutaneous fat and sebaceous gland content. The columella of the nose falls in which one of the following zone?

A. Zone 1
B. Zone 2
C. Zone 3
D. Zone 4
E. Zone 5

116. The nose is divided into separate zones based on texture, subcutaneous fat and sebaceous gland content. The soft triangle of the nose falls in which one of the following zone?

A. Zone 1
B. Zone 2
C. Zone 3
D. Zone 4
E. Zone 5

117. The nose is divided into separate zones based on texture, subcutaneous fat and sebaceous gland content. The highest sebaceous gland content exists in the skin of which one of the following zone?

A. Zone 1
B. Zone 2
C. Zone 3
D. Zone 4
E. Zone 5

118. Which one of the following is the correct definition of orthognathic aesthetic surgery?

A. Surgery of developmental deformities of maxilla and mandible
B. Surgery of congenital deformities of maxilla and mandible
C. Surgery of traumatic deformities of maxilla and mandible
D. Surgery of syndromic deformities of maxilla and mandible

119. Which teeth in the maxilla and the mandible help in defining the type of malocclusion?

A. First molar
B. Premolar
C. Canine
D. Incisor
E. Second molar

120. In the normal class I occlusion, which parts of the molars come in contact with each other?

A. Mesiobuccal cusp of first maxillary molar in the buccal groove of the first mandibular molar
B. Mesiobuccal groove of the first maxillary molar in the buccal cusp of the first mandibular molar
C. Mesiopalatal cusp of first maxillary molar in the buccal groove of the first mandibular molar
D. Mesiopalatal groove of the first maxillary molar in the buccal cusp of the first mandibular molar
E. Mesiopalatal cusp of first mandibular molar in the buccal groove of the first maxillary molar

121. In Class II malocclusion what is the relationship of the maxillary first and mandibular molar with each other?

A. Mandibular molar is posterior to the maxillary molar
B. Mandibular molar is anterior to the maxillary molar
C. Mandibular molar is in buccal cross bite relationship to maxillary molar
D. Maxillary molar is in buccal cross bite relationship to mandibular molar
E. Maxillary molar is in lingual cross bite relationship to mandibular molar

122. In Class III malocclusion what is the relationship of the maxillary first and mandibular molar with each other?

A. Mandibular molar is posterior to the maxillary molar
B. Mandibular molar is anterior to the maxillary molar
C. Mandibular molar is in buccal cross bite relationship to maxillary molar
D. Maxillary molar is in buccal crossbite relationship to mandibular molar
E. Maxillary molar is in lingual crossbite relationship to mandibular molar

123. Sagittal split ramus osteotomy was described for the first time by which one of the following ?

A. Angle
B. Dingman
C. Caldwell and Letterman
D. Trauner and Obwegeser
E. Gillies

124. Which one of the following correctly defines the 'Wassmund osteotomy'?

A. Sagittal split osteotomy of the mandible
B. Segmental osteotomy of the mandible
C. Segmental osteotomy of the maxilla
D. LeFort II osteotomy of the maxilla
E. Combined maxillary and mandibular osteotomy

125. A patient with class I occlusion has anterior open bite. Name the procedure of choice for his treatment:

A. LeFort I
B. LeFort II
C. LeFort III
D. Any of the above
E. All of the above

126. A patient with class II malocclusion has an open bite deformity. Which one of the following procedure is likely to benefit this patient?

A. LeFort I osteotomy
B. LeFort II osteotomy
C. Sagittal split osteotomy
D. Wassmund osteotomy
E. Kole osteotomy

127. A patient with class III malocclusion has anterior deep bite deformity. Which of the following procedure is likely to benefit this patient?

A. LeFort I
B. LeFort II
C. Sagittal split osteotomy
D. Wassmund osteotomy
E. Kole osteotomy

128. A patient has a gummy smile. Her probable diagnosis is vertical maxillary excess. The procedure of choice for her treatment would be which one of the following?

A. LeFort I osteotomy
B. LeFort II osteotomy
C. Saggital split osteotomy
D. Wassmund osteotomy
E. Kole osteotomy

129. An individual who has an absence of incisor show on smiling is a case of 'Short face syndrome' which is characterised by the following features except which one of the following?

A. Wide oral commissure
B. Everted lip
C. Deep labiomental folds
D. Jowls
E. Class III malocclusion

130. The total number of hairs on the scalp in adult males is which one of the following?

A. 1.0 lac
B. 1.5 lac
C. 2.0 lac
D. 2.5 lac
E. 3.0 lac

131. Baldness has been classified by Norwood into seven types. The occipital baldness will be classified as which one of the following?

A. Type I
B. Type II
C. Type III
D. Type IV
E. Type V

132. A patient having a bridge of hair between the frontal and the occipital baldness as per Norwood classification would be classified into which one of the following type?

A. Type I
B. Type II
C. Type III
D. Type IV
E. Type V

133. Select the procedure of choice used for hair transplantation in a case of frontal baldness:

A. Punch grafts
B. Flaps
C. Micro, Mini or Follicular hair grafts
D. Tissue expanders
E. Bucket handle flaps

134. The follicular unit grafts used in hair transplantation 'are' composed of how many units?

A. One
B. Two
C. Three
D. One to three or more
E. Any combination

135. The 'double chin' can be reliably treated using a submental incision. This incision should be given at which of the following location?

A. Along the submental crease
B. Posterior to the submental crease
C. Anterior to the submental crease
D. Any of the above

136. The type of graft used to support the ala or the side wall of the nose is which one of the following?

A. Strut graft
B. Batten graft
C. Spreader graft
D. Shield graft
E. Sheen graft

137. Which type of graft should be used to support the columella?

A. Strut graft
B. Batten graft
C. Spreader graft
D. Shield graft
E. Sheen graft

138. Which type of graft should be used for widening an air passage and improving the competency of the nasal valve?

A. Strut graft
B. Batten graft
C. Spreader graft
D. Shield graft
E. Sheen graft

139. Which type of graft should be used to improve the shape of the nasal tip?

A. Strut graft
B. Batten graft
C. Spreader graft
D. Shield graft

140. Hering's law of equal innervations applies to which one of the following ocular muscle ?

A. Superior rectus
B. Inferior rectus
C. Levator palpebrae superioris
D. Inferior rectus
E. Superior oblique

141. Name the site to which the lateral canthal tendon is attached :

A. Margin of the frontal bone
B. Margin of the zygomatic bone
C. Frontozygomatic suture
D. Whitnall's tubercle
E. Annulus of Zinn

142. The lateral retinaculum is formed by contributions from all of the following except which one of the following?

A. Lateral part of the levator palpebrae superioris
B. Lateral part of the orbicularis oculi muscle
C. Lockwood ligament
D. Lateral rectus
E. Inferior rectus

143. Which one of the following is true regarding correct site of drill hole fixation for lateral canthropexy?

A. At level of orbital rim
B. 1 mm inferior to the orbital rim
C. 4 mm posterior to the orbital rim
D. 4 mm anterior to the orbital rim
E. At level of the median canthal tendon

144. A 42-year-old gentleman presented with increasing dryness and tearing from the right eye 6 months after sustaining a comminuted fracture of the orbital rim and floor in a motor vehicle accident (photo shown). He had underwent surgical exploration and wire fixation of the fracture through a subciliary incision. Currently he has epiphora, 8 mm of scleral show with ectropion and scarring of the lower eyelid to the infraorbital rim. Which of the following is the most appropriate management for him?

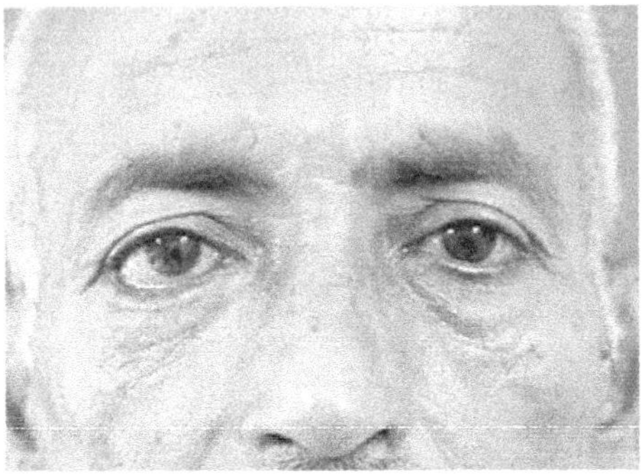

A. Corticosteroid injection into the visible lower eyelid scar
B. Central tarsorrhaphy
C. Massage and closure of the lower eyelid with tape sutures
D. Surgical exploration of the orbital floor and removal of wire fixation
E. Scar release, grafting, and tightening of the lower eyelid

145. A 23-year-old male presented with severe grade of bilateral enlargement of the breast which was making it difficult for him to participate in outdoor sports. He has no history of specific drug use and the hormonal profile is under normal limits. This can be surgically treated by which of the following?

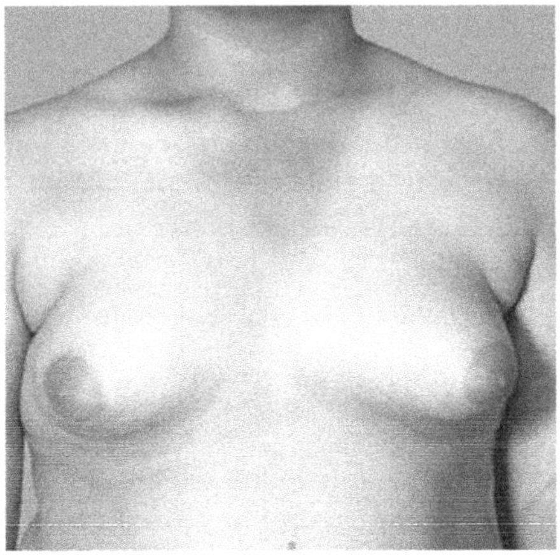

A. Total mastectomy with free nipple grafting
B. Dermal pedicle reduction mammaplasty
C. Skin resection with suction assisted lipectomy
D. Skin reduction with subcutaneous mastectomy with nipple grafting
E. All of the above

ANSWERS, EXPLANATIONS AND REFERENCES

1. The correct response is C.

Trichion is the point in the midline, where the forehead skin joins the hairline. Trichion is a Greek word meaning 'hair'. Vertex is the highest seen point on the head with the head in Frankfort horizontal. Nasion is the midline point of the junction of frontonasal suture and the superior part of nasal bones. Gnathion is the most inferior point of the lower border of the mandible, also called menton.

Reference:

1. *Vegter F, Hage JJ. Clinical anthropometry and canons of the face in historical perspective. Plast Reconstr Surg 2000; 106: 1090-1096.*
2. *Farkas LG, Hreczko TA, Kolar JC, Munro IR. Vertical and horizontal proportions of the face in young adult North American Caucasians: revision of neoclassical canons. Plast Reconstr Surg 1985; 75: 328-337.*

2. The correct response is E.

Glabella is the most prominent point of the forehead between the eyebrows. Trichion is the point in the midline, where the forehead skin joins the hairline. Trichion is a Greek word meaning 'hair'. Vertex is the highest seen point on the head with the head in Frankfort horizontal. Nasion is the midline point of the junction of frontonasal suture and the superior part of nasal bones. Gnathion is the most inferior point of the lower border of the mandible, also called menton.

Reference:

1. Vegter F, Hage JJ. Clinical anthropometry and canons of the face in historical perspective. Plast Reconstr Surg 2000; 106: 1090-1096.
2. Farkas LG, Hreczko TA, Kolar JC, Munro IR. Vertical and horizontal proportions of the face in young adult North American Caucasians: revision of neoclassical canons. Plast Reconstr Surg 1985; 75: 328-337.

3. The correct response is B.

Nasion is the midline point of the junction of frontonasal suture and the superior nasal bones. Glabella is the most prominent point of the forehead between the eyebrows. Trichion is the point in the midline, where the forehead skin joins the hairline. Trichion is a Greek word meaning 'hair'. Vertex is the highest seen point on the head with the head in Frankfort horizontal. Gnathion is the most inferior point of the lower border of the mandible, also called menton.

Reference:

1. *Vegter F, Hage JJ. Clinical anthropometry and canons of the face in historical perspective. Plast Reconstr Surg 2000; 106: 1090-1096.*
2. *Farkas LG, Hreczko TA, Kolar JC, Munro IR. Vertical and horizontal proportions of the face in young adult North American Caucasians: revision of neoclassical canons. Plast Reconstr Surg 1985; 75: 328-337.*

4. The correct response is A.

It is called 'Porion'. It is derived from the Greek word 'Poros'-which means 'Passage' and it is the most superior point of the external auditory meatus. Nasion is the midline point of the junction of frontonasal suture and the superior part of nasal bones. Glabella is the most prominent point of the forehead between the eyebrows. Trichion is the point in the midline, where the forehead skin joins the hairline. Trichion is a Greek word meaning 'hair'. Vertex is the highest seen point on the head with the head in Frankfort horizontal. Gnathion is the most inferior point of the lower border of the mandible, also called menton.

Reference:

1. *Vegter F, Hage JJ. Clinical anthropometry and canons of the face in historical perspective. Plast Reconstr Surg 2000; 106:1090-1096.*
2. *Farkas LG, Hreczko TA, Kolar JC, Munro IR. Vertical and horizontal proportions of the face in young adult North American Caucasians: revision of neoclassical canons. Plast Reconstr Surg 1985; 75: 328-337.*

5. The correct response is C.

Orbitale is the palpable point of the lowest margin of the inferior orbital rim. Nasion is the midline point of the junction of frontonasal suture and the superior nasal bones. Glabella is the most prominent point of the forehead between the eyebrows. Trichion is the point in the midline, where the forehead skin joins the hairline. Trichion is a Greek word meaning 'hair'. Vertex is the highest seen point on the head with the head in Frankfort horizontal. Gnathion is the most inferior point of the lower border of the mandible, also called menton.

Reference:

1. *Vegter F, Hage JJ. Clinical anthropometry and canons of the face in historical perspective. Plast Reconstr Surg 2000; 106: 1090-1096.*
2. *Farkas LG, Hreczko TA, Kolar JC, Munro IR. Vertical and horizontal proportions of the face in young adult North American Caucasians: revision of neoclassical canons. Plast Reconstr Surg 1985; 75: 328-337.*

6. The correct response is D.

The Frankfort horizontal joins the porion with orbitale. It is a bony landmark seen on radiological examination and this line is parallel to the floor for anthropometric measurements. It is an approximation of neutral head position in straight gaze.

Reference:

1. *Vegter F, Hage JJ. Clinical anthropometry and canons of the face in historical perspective. Plast Reconstr Surg 2000; 106: 1090-1096.*
2. *Farkas LG, Hreczko TA, Kolar JC, Munro IR. Vertical and horizontal proportions of the face in young adult North American Caucasians: revision of neoclassical canons. Plast Reconstr Surg 1985; 75: 328-337.*

7. The correct response is B.

Pronasale is the most prominent point of the nasal tip. Subnasale is the deepest point at the junction of the base of the columella and the upper lip in the midline. Glabella is the most prominent point of the forehead between the eyebrows. The other options are not valid options.

Reference:

1. *Vegter F, Hage JJ. Clinical anthropometry and canons of the face in historical perspective. Plast Reconstr Surg 2000; 106: 1090-1096.*
2. *Farkas LG, Hreczko TA, Kolar JC, Munro IR. Vertical and horizontal proportions of the face in young adult North American Caucasians: revision of neoclassical canons. Plast Reconstr Surg 1985; 75: 328-337.*

8. The correct response is D.

Subnasale is the deepest point at the junction of the base of the columella and the upper lip in the midline. Pronasale is the most prominent point of the nasal tip. Glabella is the most prominent point of the forehead between the eyebrows. The other options are not valid options.

Reference:

1. *Vegter F, Hage JJ. Clinical anthropometry and canons of the face in historical perspective. Plast Reconstr Surg 2000; 106: 1090-1096.*
2. *Farkas LG, Hreczko TA, Kolar JC, Munro IR. Vertical and horizontal proportions of the face in young adult North American Caucasians: revision of neoclassical canons. Plast Reconstr Surg 1985; 75: 328-337.*

9. The correct response is D.

Porion is the most superior point of the external auditory meatus. Nasion is the midline point of the junction of frontonasal suture and the superior part of nasal bones. Orbitale is the palpable point of the lowest margin of the inferior orbital rim. Gnathion is the most inferior point of the lower border of the mandible, also called menton. Glabella is the most prominent point of the forehead between the eyebrows.

Reference:

1. *Vegter F, Hage JJ. Clinical anthropometry and canons of the face in historical perspective. Plast Reconstr Surg 2000; 106: 1090-1096.*
2. *Farkas LG, Hreczko TA, Kolar JC, Munro IR. Vertical and horizontal proportions of the face in young adult North American Caucasians: revision of neoclassical canons. Plast Reconstr Surg 1985; 75: 328-337.*

10. The correct response is C.

Pogonion is the most prominent point of the chin in the midline. Porion is the most superior point of the external auditory meatus. Nasion is the midline point of the junction of frontonasal suture and the superior nasal bones. Gnathion is the most inferior point of the lower border of the mandible, also called menton. Glabella is the most prominent point of the forehead between the eyebrows.

Reference:

1. *Vegter F, Hage JJ. Clinical anthropometry and canons of the face in historical perspective. Plast Reconstr Surg 2000; 106: 1090-1096.*
2. *Farkas LG, Hreczko TA, Kolar JC, Munro IR. Vertical and horizontal proportions of the face in young adult North American Caucasians: revision of neoclassical canons. Plast Reconstr Surg 1985; 75: 328-337.*

11. The correct response is C.

Stomion is the midline point where the upper lip touches the lower lip. Sublabiale is the midline point at the junction of the lower border of the lower lip and the superior border of the chin. Gnathion is the most inferior point of the lower border of the mandible, also called menton.

Reference:

1. *Vegter F, Hage JJ. Clinical anthropometry and canons of the face in historical perspective. Plast Reconstr Surg 2000; 106: 1090-1096.*
2. *Farkas LG, Hreczko TA, Kolar JC, Munro IR. Vertical and horizontal proportions of the face in young adult North American Caucasians: revision of neoclassical canons. Plast Reconstr Surg 1985; 75: 328-337.*

12. The correct response is B.

Sublabiale is the midline point at the junction of the lower border of the lower lip and the superior border of the chin. It is the deepest point of the labiomental groove. Gnathion is the most inferior point of the lower border of the mandible, also called menton. The other options are not valid points on the face.

Reference:

1. *Vegter F, Hage JJ. Clinical anthropometry and canons of the face in historical perspective. Plast Reconstr Surg 2000; 106: 1090-1096.*
2. *Farkas LG, Hreczko TA, Kolar JC, Munro IR. Vertical and horizontal proportions of the face in young adult North American Caucasians: revision of neoclassical canons. Plast Reconstr Surg 1985; 75: 328-337.*

13. The correct response is D.

Endocanthion is the point of the medial canthus where the upper and lower lids join. Caruncle, canthion, limbus and medial canthus are not anthropometric points.

Reference:

1. *Vegter F, Hage JJ. Clinical anthropometry and canons of the face in historical perspective. Plast Reconstr Surg 2000; 106: 1090-1096.*
2. *Farkas LG, Hreczko TA, Kolar JC, Munro IR. Vertical and horizontal proportions of the face in young adult North American Caucasians: revision of neoclassical canons. Plast Reconstr Surg 1985; 75: 328-337.*

14. The correct response is B.

The concept of facial proportions is based on neoclassical canons introduced by Renaissance artists to define ideal facial form in art. The canons are easy to remember and allow objective evaluation of facial proportions. According to the three section canon, the heights of trichion to nasion, nasion to subnasale and subnasale to gnathion are equal.

Reference:

1. *Vegter F, Hage JJ. Clinical anthropometry and canons of the face in historical perspective. Plast Reconstr Surg 2000; 106:1090-1096.*
2. *Farkas LG, Hreczko TA, Kolar JC, Munro IR. Vertical and horizontal proportions of the face in young adult North American Caucasians: revision of neoclassical canons. Plast Reconstr Surg 1985; 75: 328-337.*

15. The correct response is B.

The length of the nose is equal to the height of the ear according to the nasoaural proportion canon.

Reference:

1. *Vegter F, Hage JJ. Clinical anthropometry and canons of the face in historical perspective. Plast Reconstr Surg 2000; 106: 1090-1096.*
2. *Farkas LG, Hreczko TA, Kolar JC, Munro IR. Vertical and horizontal proportions of the face in young adult North American Caucasians: revision of neoclassical canons. Plast Reconstr Surg 1985; 75: 328-337.*

16. The correct response is D.

The concept of facial proportions is based on neoclassical canons introduced by Renaissance artists to define ideal facial form in art. The canons are easy to remember and allow objective evaluation of facial proportions. The distance between the medial canthi equals to width of the ala. The other options are incorrect.

Reference:

1. *Vegter F, Hage JJ. Clinical anthropometry and canons of the face in historical perspective. Plast Reconstr Surg 2000; 106: 1090-1096.*
2. *Farkas LG, Hreczko TA, Kolar JC, Munro IR. Vertical and horizontal proportions of the face in young adult North American Caucasians: revision of neoclassical canons. Plast Reconstr Surg 1985; 75: 328-337.*

17. The correct response is B.

The concept of facial proportions is based on neoclassical canons introduced by Renaissance artists to define ideal facial form in art. The canons are easy to remember and allow objective evaluation of facial proportions. The width of the mouth equals 1 ½ the width of ala. The other options are incorrect.

Reference:

1. *Vegter F, Hage JJ. Clinical anthropometry and canons of the face in historical perspective. Plast Reconstr Surg 2000; 106: 1090-1096.*
2. *Farkas LG, Hreczko TA, Kolar JC, Munro IR. Vertical and horizontal proportions of the face in young adult North American Caucasians: revision of neoclassical canons. Plast Reconstr Surg 1985; 75: 328-337.*

18. The correct response is D.

Vertical overlap of maxillary incisors over the mandibular incisors is termed as overbite. Horizontal overlap of maxillary incisors over the mandibular incisors is termed as overjet.

Reference:

Mohl ND, Zarb GA, Carlson GE, Rugh JD. A textbook of occlusion. Chicago, Quintessence, 1988.

19. The correct response is E.

Cephalometry is used to assess the bone relationships of the face and the relationships of the jaws and teeth. This information is useful for planning orthodontic and surgical treatment and also for performing growth studies of the face. The technique involves making a standardised lateral head radiograph by keeping the X-ray beam, subject and the film distances constant. The cephalogram shows the skull bones, teeth, and also the shadows of the pharynx and the soft tissue profile.

Reference:

Zide B, Grayson B, McCarthy JG. Cephalometric analysis: part 1. Plast Reconstr Surg 1981; 68: 816-823.

20. The correct response is E.

Cephalometry is used to assess the bone relationships of the face and the relationships of the jaws and teeth. This information is useful for planning orthodontic and surgical treatment and also for performing growth studies of the face. The technique involves making a standardised lateral head radiograph by keeping the x-ray beam, subject and the film distances constant. The cephalogram shows the skull bones, teeth, and also the shadows of the pharynx and the soft tissue profile.

Sella menton (SM) is not a standard cephalometic plane. The rest of the options are standard planes.

Reference:

Zide B, Grayson B, McCarthy JG. Cephalometric analysis: part 1. Plast Reconstr Surg 1981; 68: 816-823.

21. The correct response is C.

The normal range of angle of SNA is 82 ± 4 degrees for men and women. It is helpful in evaluating the antero-posterior relationship of the maxilla relative to the cranial base.

Reference:

Zide B, Grayson B, McCarthy JG. Cephalometric analysis: part 1. Plast Reconstr Surg 1981; 68: 816-823.

22. The correct response is A.

The normal range of angle of SNB is 79 ± 4 degrees for men and women. It is helpful in evaluating the antero-posterior relationship of the mandible relative to the cranial base.

Reference:

1. Zide B, Grayson B, McCarthy JG. Cephalometric analysis: part 1. Plast Reconstr Surg 1981; 68: 816-823.
2. Wolford LM, Bates JD. Surgical modification for the correction of chin deformities. Oral Surg Oral Med Oral Pathol 1988; 66: 279-286.

23. The correct response is A.

The cranial base is an important measurement for analysis of craniofacial deformities. It is the measurement of sella to nasion and not subnasale. The average range for men is 83 ± 4 mm and 77 ± 4 mm in women. The Frankfort horizontal makes an angle of approximately 5-9 degrees inferior to this plane. The cranial base can be increased by monobloc Le Fort III advancement and also by distraction.

Reference:

1. Zide B, Grayson B, McCarthy JG. Cephalometric analysis: part 1. Plast Reconstr Surg 1981; 68: 816-823.
2. Wolford LM, Bates JD. Surgical modification for the correction of chin deformities. Oral Surg Oral Med Oral Pathol 1988; 66: 279-286.
3. Bell WH, Proffit WR, White RP. Surgical correction of Dentofacial Deformities, vol 1. Philadelphia, WB Saunders, 1980.

24. The correct response is E.

It is important to recognise the category of patients who are likely to remain troublesome after surgery and are hence not good candidates for surgery. All of the categories listed exemplify patients that are not good candidates for surgery.

Reference:

1. *Gorney M. Patient selection criteria. In Gradinger G, Kaye B, eds: Symposium on Problem and Complications in Aesthetic Plastic Surgery of the Face. St. Louis, Mosby, 1984: 12.*
2. *Goldwyn RM. Patient selection: the importance of being cautious. In Courtiss EH, ed: Aesthetic Surgery: Trouble, How to Avoid It and How to Treat It. St. Louis, Mosby, 1978: 15.*

25. The correct response is B.

Aesthetic brow position includes the medial brow which begins at a line perpendicular to the alar base. It should be at the level of superior orbital rim and should arch slightly superiorly when followed laterally from its medial border.

Reference:

1. *Gunter JP, Antrobus SD. Aesthetic analysis of the eyebrows. Plast Reconstr Surg 1997; 99: 1808.*
2. *Ellenbogen R. Transcoronal eyebrow lift with concomitant upper blepharoplasty. Plast Reconstr Surg 1983; 71: 490.*

26. The correct response is C.

Aesthetic brow position includes the medial brow which begins at a line perpendicular to the alar base. It should be at the level of superior orbital rim and should arch slightly superiorly when followed laterally from its medial border. The peak of the brow should be approximately at the junction of its medial two thirds and lateral third. In terms of the midpupillary line, the aesthetic location of the peak should be either at level of this line or lateral to this line.

Reference:

1. *Gunter JP, Antrobus SD. Aesthetic analysis of the eyebrows. Plast Reconstr Surg 1997; 99: 1808.*
2. *Ellenbogen R. Transcoronal eyebrow lift with concomitant upper blepharoplasty. Plast Reconstr Surg 1983; 71: 490.*
3. *Flowers RS. The art of eyelid and orbital aesthetics: multiracial surgical considerations. Clin Plast Surg 1987; 14: 703.*

27. The correct response is B

Aging of the skin and aging of the frontalis accounts for the transverse lines on the forehead. These result from tonic frontalis contractions. Galea is not primarily responsible for forehead rhytids. Procerus and the supercilii muscles are responsible for the displacements and movements of the brow and nose region.

Reference:

1. *Flowers RS. The biomechanics of brow and frontalis function and its effects on blepharoplasty. Clin Plast Surg 1993; 20: 255.*
2. *Ellenbogen R. Transcoronal eyebrow lift with concomitant upper blepharoplasty. Plast Reconstr Surg 1983; 71: 490.*
3. *Flowers RS. The art of eyelid and orbital aesthetics: multiracial surgical considerations. Clin Plast Surg 1987;14:703.*

28. The correct response is C.

Procerus is responsible for transverse nose lines. It arises from the nasal bones and inserts into the glabella and skin of the forehead in the nearby area. Frontalis is responsible for the transverse lines on the forehead. These result from tonic frontalis contractions. Galea is not primarily responsible for nose rhytids. Supercilii muscles are responsible for the displacements and movements of the brow.

Reference:

1. *Flowers RS. The biomechanics of brow and frontalis function and its effects on blepharoplasty. Clin Plast Surg 1883; 20: 155.*
2. *Knize DM. Muscles that act on glabellar skin: a closer look. Plast Reconstr Surg 2000; 105: 350.*
3. *Flowers RS. The art of eyelid and orbital aesthetics: multiracial surgical considerations. Clin Plast Surg 1987; 14: 703.*

29. The correct response is B.

Corrugator supercilli. It arises from the frontal bone by a transverse and an oblique head. The muscle fibres move laterally and get inserted into the dermis. The muscle fibres may pass through orbicularis and frontalis muscle. This muscle is responsible for producing vertical and oblique lines in the upper part of the nose. Procerus is responsible for nose lines. Frontalis is responsible for the transverse lines on the forehead.

Reference:

1. *Flowers RS. The biomechanics of brow and frontalis function and its effects on blepharoplasty. Clin Plast Surg 1883; 20: 155.*
2. *Knize DM. Muscles that act on glabellar skin: a closer look. Plast Reconstr Surg 2000; 105: 350.*

30. The correct response is E.

Endoscopic brow lift would produce minimal scarring as it involves the least skin incision among all the options listed. It involves a 2-cm midline incision, posterior to the hairline along with paramedian ports. The rest of the procedures wider exposure.

Reference:

1. *Ramirez OM. Endoscopically assisted biplanar forehead lift. Plast Reconstr Surg 1995; 96: 323.*
2. *Bostwick J, Eaves FF, Nahai F. Endoscopic Plastic Surgery. St. Louis, Quality Medical Publishers, 1995.*

31. The correct response is E.

Depigmentation usually is not associated with Botox injections. The rest are associated with this therapy. Botox is an exotoxin, produced by Clostridium botulinum. It is available in vial of 100 MU (Mouse Units). It is kept frozen. For use, it is diluted with saline 2-4 cc and used for local injection using tuberculin syringe. 5-30 MU are injected locally for the desired temporary response. Complications of Botox are few and are fully reversible.

Reference:

1. *Huan W, Foster JA, Rogachefsky AS. Pharmacology of botulinum toxin. J Am Acad Dermatol 2000;43(pt 1):249.*
2. *Fagien S. Botox for the treatment of dynamic and hyperkinetic facial lines and furrows: adjunctive use in facial aesthetic surgery. Plast Reconstr Surg 1999; 103: 701.*

32. The correct response is D.

Mouse units is the standard measure of Botox activity, the toxic dose for a mouse on intraperitoneal injection. Botox is available in vial of 100 MU (Mouse Units). It is kept frozen. For use, it is diluted with saline 2-4 cc and used for local injection using tuberculin syringe. 5-30 MU are injected locally for the desired temporary response. The other options are not valid measures for Botox activity.

Reference:

1. *Huan W, Foster JA, Rogachefsky AS. Pharmacology of botulinum toxin. J Am Acad Dermatol 2000; 43(pt 1): 249.*
2. *Fagien S. Botox for the treatment of dynamic and hyperkinetic facial lines and furrows: adjunctive use in facial aesthetic surgery. Plast Reconstr Surg 1999; 103: 701.*

33. The correct response is D.

A beautiful eye irrespective of ethnicity is characterised by all of the following features except the lower lid (1- 1.5 mm) below the cornea. The lower lid should ideally be at the lower limbus. The rest of the features are synonymous with beautiful eyes.

Reference:

1. *Flowers RS. Cosmetic blepharoplasty-state of the art. Adv Plast Surg 1992; 8: 31.*
2. *Flowers RS. The art of eyelid and orbital aesthetics: multiracial surgical considerations. Clin Plast Surg 1987; 14: 703.*

34. The correct response is B.

The orbits are pyramids formed by the frontal, sphenoid, maxillary, zygomatic, lacrimal, palatine and ethmoid bones. The lacrimal is the smallest of the bones comprising the orbital cone.

Reference:

1. *Dutton JJ. Atlas of Clinical and Surgical Orbital Anatomy. Philadelphia, WB Saunders, 1994.*
2. *McCord CD, Tanenbaum M. Oculoplastic Surgery. New York, Raven Press, 1987: 42.*

35. The correct response is B.

The medial canthal ligament is attached to the anterior and posterior lacrimal crests of the lacrimal bone. The rest of the bones do not have attachment of this ligament.

Reference:

1. *Dutton JJ. Atlas of Clinical and Surgical Orbital Anatomy. Philadelphia, WB Saunders, 1994.*
2. *McCord CD, Tanenbaum M. Oculoplastic Surgery. New York, Raven Press, 1987: 42.*

36. The correct response is A.

The lateral canthal ligament is attached to the Whitnall's tubercle located on the zygomatic bone. It is located about 3-4 mm inside the lateral orbital rim.

Reference:

1. *Dutton JJ. Atlas of Clinical and Surgical Orbital Anatomy. Philadelphia, WB Saunders, 1994.*
2. *McCord CD, Tanenbaum M. Oculoplastic Surgery. New York, Raven Press, 1987: 42.*
3. *Gioia VM, Linberg JV, McCormick SA. The anatomy of the lateral canthal tendon. Arch Ophthalmol 1987; 105: 529.*

37. The correct response is E.

Muller's muscle or the supratarsal muscle originates on the deep surface of the levator and inserts into the superior tarsus. It is not a part of lateral retinaculum. The lateral retinaculum is composed of a labyrinth of soft tissue structures viz. lateral canthal tendon, lateral part of levator aponeurosis, Lockwood's ligament, Whitnall's ligament and check ligaments of the lateral rectus muscle. It supports the globe and eyelid as a hammock.

Reference:

1. *Dutton JJ. Atlas of Clinical and Surgical Orbital Anatomy. Philadelphia, WB Saunders, 1994.*
2. *McCord CD, Tanenbaum M. Oculoplastic Surgery. New York, Raven Press, 1987: 42.*
3. *Gioia VM, Linberg JV, McCormick SA. The anatomy of the lateral canthal tendon. Arch Ophthalmol 1987; 105: 529.*

38. The correct response is C.

Corrugator supercilii. The frontalis pulls the eyebrows upwards and outwards. Procerus pulls the medial brow down. Corrugator pulls the eyebrow medially and downwards. It protects the eye against bright sun light. It helps in frowning. Orbicularis pulls the entire eyebrow down.

Reference:

1. *Dutton JJ. Atlas of Clinical and Surgical Orbital Anatomy. Philadelphia, WB Saunders, 1994.*
2. *McCord CD, Tanenbaum M. Oculoplastic Surgery. New York, Raven Press, 1987: 42.*

39. The correct response is B.

Three. The fat compartments are nasal, central and lateral. The structures which lie anterior to the orbital fat are skin, orbicularis oculi, and orbital septum. The structures which lie behind the orbital fat in the upper eyelid are levator muscle, levator aponeurosis, Muller's muscle and lateral retinaculum.

Reference:

1. *Dutton JJ. Atlas of Clinical and Surgical Orbital Anatomy. Philadelphia, WB Saunders, 1994.*
2. *McCord CD, Tanenbaum M. Oculoplastic Surgery. New York, Raven Press, 1987: 42.*

40. The correct response is B.

Superior tarsus. Muller's muscle originates on the deep surface of the levator near the point where the muscle becomes aponeurotic and inserts into the superior tarsus. It is an important muscle in surgery for ptosis correction.

Reference:

1. *Dutton JJ. Atlas of Clinical and Surgical Orbital Anatomy. Philadelphia, WB Saunders, 1994.*
2. *McCord CD, Tanenbaum M. Oculoplastic Surgery. New York, Raven Press, 1987: 42.*

41. The correct response is C.

The frontalis muscle arises from the galea and is attached to the medial two-third of the brow. It is directed downwards and medially. There is a V- Shaped gap between the medial fibres of the frontalis muscles of the two sides. The apex of the V- is towards the nasion.

The central part of the forehead is without any muscles and has therefore no mobility. It is eminently suited for a Tilak or a Bindi on the forehead.

Reference:

1. *Dutton JJ. Atlas of Clinical and Surgical Orbital Anatomy. Philadelphia, WB Saunders, 1994.*
2. *Flowers RS. The biomechanics of brow and frontalis function and its effects on blepharoplasty. Clin Plast Surg 1993; 20: 255.*

42. The correct response is D.

When the upper eyelid skin hangs down to cover the lid margin, then it is called pseudoptosis and hence is not a characteristic feature of true ptosis. The other options show features of true ptosis.

Reference:

1. *Dutton JJ. Atlas of Clinical and Surgical Orbital Anatomy. Philadelphia, WB Saunders, 1994.*
2. *Flowers RS. The biomechanics of brow and frontalis function and its effects on blepharoplasty. Clin Plast Surg 1993; 20: 255.*
3. *Putterman AM. Cosmetic Oculoplastic Surgery: Eyelid, Forehead, and Facial Techniques, 3rd ed. Philadelphia, WB Saunders, 1999.*

43. The correct response is A.

The anchor or invagination blepharoplasty allows creation of precise, crisp lid folds which persist for a long time. It also avoids lid skin excision and preserves the skin for normal lid function. The disadvantage of this procedure is that it is technically demanding and requires greater surgical skill and expertise.

Reference:

1. *Flowers RS. Upper blepharoplasty by eyelid invagination: anchor blepharoplasty. The biomechanics of brow and frontalis function and its effects on blepharoplasty. Clin Plast Surg 1993; 20: 193.*
2. *Flowers RS. The biomechanics of brow and frontalis function and its effects on blepharoplasty. Clin Plast Surg 1993; 20: 255.*

44. The correct response is C.

The V–W epicanthoplasty is the procedure of choice for correction of epicanthal folds.

Reference:

1. *Flowers RS. Upper blepharoplasty by eyelid invagination: anchor blepharoplasty. The biomechanics of brow and frontalis function and its effects on blepharoplasty. Clin Plast Surg 1993; 20: 193.*
2. *Flowers RS. Surgical treatment of the epicanthal fold [invited essay]. Plast Reconstr Surg 1983; 73: 571.*

45. The correct response is D.

The upper lid blepharoplasty is not included in coronocanthopexy. The operation of coronocanthopexy' aims at correcting the position of the lower eyelid. The four procedures as mentioned above are all done together as part of coronocanthopexy for periorbital aesthetic rejuvenation.

Reference:

1. *Flowers RS. Upper blepharoplasty by eyelid invagination: anchor blepharoplasty. The biomechanics of brow and frontalis function and its effects on blepharoplasty. Clin Plast Surg 1993; 20: 193.*
2. *Flowers RS. Surgical treatment of the epicanthal fold [invited essay]. Plast Reconstr Surg 1983; 73: 571.*
3. *Flowers RS. Corono-canthopexy: our most rejuvenating operation (and associated procedures}. Instructional Course, American Society of Plastic Surgeons Annual Meeting. October 2003.*

46. The correct response is E.

Spastic pathology does not contribute to ptosis. The rest are various common conditions in the aetiology of ptosis.

Reference:

1. *Carraway JH. Combining blepharoplasty with upper eyelid ptosis correction. Aesthetic Surg J 2003; 23: 59.*
2. *Jelks GW, Smith BC. Reconstruction of the eyelids and associated structures. In McCarthy JG, ed: Plastic Surgery. Philadelphia, WB Saunders, 1990:1679.*

47. The correct response is B.

Muller's muscle is involuntary and can lift the eye for about 2-3 mm. It is supplied by sympathetic nerves through the vasculature in that area. The levator palpabrae superioris muscle is voluntary and is supplied by the oculomotor nerve. This is the main muscle which lifts the eye upwards.

Reference:

1. *Carraway JH. Combining blepharoplasty with upper eyelid ptosis correction. Aesthetic Surg J 2003; 23: 59.*
2. *Jelks GW, Smith BC. Reconstruction of the eyelids and associated structures. In McCarthy JG, ed: Plastic Surgery. Philadelphia, WB Saunders, 1990: 1679.*

48. The correct response is B.

Muller's muscle is attached to the upper border of the tarsal plate. Levator palpebrae superioris is attached to the anterior surface of the tarsal plate. The tarsal plate is the solid structure of the upper lid that gives it integrity and allows the lash follicles to seat themselves for stability.

Reference:

1. *Carraway JH. Combining blepharoplasty with upper eyelid ptosis correction. Aesthetic Surg J 2003; 23: 59.*
2. *Jelks GW, Smith BC. Reconstruction of the eyelids and associated structures. In McCarthy JG, ed: Plastic Surgery. Philadelphia, WB Saunders, 1990:1679.*

49. The correct response is A.

Levator palpebrae superioris is attached to the anterior surface of the tarsal plate. The tarsal plate is the solid structure of the upper lid that gives it integrity and allows the lash follicles to seat themselves for stability. The Muller's muscle is attached to the upper border of the tarsal plate.

Reference:

1. *Carraway JH. Combining blepharoplasty with upper eyelid ptosis correction. Aesthetic Surg J 2003; 23: 59.*
2. *Jelks GW, Smith BC. Reconstruction of the eyelids and associated structures. In McCarthy JG, ed: Plastic Surgery. Philadelphia, WB Saunders, 1990: 1679.*

50. The correct response is D.

Frontalis sling procedure is indicated in patients with ptosis with no levator function. A sling is placed from the frontalis muscle to the tarsal margin. Levator based procedures are not indicated due to non-functional muscle.

Reference:

1. *Jelks GW, Smith BC. Reconstruction of the eyelids and associated structures. In McCarthy JG, ed: Plastic Surgery. Philadelphia, WB Saunders, 1990:1679.*
2. *Jelks GW, Jelks EB. Preoperative evaluation of the blepharoplasty patient. Bypassing the pitfalls. Clin Plast Surg 1993; 20: 213.*

51. The correct response is B.

Stenting would make the lower lid heavy and hence should not be used for correction of ptosis. The rest of the procedures may be used in different indications.

Reference:

1. *Jelks GW, Smith BC. Reconstruction of the eyelids and associated structures. In McCarthy JG, ed: Plastic Surgery. Philadelphia, WB Saunders, 1990: 1679.*
2. *Bilyk JR. Periorbital reconstruction using novel alloplastic material. Ophthalmol Clin North Am 2000; 13: 571.*

52. The correct response is B.

The nasojugal groove occurs along the attachment of the arcus marginalis. The undersurface of the orbicularis oculi of the lower lid has a fascial attachment to the lower orbital rim. Over time, the orbital septum weakens and periocular fat herniation occurs. Whitnall's ligament, Muller's muscle and canthal ligament have no relationship to aetiology of nasojugal groove.

Reference:

1. *Jelks GW, Smith BC. Reconstruction of the eyelids and associated structures. In McCarthy JG, ed: Plastic Surgery. Philadelphia, WB Saunders, 1990: 1679.*
2. *Rizk SS, Matarasso A. Lower eyelid blepharoplasty: analysis of indications and treatment of 100 patients. Plast Reconstr Surg 2003; 111: 1299.*

53. The correct response is B.

SMAS is superficial musculoaponeurotic system. It is a discrete layer. It is under the skin and the subcutaneous fat. SMAS is the anatomical plane of dissection for the face lift. The parotido-masseteric fascia is deep to it. It was described by Mitz and Peyronie based on their study of cadaveric dissections to define its limits.

Reference:

1. *Mitz V, Peyronie M. The superficial musculoaponeurotic system (SMAS) in the parotid and cheek area. Plast Reconstr Surg 1976; 58: 80.*
2. *Hunt HL. Plastic Surgery of the Head, Face and Neck. Philadelphia, Lea and Febiger, 1926.*

54. The correct response is B.

All the superficial group of muscles get their nerve supply from the facial nerve, which enters these muscles on their under surfaces. These are orbicularis oculi, zygomaticus major, zygomaticus minor, platysma and risorius. The deeper muscles which lie deep to the plane of the facial nerve are innervated along their superficial surfaces.

Reference:

1. *Mitz V, Peyronie M. The superficial musculoaponeurotic system (SMAS) in the parotid and cheek area. Plast Reconstr Surg 1976; 58: 80.*
2. *Freilinger G, Gruber H, Happak W, Pechmann U. Surgical anatomy of the mimic muscle system and the facial nerve: Importance for reconstructive and aesthetic surgery. Plast Reconstr Surg 1987; 80: 686.*

55. The correct response is A.

The deep group of muscles encountered in a face lift procedure get their nerve supply from the superficial surface as they lie deep to the plane of the facial nerve. These muscles are buccinator, mentalis and levator anguli oris.

Reference:

1. *Mitz V, Peyronie M. The superficial musculoaponeurotic system (SMAS) in the parotid and cheek area. Plast Reconstr Surg 1976; 58: 80.*
2. *Freilinger G, Gruber H, Happak W, Pechmann U. Surgical anatomy of the mimic muscle system and the facial nerve: Importance for reconstructive and aesthetic surgery. Plast Reconstr Surg 1987; 80: 686.*

56. The correct response is A.

Cervical branches of facial nerve supply the platysma. These enter through the gap between the angle of the mandible and the sternocleidomastoid muscle. The other options are not the correct nerve supply for the platysma muscle.

Reference:

Guerrero-Santos J. The role of the platysma muscle in rhytidoplasty. Clin Plast Surg 1978; 5: 29.

57. The correct response is E.

The platysma takes origin from the fascia covering the pectoralis major, deltoid muscle, mastoid process and the occipital bone. It does not take attachment from the hyoid cartilage.

Reference:

Guerrero-Santos J. The role of the platysma muscle in rhytidoplasty. Clin Plast Surg 1978; 5: 29.

58. The correct response is E.

The platysma is inserted into all the above. The muscle is used in expressions of horror, surprise, anger, yelling and shouting. It also helps in deep inspiration. The external jugular vein lies deep to the muscle from the angle of the mandible to the middle of the clavicle. Its contracture may lead to deformities of the lower lip and lower jaw.

Reference:

Guerrero-Santos J. The role of the platysma muscle in rhytidoplasty. Clin Plast Surg 1978; 5: 29.

59. The correct response is B.

Parotid duct and the facial nerve lie deep to the parotid- masseteric fascia, and hence are safe during the facelift surgery because the elevation of the SMAS flap is superficial to this fascia. Beyond it, medial to the masseter, these structures come to lie in more superficial plane and overlie the buccal pad of fat and are prone to injury. It pierces the fat and the buccinator muscle opposite the 3rd molar and finally opens into the buccal cavity opposite the upper 2nd molar.

They are not related to the midbelly of the sternocleidomastoid muscle 6.5 cm inferior to the external auditory canal which is the classic landmark for the great auricular nerve.

Reference:

1. *Mitz V, Peyronie M. The superficial musculoaponeurotic system (SMAS) in the parotid and cheek area. Plast Reconstr Surg 1976; 58: 80.*
2. *Freilinger G, Gruber H, Happak W, Pechmann U. Surgical anatomy of the mimic muscle system and the facial nerve: Importance for reconstructive and aesthetic surgery. Plast Reconstr Surg 1987; 80: 686.*

60. The correct response is A.

The temporal branch of the facial nerve is at risk of injury in the temporal region where an incision through the SMAS can produce a direct injury to the nerve. It would not be injured by a more superficial incision over the skin and subcutaneous tissue. As an anatomic landmark, it travels along a line connecting the base of the tragus to a point 1.5 cm above the eyebrow. Anatomically, multiple branches of this nerve may be observed crossing the zygomatic arch. The nerve can exhibit multiple branching patterns crossing the zygomatic arch. The nerve is located medial and inferior to the frontal branch of the superficial temporal artery

Reference:

1. *Baker TJ, Gordon HL, Stuzin JM. Surgical Rejuvenation of the Face. 2nd ed. St. Louis, Mosby-year Book, 1996:167.*
2. *Pitanguy I, Ramos AS. The frontal branch of the facial nerve: the importance of its variations in face lifting. Plast Reconstr Surg 1966; 38: 352.*

61. The correct response is D.

The marginal mandibular nerve crosses the facial vessels at the anterior border of the masseter where the nerve is superficial and is vulnerable to injury. The facial artery and vein lie deep to the marginal mandibular nerve at the anterior border of the masseter which serves as a useful landmark for these vessels. The other options are incorrect.

Reference:

1. *Baker TJ, Gordon HL, Stuzin JM. Surgical Rejuvenation of the Face. 2nd ed. St. Louis, Mosby-year Book, 1996: 167.*
2. *Dingman RO, Grabb WG. Surgical anatomy of the mandibular ramus of the facial nerve based on the dissection of 100 facial halves. Plast Reconstr Surg 1962; 29: 266.*

62. The correct response is E.

The parotid duct does not cross the zygomaticus minor. The duct after emerging from the parotid gland lies on the surface of the masseter muscle and then dips in to pass through all the above three structures. A line joining the tragus with the oral commissure overlies the parotid duct in its posterior half.

Reference:

1. *Baker TJ, Gordon HL, Stuzin JM. Surgical Rejuvenation of the Face. 2nd ed. St. Louis, Mosby-year Book, 1996: 167.*
2. *Stuzin JM, Wagstrom L, Kawamoto HK, et al. The anatomy and clinical applications of the buccal fat pad. Plast Reconstr Surg 1990; 85: 29.*

63. The correct response is C.

There are four retaining ligaments. These are zygomatic, mandibular, parotid cutaneous ligament and masseteric ligament.

Reference:

1. *Baker TJ, Gordon HL, Stuzin JM. Surgical Rejuvenation of the Face. 2nd ed. St. Louis, Mosby-year Book, 1996: 167.*
2. *Stuzin JM, Baker TJ, Gordon HL. The relationship of the superficial and deep facial fascias: relevance to rhytidectomy and aging. Plast Reconstr Surg 1992; 89: 441.*

64. The correct response is C.

The great auricular nerve lies 6.5 cm below the external auditory canal. It is likely to get damaged during the facelift procedure if attention is not given to this location of the nerve during dissection. Injury to the nerve would produce the following:

1. Loss of sensation to the ear
2. Loss of sensation to the adjoining cheek
3. Possibility of neuroma

The nerve crosses the sternocleidomastoid muscle above the external jugular vein and can be easily seen deep to the platysma.

Reference:

1. *Baker TJ, Gordon HL, Stuzin JM. Surgical Rejuvenation of the Face. 2nd ed. St. Louis, Mosby-year Book, 1996: 167.*
2. *McKinney P, Katrana DJ. Prevention of injury to the great auricular nerve during rhytidectomy. Plast Reconstr Surg 1980; 66: 675.*

65. The correct response is A.

The great auricular nerve is the major sensory nerve which is most commonly injured in rhytidectomy. It lies 6.5 cm below the external auditory canal. Special care must be taken during the facelift procedure while elevating the cervical flap to avoid injury to this structure. The nerve if injured should be repaired primarily and this usually leads to good return of function.

The other options are motor nerves of the face.

Reference:

1. *Baker TJ, Gordon HL, Stuzin JM. Surgical Rejuvenation of the Face. 2nd ed. St. Louis, Mosby-year Book, 1996:167.*
2. *McKinney P, Katrana DJ. Prevention of injury to the great auricular nerve during rhytidectomy. Plast Reconstr Surg 1980; 66: 675.*

66. The correct response is B.

The buccal branch of facial nerve is the most commonly injured motor nerve in rhytidectomy. The great auricular nerve is the major sensory nerve which is most commonly injured in rhytidectomy. It lies 6.5 cm below the external auditory canal. Special care must be taken during the facelift procedure while elevating the cervical flap to help avoid injury to this structure. The nerve if injured should be repaired primarily and this usually leads to good return of function.

Reference:

1. *Baker TJ, Gordon HL, Stuzin JM. Surgical Rejuvenation of the Face. 2nd ed. St. Louis, Mosby-year Book, 1996: 167.*
2. *Baker DC, Conley J. Avoiding facial nerve injuries in rhytidectomy: anatomic variations and pitfalls. Plast Reconstr Surg 1979; 64: 781.*

67. The correct response is D.

Ptosis would not be produced in case the frontal nerve is damaged. The rest are signs of neurologic injury to the frontal branch of the facial nerve. The recovery following neuropraxia to this nerve takes from 2-6 months time.

Reference:

1. *Baker TJ, Gordon HL, Stuzin JM. Surgical Rejuvenation of the Face, 2nd ed. St. Louis, Mosby-Year Book, 1996: 360-361.*
2. *Baker DC, Conley J. Avoiding facial nerve injuries in rhytidectomy: anatomic variations and pitfalls. Plast Reconstr Surg 1979; 64: 781.*

68. The correct response is B.

The insertion of the intermediate temporal fascia and of the deep temporal fascia is directly onto the zygoma only in the central part. The deep temporal fascia and intermediate temporal fascia coalesce into the periosteum of the zygoma at the anterior and posterior thirds of the zygoma only. In endoscopic brow lifts, the plane of dissection is superficial to the intermediate temporal fascia until just before its insertion onto the zygoma when this fascia needs to be divided to gain access into the space occupied by the temporal fat pad.

Reference:

1. *Campiglio GL, Candiani P. Anatomical study on the temporal fascial layers and their relationships with the faci al nerve. Aesthet Plast Surg 1997; 21: 72.*
2. *Baker TJ, Gordon HL, Stuzin JM. Surgical Rejuvenation of the Face, 2nd ed. St. Louis, Mosby-Year Book, 1996: 360-361.*

69. The correct response is A.

The term 'SOOF' is used for suborbicularis oculi fat in relation to redraping of the orbicularis arc for the treatment of lower lid ectropion in patients with midfacial aging. The other options are not valid terms.

Reference:

McCord CD, Codner MA, Hester TR. Redraping the inferior orbicularis arc. Plast Reconstr Surg 1998; 102: 2471.

70. The correct response is D.

The infraorbital hollow region is particularly unsuitable for routine fat injection as the deposited fat may be visible as a subcutaneous irregularity. It can also form calcific nodules which may require direct excision. The other locations are relatively safer locations for fat injection.

Reference:

Baker TJ, Gordon HL, Stuzin JM. Surgical Rejuvenation of the Face, 2nd ed. St. Louis, Mosby-Year Book, 1996: 360-361.

71. The correct response is D.

Crow's feet are lateral periorbital wrinkles due to muscle hyperactivity combined with senile degeneration of the overlying skin. They can be treated temporarily using Botox injection therapy but definitive treatment may require suborbicularis midfacial elevation.

The rest of the options are incorrect.

Reference:

1. *Baker TJ, Gordon HL, Stuzin JM. Surgical Rejuvenation of the Face, 2nd ed. St. Louis, Mosby-Year Book, 1996: 360-361.*
2. *Fogli AL. Orbicularis muscleplasty and facelift: a better orbital contour. Plast Reconstr Surg 1995; 96: 1560.*

72. The correct response is C.

Otto Bames described the continuous periauricular and hairline incision for facelift. Previously segmental resection of strips of skin was being done in the preauricular and postauricular hairline areas with closure under tension.

Reference:

Bames OH. Truth and fallacies of face peeling and face lifting. Med J Reconstr 1927; 126: 86.

Larson DL. An historical glimpse of the evaluation of rhytidectomy. Clin Plast Surg 1995; 22: 207.

73. The correct response is D.

The term 'malar fat pad' was introduced by Owsley. Descent of the malar fat pad along with overlying attached skin is the dominant anatomic change of midfacial aging. It is triangular in shape with its base along the nasolabial fold.

Reference:

1. *Owsley JQ Jr, Fiala TGS. Update: lifting the malar fat pad for correction of prominent nasolabial folds. Plast Reconstr Surg 1997; 100: 715.*
2. *Owsley JQ Jr. Lifting the malar fat pad for correction of prominent nasolabial folds. Plast Reconstr Surg 1993; 91: 463.*

74. The correct response is C.

The zygomaticus and levator muscles that are invested by the SMAS lie beneath the malar fat pad. The localised fat pad presumably provides protective cushioning for the underlying thin walled maxillary sinus.

The rest of the muscles do not lie directly underneath the fat pad.

Reference:

1. *Owsley JQ Jr, Fiala TGS. Update: lifting the malar fat pad for correction of prominent nasolabial folds. Plast Reconstr Surg 1997; 100: 715.*
2. *Owsley JQ Jr. Lifting the malar fat pad for correction of prominent nasolabial folds. Plast Reconstr Surg 1993; 91: 463.*

75. The correct response is B.

The term 'malar fat pad' was introduced by Owsley. Descent of the malar fat pad along with overlying attached skin is the dominant anatomic change of midfacial aging. It is triangular in shape with its base along the nasolabial fold. The zygomaticus and levator muscles that are invested by the SMAS lie beneath the malar fat pad. The localised fat pad presumably provides protective cushioning for the underlying thin walled maxillary sinus.

Reference:

1. *Owsley JQ Jr, Fiala TGS. Update: lifting the malar fat pad for correction of prominent nasolabial folds. Plast Reconstr Surg 1997; 100: 715.*
2. *Owsley JQ Jr. Lifting the malar fat pad for correction of prominent nasolabial folds. Plast Reconstr Surg 1993; 91: 463.*

76. The correct response is D.

Lateral orbital wrinkles along with infraorbital flattening and prominent nasolabial folds completes the triad of midfacial aging. This triad is produced by the active contraction of the levator muscles.

Reference:

1. *Owsley JQ Jr, Fiala TGS. Update: lifting the malar fat pad for correction of prominent nasolabial folds. Plast Reconstr Surg 1997; 100: 715.*
2. *Owsley JQ Jr. Lifting the malar fat pad for correction of prominent nasolabial folds. Plast Reconstr Surg 1993; 91: 463.*
3. *Gosain AK, Amarante MTJ, Hyde JS, Yousif NJ. A dynamic analysis of changes in the nasolabial fold using magnetic resonance imaging: implications for facial rejuvenation and facial animation surgery. Plast Reconstr Surg 1996; 98: 622.*

77. The correct response is B.

The subperiosteal midface lift is a complete mobilisation of all of the facial soft tissue structures using subperiosteal dissection over the zygoma and maxilla. This technique is based on the established principles of midface craniofacial surgery.

The other options listed do not accomplish this goal. The submalar implant augments the inferior medial zygoma and the maxilla upto the region of the pyriform margin. Its function is to disguise the deformity.

Reference:

1. *Owsley JQ Jr, Fiala TGS. Update: lifting the malar fat pad for correction of prominent nasolabial folds. Plast Reconstr Surg 1997; 100: 715.*
2. *Little JW. Three dimensional rejuvenation of the mid face: volumetric resculpture by mala imbrications. Plast Reconstr Surg 2000; 105: 267.*

78. The correct response is E.

Perioral rhytids occur due to a combination of all of the above factors. Frequent perioral motion, subcutaneous atrophy and loss of skin elasticity contribute to perioral rhytids. They are accentuated in smokers and are especially visible in thin skinned and light skinned women.

Reference:

1. *Baker TJ, Gordon HL, Stuzin JM. Surgical Rejuvenation of the Face, 2nd ed. St. Louis, Mosby-Year Book, 1996: 360-361.*
2. *Sigal RK, Poindexter B, Weston GW, et al. Rejuvenating the aged face. Perspect Outlook Plast Surg 2000; 14:1.*

79. The correct response is E.

The masseter muscle does not contribute to the formation of the nasolabial fold. The rest of the muscles contribute to the formation of the nasolabial fold.

Reference:

1. *Baker TJ, Gordon HL, Stuzin JM. Surgical Rejuvenation of the Face, 2nd ed. St. Louis, Mosby-Year Book, 1996: 360-361.*
2. *Walker LR, Mudrovich S, Epker BN. The nasolabial fold: applied surgical anatomy and histology. Am J Cosmet Surg 1991; 8: 217.*

80. The correct response is D.

Direct neck lift is the procedure of choice in elderly patients (70 years and older) as they are usually either unwilling or unfit to undergo the regular facelift operations. Moreover this group would not be ideally treated with the standard facelift as the redundant neck skin will recur fairly early. Removal of skin excess by direct approach will also achieve a better profile for them.

Reference:

1. *Baker TJ, Gordon HL, Stuzin JM. Surgical Rejuvenation of the Face, 2nd ed. St. Louis, Mosby-Year Book, 1996: 360-361.*
2. *Gradinger GP. Anterior cervicoplasty in the male patient. Plast Reconstr Surg 2000; 106: 1146.*

81. The correct response is B.

The corset platysmaplasty was described by Feldman and utilises a vertical skin incision with a small horizontal limb on the cranial border of the incision. The horizontal arc shaped submental incision is another common incision used for platysmaplasty. The Gradinger technique uses a 'Z' plasty on the platysma as well as the skin.

Reference:

1. *Feldman JJ. Corset platysmaplasty. Clin Plast Surg 1992; 19: 369.*
2. *Feldman JJ. Corset platysmaplasty. Plast Reconstr Surg 1990; 85: 333.*
3. *Gradinger GP. Anterior cervicoplasty in the male patient. Plast Reconstr Surg 2000; 106: 1146.*

82. The correct response is C.

The submandibular gland is the one that requires consideration for ptosis in neck rejuvenation. Many techniques have been described for correction of ptosis of this gland. Gore-tex suture suspension from the midline to the sternocleidomastoid fascia has been described. Alternatively, vertical plication of the platysma over the ptotic submandibular gland may be performed as described by Feldman in corset platysmaplasty.

The other glands described do not qualify for this consideration in this situation. Branchial cyst is a pathological finding.

Reference:

1. *Singer DP, Sullivan PK. Submandibular gland. An anatomic evaluation. Plast Reconstr Surg 2003; 15: 112.*
2. *Feldman JJ. Corset platysmaplasty. Plast Reconstr Surg 1990; 85: 333.*

83. The correct response is B.

'Jowls' develop in relation to the lower jaw line posteriorly near the angle of the mandible as a result of tissue laxity. They are not located near any other bone of the face.

Reference:

Baker TJ, Gordon HL, Stuzin JM. Surgical Rejuvenation of the Face, 2nd ed. St. Louis, Mosby-Year Book, 1996: 360-361.

84. The correct response is E.

The buccal nerve is the only structure which is deep to the parotid gland. All the other structures as mentioned above lie superficial to the parotid gland.

Reference:

1. *Baker TJ, Gordon HL, Stuzin JM. Surgical Rejuvenation of the Face, 2nd ed. St. Louis, Mosby-Year Book, 1996: 360-361.*
2. *Castanares S. Facial nerve paralysis coincident with or subsequent to rhytidectomy. Plast Reconstr Surg 1974; 54: 637.*

85. The correct response is E.

The vagus nerve does not lie on the surface of the sternocleidomastoid muscle. It lies deep to it. The rest of the structures lie superficial to the muscle.

Reference:

1. *Baker TJ, Gordon HL, Stuzin JM. Surgical Rejuvenation of the Face, 2nd ed. St. Louis, Mosby-Year Book, 1996: 360-361.*
2. *Castanares S. Facial nerve paralysis coincident with or subsequent to rhytidectomy. Plast Reconstr Surg 1974; 54: 637.*

86. The correct response is C.

The marginal mandibular nerve is not a sensory nerve. It exits the anterior caudal margin of the parotid gland near the angle of the mandible and penetrates the deep cervical fascia. It then crosses superficial to the anterior facial artery to enter the buccal space where it provides branches to the depressor labii inferioris and mentalis. It does not supply either the buccinator or the platysma muscle.

Reference:

1. *Baker DC, Conley J. Avoiding facial nerve injuries in rhytidectomy. Anatomic variations and pitfalls. Plast Reconstr Surg 1979; 64: 781.*
2. *Castanares S. Facial nerve paralysis coincident with or subsequent to rhytidectomy. Plast Reconstr Surg 1974; 54: 637.*

87. The correct response is A.

Injury to a motor branch of the facial nerve is the most dreaded complication of a facelift surgery. There are no facial nerve branches in the superficial subcutaneous plane. Sub-SMAS plane runs the maximum risk of injury to the branches of the facial nerve. Frontal nerve injury is common in the subperiosteal plane.

Reference:

1. *Baker DC, Conley J. Avoiding facial nerve injuries in rhytidectomy. Anatomic variations and pitfalls. Plast Reconstr Surg 1979; 64: 781.*
2. *Castanares S. Facial nerve paralysis coincident with or subsequent to rhytidectomy. Plast Reconstr Surg 1974; 54: 637.*

88. The correct response is C.

Injury to marginal mandibular nerve paralyses the depressors of the lip. The patient will not be able to depress the lower lip down due to loss of supply to the lower lip and chin. The lip would cover the lower teeth from view and hence the patient will not be able to have a full denture smile.

Reference:

1. *Owsley JQ Jr. Aesthetic Facial Surgery. Philadelphia. WB Saunders, 1994: 184.*
2. *Matarasso A, Elkwood A, Rankin M, Elkowitz M. National Plastic Surgery Survey: Face lift techniques and complications. Plast Reconstr Surg 2000; 106: 1185.*

89. The correct response is B.

The mentalis is the one that is supplied by the marginal mandibular nerve. The rest are not supplied by marginal mandibular nerve. The patient is asked to perform the act of 'blowing'. If the mentalis muscle is having an intact nerve supply, then there would be dimpling of the skin in front of the chin.

Reference:

1. *Owsley JQ Jr. Aesthetic Facial Surgery. Philadelphia. WB Saunders, 1994: 184.*
2. *Matarasso A, Elkwood A, Rankin M, Elkowitz M. National Plastic Surgery Survey: Face lift techniques and complications. Plast Reconstr Surg 2000; 106: 1185.*

90. The correct response is E.

The Fitzpatick classification is a universally accepted classification of skin based on skin colour and reaction to first yearly sun exposure. The dark brown skin falls in Type V while light brown skin falls in Type IV category.

Reference:

Fitzpatrick RE, Goldman MP, Satur NM et al. Pulsed carbon dioxide laser resurfacing of photo-aged facial skin. Arch Dermatol 1996; 132: 395-402.

91. The correct response is C.

The laser energy produces its effect by selective 'photothermolysis'. This is the basis for use of lasers in clinical practice.

Reference:

1. *Goldman L, Rockwell RJ Jr. Lasers in Medicine. New York, Gordon and Breech, 1971.*
2. *Anderson RR, Parish JA. Selective photothermolysis: precise microsurgery by selective absorption of pulsed radiation. Science 1983; 22: 524.*

92. The correct response is D.

Fluence is a measure of laser energy and is expressed as energy (joules) per surface area of tissue (cm^2). The energy density required to cause ablation of a given tissue is the ablation threshold.

Reference:

1. *Goldman L, Rockwell RJ Jr. Lasers in Medicine. New York, Gordon and Breech, 1971.*
2. *Roberts TL, Pozner JN. Lasers, facelifting, and the future. Clin Plast Surg 2000; 27: 298.*

93. The correct response is D.

The nose does not need any special protection from laser. The rest need protection from laser. The eyes are protected by the eye shield, teeth by the wet gauze and endotracheal tube also needs to be covered by a wet gauze.

Reference:

1. *Goldman L, Rockwell RJ Jr. Lasers in Medicine. New York, Gordon and Breech, 1971.*
2. *Rohrich RJ, Gyimesi IM, Clark P, et al. CO_2 laser safety considerations in facial skin resurfacing. Plast Reconstr Surg 1997; 100: 1285.*

94. The correct response is E.

Hypertrophic scarring is one complication that may require further treatment, possibly in the form of a surgical intervention. The rest of the listed complications do not require surgical intervention and respond to medical treatment.

Reference:

1. *Goldman L, Rockwell RJ Jr. Lasers in Medicine. New York, Gordon and Breech, 1971.*
2. *Schwartz RJ, Burns AJ, Rohrich RJ, et al. Long–term assessment of CO_2 facial laser resurfacing aesthetic results and complications. Plast Reconstr Surg 1999; 103: 592.*

95. The correct response is A

Out of all the options listed, laser therapy would be the best choice as it will give the least possible scarring.

Reference:

1. *Goldman L, Rockwell RJ Jr. Lasers in Medicine. New York, Gordon and Breech, 1971.*
2. *Alster T. Manual of Cutaneous Laser Techniques, 2nd ed. Philadelphia, Lippincott Williams and Wilkins, 2000.*

96. The correct response is E.

Vitamin A helps in rejuvenation of the skin out of the listed actions.

Reference:

1. *Orfanos CE, Zouboules CC, Almond-Rocoler B, et al. Current use and future potential role of retinoids in dermatology. Drugs 1997; 53: 358-363.*
2. *Klingman AM, Grahm GF. Histologic changes in facial skin after daily application of tretinoin for 5-6 years. J Dermatol Treat 1993; 4: 113-117.*

97. The correct response is D.

Atrophy of the skin appendages does not occur with Vitamin A therapy. All the rest of the changes mentioned occur with this type of therapy.

Reference:

1. *Klingman AM, Grahm GF. Histologic changes in facial skin after daily application of tretinoin for 5-6 years. J Dermatol Treat 1993; 4: 113-117.*
2. *Orfanos CE, Zouboules CC, Almond-Rocoler B et al. Current use and future potential role of retinoids in dermatology. Drugs 1997; 53: 358-363.*

98. The correct response is D.

Alphatocopherol is the biologically active form of Vitamin E. Vitamin E is a naturally occurring lipid soluble antioxidant. It can regenerate its antioxidant properties in the presence of Vitamin C.

Reference:

1. *Mayer P. The effects of vitamin E on the skin. Cosmetics Toiletries 1993; 108: 99-109.*
2. *Keller KL, Fenske NA. Uses of vitamins A, C, and E and related compounds in dermatology: a review. J Am Acad Dermatol 1998; 39: 611-625.*

99. The correct response is B.

Silicone is chemically polysiloxane, which is a polymer formed by interlinking silicone and oxygen with methyl side groups.

Reference:

Rubin JP, Yaremchuk MJ. Complications and toxicities of implantable biomaterials used in facial reconstructive and aesthetic surgery: a comprehensive review of the literature. Plast Reconstr Surg 1997; 100: 1336.

100. The correct response is B.

In normal healthy young adults, the eye is placed at a distance of about 10 mm behind the supraorbital ridge. The infraorbital ridge is about 2-3 mm behind the overlying skin surface. This translates to a distance of 13 mm between the supraorbital and the infraorbital rim.

Reference:

Yaremchuk MJ. Infraorbital rim augmentation. Plast Reconstr Surg 2001; 107: 1585.

101. The correct response is E.

Transcolumellar scarring is the main criticism of the open approach. The rest all are advantages of the open rhinoplasty approach.

Reference:

Johnson C Jr, Toriumi DM: Open Structure Rhinoplasty. Philadelphia. WB Saunders, 1990.

102. The correct response is A.

The nasal septum is the first choice for cartilage grafts in rhinoplasty. It helps in correcting the deviation of the septum and also for performing other rhinoplastic procedures. The septum provides straight cartilage with adequate thickness which is suitable for both primary and secondary rhinoplasty. The other advantages of septal cartilage are minimal donor site morbidity, ease of harvest and local availability in the same operative field.

The other options do not offer the above advantages and MEDPOR is unsuitable as cartilage graft material.

Reference:

Gunter JP, Rohrich RJ. Management of the deviated nose-the importance of the septal reconstruction. Clin Plast Surg 1988; 15: 43.

103. The correct response is A.

Rethi was the one who first introduced the open approach in 1934. He had a case with an excessively long nose. He performed open rhinoplasty for the first time to reduce it, because it was not possible to reduce it by a closed rhinoplasty approach.

Reference:

Rethi A. Operation to shorten an excessively long nose. Rev Chir Plast 1934; 2: 85.

104. The correct response is C.

It was a case of excessively long nose for which open rhinoplasty was done for the first time by Rethi in 1934.

Reference:

Rethi A. Operation to shorten an excessively long nose. Rev Chir Plast 1934; 2: 85.

105. The correct response is B.

The normal columellar labial angle in women ranges from 100 - 108°, while in men it is 90 – 100°. An acute angle of 80 degrees is typical of a nose with drooping tip.

Reference:
Guyuron B. Nasal proportions. In Gruber RP, Peck GC, eds: Rhinoplasty: State of the Art. St. Louis, Mosby, 1993: 13-28.

106. The correct response is E.

In general the open approach is preferred when there is a need to execute complicated manoeuvres such as tip work, difficult septal work, placement of grafts etc. Hump reduction requires simple rasping which can be accomplished by a closed approach.

Reference:
Johnson CM Jr, Toriumi DM. Open Structure Rhinoplasty. Philadelphia, WB Saunders, 1990: 99-107.

107. The correct response is B.

The interdomal suture is used for providing better definition to the tip of the nose. Transdomal suture is used for correcting the domes of either side. Intercrural suture is used for correcting the flare of the medial crus. Lateral crural suture is used for correcting the curvature of the lateral crus and columellar-septal suture is used for fixing the columellar struts.

Reference:
1. *Tebbetts JB. Shaping and positioning the nasal tip without structural disruption: a new systemic approach. Plast Reconstr Surg 1994; 94: 61-77.*
2. *Johnson CM Jr, Toriumi DM. Open Structure Rhinoplasty. Philadelphia, WB Saunders, 1990: 99-107.*

108. The correct response is E.

All of the above may be responsible for producing the oversized nose. The treatment lies in identifying the correct causative structural abnormality. This can be done by studying the angle of the nose, labiocolumellar angle, basal view, side view of the nose and other parameters like the length of the nose, width of the nose and height of the nose. The treatment of this deformity lies in reducing the oversized cartilage by 3-5 mm as required.

Reference:
1. *Guntur JP. Decreasing tip projection in rhinoplasty: and algorithm. Dallas Rhinoplasty Symposium, Dallas, Texas, 1996.*
2. *Tebbetts JB. Shaping and positioning the nasal tip without structural disruption: a new systemic approach. Plast Reconstr Surg 1994; 94: 61-77.*

109. The correct response is E.

All of the above are correct.

Reference:
Gillies HD, Millard DR. The principles and art of plastic surgery. Boston, Little Brown, 1957: 48-54.

110. The correct response is D.

The time honoured turn over flaps are usually based on scarred skin or skin graft placed along the edge of the defect. They thus form a stiff lining and their length is also limited by their tenous blood supply. The rest of the flaps are based on healthy skin.

Reference:
1. *Millard DR Jr. Reconstructive rhinoplasty for the lower half of a nose. Plast Reconstr Surg 1974; 53: 133-139.*
2. *Kazanjian VH. Reconstruction of the ala using a septal flap. Trans Am Acad Ophthalmol Otolaryngol 1937; 42: 338.*

111. The correct response is B.

Zone 2 skin is stiff, thick and filled with sebaceous glands. The only skin donor site that matches the colour and texture of this zone is the forehead and local skin. Hence a bilobed flap is the flap of choice as it moves local skin into the defect without causing dog ears.

Reference:
1. *Jackson IT. Local flaps in head and neck reconstruction. St. Louis, Mosby, 1985.*
2. *Zitelli JA. The bilobed flap for nasal reconstruction. Arch Dermatol 1989; 125: 957-959.*

112. The correct response is C.

Bilobed flaps were first described by Esser in 1918 for defects of the nose. Later Zitelli suggested improvements in the bilobed flap.

Reference:

1. *Jackson IT. Local flaps in head and neck reconstruction. St. Louis, Mosby, 1985.*
2. *Zitelli JA. The bilobed flap for nasal reconstruction. Arch Dermatol 1989; 125: 957-959.*

113. The correct response is B.

The nose is divided into separate zones based on texture, subcutaneous fat and sebaceous gland content. The nose tip falls majorly in zone 2.

Zone 1 covers the upper dorsum and sidewalls of the nose. Its skin is smooth, thin and non-sebaceous and glides easily over the underlying bone and cartilage. Zone 2 begins about 1.5 cm above the supratip area and covers most of the nasal tip and alar lobules. The skin is thick and filled with sebaceous glands. Zone 3 includes a 4 mm strip along the alar margin, the soft triangles, the lower half of the infratip lobule and the columella. The skin is fixed to the deep cartilage.

Zones 4 and 5 do not exist.

Reference:

1. *Burget GC, Menick FJ. Aesthetic reconstruction of the nose. St. Louis, Mosby, 1994: ix.*
2. *Burget GC. Aesthetic reconstruction of the tip of the nose. Dermatol Surg 1995; 2: 419–429.*

114. The correct response is A.

The nose is divided into separate zones based on texture, subcutaneous fat and sebaceous gland content. The sidewall falls in zone 1.

Zone 1 covers the upper dorsum and sidewalls of the nose. Its skin is smooth, thin and non-sebaceous and glides easily over the underlying bone and cartilage. Zone 2 begins about 1.5 cm above the supratip area and covers most of the nasal tip and alar lobules. The skin is thick and filled with sebaceous glands. Zone 3 includes a 4 mm strip along the alar margin, the soft triangles, the lower half of the infratip lobule and the columella. The skin is fixed to the deep cartilage.

Zones 4 and 5 do not exist.

Reference:

1. *Burget GC, Menick FJ. Aesthetic reconstruction of the nose. St. Louis, Mosby, 1994: ix.*
2. *Burget GC. Aesthetic reconstruction of the tip of the nose. Dermatol Surg 1995; 2: 419-429.*

115. The correct response is C.

The nose is divided into separate zones based on texture, subcutaneous fat and sebaceous gland content. The columella falls in zone 3.

Zone 1 covers the upper dorsum and sidewalls of the nose. Its skin is smooth, thin and non-sebaceous and glides easily over the underlying bone and cartilage. Zone 2 begins about 1.5 cm above the supratip area and covers most of the nasal tip and alar lobules. The skin is thick and filled with sebaceous glands. Zone 3 includes a 4 mm strip along the alar margin, the soft triangles, the lower half of the infratip lobule and the columella. The skin is fixed to the deep cartilage.

Zones 4 and 5 do not exist.

Reference:

1. *Burget GC, Menick FJ. Aesthetic reconstruction of the nose. St. Louis, Mosby, 1994: ix.*
2. *Burget GC. Aesthetic reconstruction of the tip of the nose. Dermatol Surg 1995; 2: 419-429.*

116. The correct response is C.

The nose is divided into separate zones based on texture, subcutaneous fat and sebaceous gland content. The soft triangle falls in zone 3.

Zone 1 covers the upper dorsum and sidewalls of the nose. Its skin is smooth, thin and non-sebaceous and glides easily over the underlying bone and cartilage. Zone 2 begins about 1.5 cm above the supratip area and covers most of the nasal tip and alar lobules. The skin is thick and filled with sebaceous glands. Zone 3 includes a 4 mm strip along the alar margin, the soft triangles, the lower half of the infratip lobule and the columella. The skin is fixed to the deep cartilage.

Zones 4 and 5 do not exist.

Reference:

1. *Burget GC, Menick FJ. Aesthetic reconstruction of the nose. St. Louis, Mosby, 1994: ix.*
2. *Burget GC. Aesthetic reconstruction of the tip of the nose. Dermatol Surg 1995; 2: 419-429.*

117. The correct response is B.

The nose is divided into separate zones based on texture, subcutaneous fat and sebaceous gland content. The highest sebaceous gland content is in zone 2.

Zone 1 covers the upper dorsum and sidewalls of the nose. Its skin is smooth, thin and non-sebaceous and glides easily over the underlying bone and cartilage. Zone 2 begins about 1.5 cm above the supratip area and covers most of the nasal tip and alar lobules. The skin is thick and filled with sebaceous glands. Zone 3 includes a 4 mm strip along the alar margin, the soft triangles, the lower half of the infratip lobule and the columella. The skin is fixed to the deep cartilage.

Zones 4 and 5 do not exist.

Reference:

1. *Burget GC, Menick FJ. Aesthetic reconstruction of the nose. St. Louis, Mosby, 1994: ix.*
2. *Burget GC. Aesthetic reconstruction of the tip of the nose. Dermatol Surg 1995; 2: 419-429.*

118. The correct response is A.

Surgery of developmental deformities of maxilla and mandible due to genetic and environmental aetiology is orthognathic surgery. Deformities caused by congenital, traumatic and syndromic causes are excluded.

Reference:

Rosen HM. Aesthetics in facial skeletal surgery. Perspect Plast Surg. 1993; 6:1.

119. The correct response is A.

The relationship of the first molars of the upper and lower jaw is considered to classify malocclusion.

In class I occlusion, the mesiobuccal cusp of the first permanent maxillary molar occludes in the buccal groove of the permanent mandibular first molar. In class II malocclusion, the mesiobuccal cusp of the first permanent maxillary molar occludes mesial to the buccal groove of the permanent mandibular first molar. In class III malocclusion, the mesiobuccal cusp of the first permanent maxillary molar occludes distal to the buccal groove of the permanent mandibular first molar.

Reference:

1. *Tompach PC, Wheeler JJ, Fridrich KL et al. Orthodontic considerations in orthognathic surgery. Int J Adult Orthod Orthognath Surg. 1995; 10: 97.*
2. *Rosen HM. Aesthetics in facial skeletal surgery. Perspect Plast Surg. 1993; 6: 1.*

120. The correct response is A.

The mesiobuccal cusp of first maxillary molar in the buccal groove of the first mandibular molar defines the state of normal occlusion.

In class I occlusion, the mesiobuccal cusp of the first permanent maxillary molar occludes in the buccal groove of the permanent mandibular first molar. In class II malocclusion, the mesiobuccal cusp of the first permanent maxillary molar occludes mesial to the buccal groove of the permanent mandibular first molar. In class III malocclusion, the mesiobuccal cusp of the first permanent maxillary molar occludes distal to the buccal groove of the permanent mandibular first molar.

The rest of the options are incorrect.

Reference:

1. *Tompach PC, Wheeler JJ, Fridrich KL et al. Orthodontic considerations in orthognathic surgery. Int J Adult Orthod Orthognath Surg. 1995; 10: 97.*
2. *Rosen HM. Aesthetics in facial skeletal surgery. Perspect Plast Surg. 1993; 6:1.*

121. The correct response is A.

The mandibular molar is posterior to the maxillary molar in class II relationship.

In class I occlusion, the mesiobuccal cusp of the first permanent maxillary molar occludes in the buccal groove of the permanent mandibular first molar. In class II malocclusion, the mesiobuccal cusp of the first permanent maxillary molar occludes mesial to the buccal groove of the permanent mandibular first molar. In class III malocclusion, the mesiobuccal cusp of the first permanent maxillary molar occludes distal to the buccal groove of the permanent mandibular first molar.

The rest of the options are incorrect.

Reference:

1. *Tompach PC, Wheeler JJ, Fridrich KL et al. Orthodontic considerations in orthognathic surgery. Int J Adult Orthod Orthognath Surg. 1995; 10: 97.*
2. *Rosen HM. Aesthetics in facial skeletal surgery. Perspect Plast Surg. 1993; 6: 1.*

122. The correct response is B.

The mandibular molar is anterior to the maxillary molar.

In class I occlusion, the mesiobuccal cusp of the first permanent maxillary molar occludes in the buccal groove of the permanent mandibular first molar. In class II malocclusion, the mesiobuccal cusp of the first permanent maxillary molar occludes mesial to the buccal groove of the permanent mandibular first molar. In class III malocclusion, the mesiobuccal cusp of the first permanent maxillary molar occludes distal to the buccal groove of the permanent mandibular first molar.

The rest of the options are incorrect.

Reference:

1. *Tompach PC, Wheeler JJ, Fridrich KL et al. Orthodontic considerations in orthognathic surgery. Int J Adult Orthod Orthognath Surg. 1995; 10: 97.*
2. *Rosen HM. Aesthetics in facial skeletal surgery. Perspect Plast Surg. 1993; 6: 1.*

123. The correct response is D.

The sagittal split ramus osteotomy was described for the first time by Trauner and Obwegeser to correct both mandibular prognathism and deficiency. Angle and Caldwell described extraoral approaches for mandibular osteotomy. Dingman employed the intraoral approach.

The sagittal split osteotomy is done to save the inferior alveolar nerve, though risk of injury to the nerve is always there.

Reference:

1. *Tompach PC, Wheeler JJ, Fridrich KL et al. Orthodontic considerations in orthognathic surgery. Int J Adult Orthod Orthognath Surg. 1995; 10: 97.*
2. *Rosen HM. Aesthetics in facial skeletal surgery. Perspect Plast Surg. 1993; 6:1.*

124. The correct response is C.

The Wassmund osteotomy is segmental osteotomy of the maxilla. It is commonly done for correction of open bite deformities.

Reference:

1. *Tompach PC, Wheeler JJ, Fridrich KL et al. Orthodontic considerations in orthognathic surgery. Int J Adult Orthod Orthognath Surg. 1995; 10: 97.*
2. *Rosen HM. Aesthetics in facial skeletal surgery. Perspect Plast Surg. 1993; 6:1.*

125. The correct response is A.

The 'LeFort 1 osteotomy' is the procedure which can allow the posterior maxilla to move up and rotate to help correct the occlusion. LeFort II and III procedures are not suitable and justifiable to correct the occlusion.

Reference:

1. *Proffit WR, Turvey TA, Phillips C et al. Orthognathic surgery: a hierarchy of stability. Int J Adult Orthod Orthognath Surg. 1996; 11: 191–204.*
2. *Proffit WR, Sarver DM. Treatment planning: optimizing benefit to the patient. In: Proffit WR, White RP, Sarver DM, eds. Contemporary Treatment of Dentofacial Deformity. St. Louis: Mosby; 2003: 213–223.*

126. The correct response is C.

A patient with class II malocclusion needs mandibular advancement to correct the deformity. Thus the sagittal split osteotomy for mandibular advancement and rotation is the procedure of choice for him. The LeFort and other osteotomies would not be helpful in this situation.

Genioplasty would provide further necessary correction as required.

Reference:

1. *Proffit WR, Turvey TA, Phillips C et al. Orthognathic surgery: a hierarchy of stability. Int J Adult Orthod Orthognath Surg. 1996; 11: 191–204.*
2. *Proffit WR, Sarver DM. Treatment planning: optimizing benefit to the patient. In: Proffit WR, White RP, Sarver DM, eds. Contemporary Treatment of Dentofacial Deformity. St. Louis: Mosby; 2003: 213–223.*

127. The correct response is C.

A patient with class III malocclusion needs mandibular set back by sagittal split osteotomy to correct the deformity. Thus the sagittal split osteotomy for mandibular setback and rotation is the procedure of choice for him. The LeFort and other osteotomies would not be helpful in this situation.

Reference:

1. *Proffit WR, Turvey TA, Phillips C et al. Orthognathic surgery: a hierarchy of stability. Int J Adult Orthod Orthognath Surg. 1996; 11: 191–204.*
2. *Proffit WR, Sarver DM. Treatment planning: optimizing benefit to the patient. In: Proffit WR, White RP, Sarver DM, eds. Contemporary Treatment of Dentofacial Deformity. St. Louis: Mosby; 2003: 213–223.*

128. The correct response is A.

This patient needs a vertical reduction of the height of the maxilla. This can be achieved by LeFort I osteotomy to reduce the excess maxillary height by removing a wedge of bone. The other procedures would not be helpful in this situation.

Reference:

1. *Proffit WR, Turvey TA, Phillips C et al. Orthognathic surgery: a hierarchy of stability. Int J Adult Orthod Orthognath Surg. 1996; 11: 191–204.*
2. *Proffit WR, Sarver DM. Treatment planning: optimizing benefit to the patient. In: Proffit WR, White RP, Sarver DM, eds. Contemporary Treatment of Dentofacial Deformity. St. Louis: Mosby; 2003: 213–223.*

129. The correct response is E.

The short face patient is an infrequently encountered problem. It is characterised by vertical facial deficiency. These patients will usually have a class II malocclusion and mandibular deficiency. Class III malocclusion is not a feature of short face syndrome.

Reference:

1. *Tompach PC, Wheeler JJ, Fridrich KL et al. Orthodontic considerations in orthognathic surgery. Int J Adult Orthod Orthognath Surg. 1995; 10: 97.*
2. *Rosen HM. Aesthetics in facial skeletal surgery. Perspect Plast Surg. 1993; 6:1.*

130. The correct response is B.

The total number of hairs on the scalp in adult males is about 1.5 lacs. It could be little less or more.

Reference:

1. *Bernstein RM, Rassman WR. Follicular transplantation, patient evaluation and surgical planning. Dermatol Surg 1997; 23: 771.*
2. *Bernstein RM, Rassman WR. The aesthetics of follicular transplantation. Dermatol Surg 1997; 23: 785.*

131. The correct response is C.

Many classifications for baldness have been advocated which compare the hair bearing with the non-hair bearing areas. The occipital baldness is classified as type III according to the Norwood classification.

Reference:

1. *Norwood OT. Male pattern baldness: classification and incidence. South Med J 1975; 68: 1359-1365.*
2. *Hamilton JB. Patterned loss of hair in man: types and incidence. Ann N Y Acad Sci 1951; 53: 708.*

132. The correct response is D.

A patient having a bridge of hair between the frontal and the occipital baldness as per Norwood classification would be classified into type IV.

Reference:

1. *Norwood OT. Male pattern baldness: classification and incidence. South Med J 1975; 68: 1359-1365.*
2. *Hamilton JB. Patterned loss of hair in man: types and incidence. Ann N Y Acad Sci 1951; 53: 708.*

133. The correct response is C.

Micro, mini or follicular hair grafts would be a very suitable procedure. The rest of the options have their own drawbacks.

Reference:

1. *Bernstein RM, Rassman WR. Follicular transplantation, patient evaluation and surgical planning. Dermatol Surg 1997; 23: 771.*
2. *Bernstein RM, Rassman WR. The aesthetics of follicular transplantation. Dermatol Surg 1997; 23: 785.*

134. The correct response is E.

The follicular unit can have one, two or three hair units. The term follicular unit basically refers to the fact that anatomically there is a clustering of two or three follicles together in units.

Reference:

1. *Bernstein RM, Rassman WR. Follicular transplantation, patient evaluation and surgical planning. Dermatol Surg 1997; 23: 771.*
2. *Bernstein RM, Rassman WR. The aesthetics of follicular transplantation. Dermatol Surg 1997; 23: 785.*

135. The correct response is B.

The submental incision for correction of the double chin should not be given directly over the submental crease as it would lead to accentuation of the crease. It should be given posterior to the crease where it prevents accentuation of the double chin and provides for easier dissection and suturing.

Reference:

1. *Connell BF, Martin TJ. Facelift. In Cohen M, ed: Mastery of Plastic and Reconstructive Surgery. Boston, Little Brown, 1994.*
2. *Martin TJ. Facelift: Planning and technique. Clin Plast Surg 1997; 24: 269.*

136. The correct response is B.

The type of grafts used to support the ala or the side wall of the nose are called 'Batten grafts' because they are "like a flat strip" and would provide support to the ala and the side wall. Strut grafts are placed in the columella, spreader grafts are placed between the nasal septum and lateral cartilage. Shield grafts are used for tip augmentation purposes.

Reference:

1. *Peck GC. Techniques in Aesthetic Rhinoplasty. New York, Thieme-Stratton, 1984.*
2. *Gunter J, Rohrich R, Adams W Jr. Dallas Rhinoplasty: Nasal Surgery by the Masters. St. Louis, Quality Medical Publishing, 2000.*

137. The correct response is A.

The "Strut graft" is like a bar and is used to provide support to columella to lift up the tip of the nose. It can be of two types, floating or fixed. The type of grafts used to support the ala or the side wall of the nose are called 'Batten grafts' because they are "like a flat strip" and would provide support to the ala and the side wall. Shield grafts are used for tip augmentation purposes.

Reference:

1. *Peck GC. Techniques in Aesthetic Rhinoplasty. New York, Thieme-Stratton, 1984.*
2. *Gunter J, Rohrich R, Adams W Jr. Dallas Rhinoplasty: Nasal Surgery by the Masters. St. Louis, Quality Medical Publishing, 2000.*

138. The correct response is C.

The "Spreader graft" is a longitudinal piece of cartilage which is placed in between the upper lateral cartilage and the septum to widen the space and thus allows more air to flow through the nostril. It helps in restoring the nasal valve.

The "Strut graft" is like a bar and is used to provide support to columella to lift up the tip of the nose. It can be of two types, floating or fixed. The type of graft used to support the ala or the side wall of the nose are called 'Batten grafts' because they are "like a flat strip" and would provide support to the ala and the side wall. Shield grafts are used for tip augmentation purposes.

Reference:

1. *Peck GC. Techniques in Aesthetic Rhinoplasty. New York, Thieme-Stratton, 1984.*
2. *Gunter J, Rohrich R, Adams W Jr. Dallas Rhinoplasty: Nasal Surgery by the Masters. St. Louis, Quality Medical Publishing, 2000.*

139. The correct response is D.

The "Shield graft" is a curved cartilage graft taken from the conchal cartilage. It is commonly used to improve the shape of the nasal tip.

The "Spreader graft" is a longitudinal piece of cartilage which is placed in between the upper lateral cartilage and the septum to widen the space and thus allows more air to flow through the nostril. It helps in restoring the nasal valve.

The "Strut graft" is like a bar and is used to provide support to columella to lift up the tip of the nose. It can be of two types, floating or fixed. The type of graft used to support the ala or the side wall of the nose are called 'Batten grafts' because they are "like a flat strip" and would provide support to the ala and the side wall. Shield grafts are used for tip augmentation purposes.

Reference:

1. *Peck GC. Techniques in Aesthetic Rhinoplasty. New York, Thieme-Stratton, 1984.*
2. *Gunter J, Rohrich R, Adams W Jr. Dallas Rhinoplasty: Nasal Surgery by the Masters. St. Louis, Quality Medical Publishing, 2000.*

140. The correct response is C.

Hering's law of equal innervation states that both the levator palpebrae superioris muscles get equal innervations from cranial nerve III even when the upper eyelid level is asymmetric. This has implications in both ptosis repair and lid retraction repair.

Reference:

Carraway JH. The impact of Hering's law on blepharoplasty and ptosis surgery. Aesthetic Surg J 2004; 24: 275.

141. The correct response is D.

The lateral retinaculum is attached to the Whitnall's tubercle, which is located just inside the orbital rim of the upper part of the zygomatic bone. It is about 1 cm below the frontozygomatic suture and 2-4 mm inside the lateral orbital margin.

Reference:

1. *Zide BM, Jelks GW. Surgical anatomy of the orbit. New York, Raven Press, 1985.*
2. *Doxanas MT, Anderson RL. Clinical orbital anatomy. Baltimore, Williams and Wilkins, 1984.*

142. The correct response is E.

The lateral ligament is not formed by fibres from the inferior rectus. The remaining structures listed in the options are part of the lateral retinaculum.

The lateral retinaculum is attached to the Whitnall's tubercle, which is located just inside the orbital rim of the upper part of the zygomatic bone. It is about 1 cm below the frontozygomatic suture and 2-4 mm inside the lateral orbital margin.

Reference:

1. *Zide BM, Jelks GW. Surgical anatomy of the orbit. New York, Raven Press, 1985.*
2. *Doxanas MT, Anderson RL. Clinical orbital anatomy. Baltimore, Williams and Wilkins, 1984.*

143. The correct response is C.

Drill hole fixation of the lateral canthropexy should be performed approximately 4 mm posterior to the lateral orbital rim. A double armed Dacron suture is used for fixation.

Reference:

1. *Zide BM, Jelks GW. Surgical anatomy of the orbit. New York, Raven Press, 1985.*
2. *Doxanas MT, Anderson RL. Clinical orbital anatomy. Baltimore, Williams and Wilkins, 1984.*

144. The correct response is E.

The most appropriate management in this gentleman is release of the scar deformity, grafting, and tightening of the lower eyelid.

Increased scleral show is frequently seen following this type of fixation as it has been suggested that the use of a subciliary incision plays a role in its development. Scar contracture and the positioning of the orbital rim are also associated with this deformity. In patients with comminuted fractures of the orbital rim and floor, the fracture segments may be displaced inferiorly and posteriorly in the absence of rigid fixation resulting in a downward stretching of the septum and lower eyelid.

Horizontal tightening or fascial suspension will stabilize the eyelid position. Full thickness skin grafting should be considered in patients with severe deformities who require replacement of one of the layers of the lower eyelid. Tarsorrhaphy may be used in combination with other techniques but will not be effective alone. Massage therapy, injection of corticosteroids, and closure using tape sutures are not recommended.

Reference:

1. *Manson PN. Facial injuries. In: McCarthy JG, ed. Plastic Surgery. Philadelphia, Pa: WB Saunders Co; 1990; 2: 867-1141.*
2. *Whitaker LA. Problems and complications in craniofacial surgery. In: Goldwyn RM, ed. The Unfavourable Result in Plastic Surgery. 2nd ed. Boston, Mass: Little, Brown and Co; 1984: 229-251.*

145. The correct response is E.

The mainstay of treatment of gynaecomastia is surgical. Several options are available depending upon the classification of gynaecomastia. This male has large Grade III gynaecomastia the treatment of which is controversial. All of the mentioned techniques have been advocated for this grade. When all the grades are evaluated, there is no significant increase in complication rates observed over increasing grade but skin resection adds to the overall rate of complications.

Reference:

1. *Wiesman IM, Lehman JA Jr, Parker MG et al. Gynaecomastia: an outcome analysis. Ann Plast Surg 2004; 53: 97-101.*
2. *Murphy TP, Ehrlichman RJ, Seckel BR. Nipple placement in simple mastectomy with free nipple grafting for severe gynaecomastia. Plast Reconstr Surg 1994; 94: 818.*
3. *Ward CM, Khalid K. Surgical treatment of grade III gynaecomastia. Ann R Coll Surg Engl 1989; 71: 226-228.*

3

HEAD AND NECK

QUESTIONS

1. **Langer's lines are due to which one of the following?**
   A. Mechanical forces from underlying muscle fibres
   B. Repeated movements of skin
   C. Ultrastructural organisation of the dermis
   D. Ultrastructural organisation of the epidermis
   E. Photoaging of the skin

2. **The Arnold nerve provides sensation to which one of the following?**
   A. Nose
   B. Ear
   C. Lips
   D. Cheeks
   E. Forehead

3. **The Erb's point located along the posterior border of the sternocleidomastoid muscle is useful to block which one of the following nerve?**
   A. Great auricular nerve
   B. Transverse cervical nerve
   C. Lesser occipital nerve
   D. Auditory branch of vagus nerve
   E. Spinal accessory nerve

4. **The scalp has five layers. Which is the most common plane of avulsion of scalp?**
   A. Skin level
   B. Subcutaneous tissue level
   C. Aponeurosis
   D. Loose areolar tissue
   E. Pericranium

5. **Which one of the following may reduce the pain associated with injection of local anaesthetic?**
   A. Using a slow injection technique
   B. Using a fast injection technique
   C. Adding epinephrine
   D. Buffering with sodium bicarbonate
   E. Adding cocaine

6. **The parotid duct is vulnerable to injury in lacerations of the face. Which one of the following correctly describes the location of the parotid duct in the face?**
   A. Lies on the middle third of a line between tragus and middle of upper lip
   B. Lies on the anterior third of a line between tragus and middle of upper lip
   C. Lies on the posterior third of a line between tragus and middle of upper lip
   D. Lies on the middle third of a line between tragus and angle of mouth
   E. Lies on the middle third of a line between tragus and middle of lower lip

7. **The lower eyelid gets its sensory innervation from which one of the following nerve?**
   A. Zygomaticofrontal
   B. Infraorbital
   C. Infratrochlear
   D. Nasociliary
   E. Supraorbital

8. Suppurative chondritis is most commonly seen in patients with ear burns. The most common organism implicated in this condition is which one of the following?

A. Streptococcus pyogenes
B. Proteus mirabilis
C. Anaerobic
D. Pseudomonas
E. Mycobacteria

9. Which one of the following will not be anaesthetised by a ring block around the ear?

A. Helix
B. Scapha
C. Lobule
D. External auditory canal
E. Tragus

10. The ear lobule receives its nerve supply from which one of the following nerve?

A. Great auricular nerve
B. Lesser occipital nerve
C. Auriculotemporal nerve
D. Facial nerve
E. Auricular branch of vagus

11. The tragus and concha receive their nerve supply from which one of the following nerve?

A. Great auricular nerve
B. Lesser occipital nerve
C. Auriculotemporal nerve
D. Facial nerve
E. Auricular branch of vagus nerve

12. Which one of the following procedures would be most suitable in a case having severe post burn contracture of the upper eyelid?

A. Release and partial thickness skin grafting
B. Release and full thickness post auricular graft
C. Local flaps from supraorbital region
D. Free radial artery forearm flap
E. Forehead flap

13. Which one of the following procedures would give a better result in a case of severe post burn contracture of the lower eyelid?

A. Release and cover by partial thickness skin graft
B. Release and cover by thick partial thickness skin graft
C. Release and cover by a postauricular graft
D. Release and cover by a thick postauricular graft
E. Release and cover by a forehead flap

14. Which one of the following procedures is suitable for treating large postburn medial canthal webs?

A. Release and full thickness grafting
B. V-M plasty
C. Z- plasty
D. Double Z -plasty
E. Any one of the above

15. Which one of the following procedures is the best technique for reconstructing a philtral dimple in severe tight post burn skin contracture of the upper lip and lower lip with loss of all contours?

A. Adequate release followed by a contoured split thickness graft
B. Adequate release followed by a contoured full thickness graft
C. Adequate release followed by a triangular fossa graft
D. Adequate release followed by reconstruction using strips of local muscle
E. Abbe flap

16. Which of the following is correct regarding residual neck webbing seen after split thickness grafting and release of neck contracture?

A. Can be prevented by using darts at time of original grafting
B. Can be prevented by using Z plasties at time of original grafting
C. Occurs at the edges of the graft
D. Correctable by using Z plasty
E. All of the above

17. Life threatening haemorrhage in adult facial fractures is defined as a condition when there is loss of:

A. 1 unit of blood
B. 2 units of blood
C. 3 units of blood
D. More than three units
E. Systolic blood pressure falls below 80 mm Hg

18. Glasgow coma scale (GCS) is a point based system. The points are given to the responses evaluated from examination of the eyes, best verbal and motor response. A higher score indicates:

A. Good prognosis
B. Bad prognosis
C. Deterioration in the condition of the patient
D. Impending coma
E. Acute herniation of the hind brain

19. **The Glasgow Coma Scale (GCS) is useful for evaluating patients with head injuries. What score would be assigned to 'confused' verbal response in this scale?**
   A. 1
   B. 2
   C. 3
   D. 4
   E. 5

20. **The Glasgow Coma Scale (GCS) is useful for evaluating patients with head injuries. What score would be assigned to spontaneous eye opening response in Glasgow Coma Scale?**
   A. 1
   B. 2
   C. 3
   D. 4
   E. 5

21. **The Glasgow Coma Scale (GCS) is useful for evaluating patients with head injuries. A patient who obeys commands and moves his body according to the given instructions would be assigned what score in Glasgow Coma Scale?**
   A. 2
   B. 4
   C. 5
   D. 6
   E. 7

22. **A patient presents with subconjunctival haemorrhage, palpebral ecchymosis and welling around the eye. He is likely to have sustained a fracture of which one of the following bone?**
   A. Frontal bone
   B. Zygoma
   C. Nasal
   D. Maxilla
   E. Anterior cranial fossa

23. **In a case of optic nerve injury, the following pupillary changes would be seen except:**
   A. The pupillary size on the injured and the normal side is equal
   B. The pupil on the injured side is less reactive to light
   C. The pupil on the injured side would dilate when light is flashed on the intact side
   D. The pupil on the injured side would constrict when light is flashed on the intact side
   E. The pupil remains the same on both the sides

24. **Facial fractures are best assessed by which one of the following modality?**
   A. Mayer view on plain radiograph
   B. Panoramic film
   C. MRI
   D. Computed tomographic scan
   E. Colour doppler

25. **Which one of the following is the weakest area of the mandible and shows the highest incidence of fractures?**
   A. Coronoid process
   B. Neck
   C. Angle
   D. Body
   E. Parasymphyseal region

26. **Which one of the following is incorrect regarding compression plating of the craniofacial skeleton?**
   A. Compression of the bone ends conceptually speeds fracture healing
   B. Compression of craniofacial fracture may result in malunion
   C. Compression in craniofacial fracture may lead to undesirable movement of well reduced fractures
   D. Compression fixation is recommended for craniofacial skeleton
   E. Only one screw on each side of the plate can be used in the compression mode

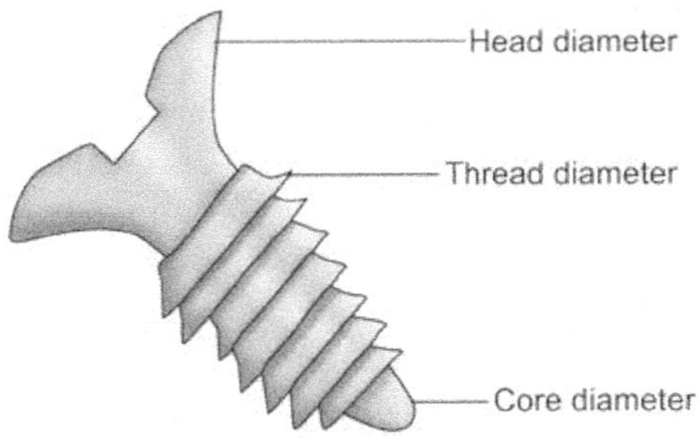

Fig. Diagram of a lag screw

27. **The distance between the two threads of a screw (shown above) used for osteosynthesis is known as which one of the following?**
   A. Flute
   B. Core
   C. Pitch
   D. Depth

3

HEAD AND NECK

28. Primary bone grafting is routinely used in management of facial fractures. These grafts help in maintaining the contour and projection of the bone in areas of severe comminution. Primary bone grafting is indicated for all of these except which one of the following?

A. Mandible comminuted fractures
B. Nasal skeleton
C. Orbital bone
D. Frontal bone
E. Orbital rim

29. Which one of the following autogenous bone graft is easiest to contour?

A. Calvarial
B. Tibial
C. Rib
D. Iliac
E. MMCA (Methylmethacrylate)

30. Which one of the following autogenous bone graft is difficult to shape to curved defects?

A. Calvarial
B. Tibial
C. Rib
D. Iliac
E. MMCA (Methylmethacrylate)

31. The clinical signs of a subcondylar fracture of the mandible are the following except which one of the following?

A. Restricted mouth opening
B. Local swelling in the subcondylar region
C. Deviation of chin to the same side on opening the mouth
D. Deviation of chin to the opposite side on opening the mouth
E. Loss of ramus height

32. The most common form of condylar head dislocation is which one of the following?

A. Lateral and posterior
B. Medial and anterior
C. Lateral and anterior
D. Medial and posterior
E. Superiorly into the intracranial fossa

33. Nasal fractures can be divided into lateral impact and frontal impact injuries. A patient with fractures involving lower half of both the nasal bones with telescoping of the septum would be classifiable into which one of the following?

A. Plane I frontal impact injury
B. Plane II frontal impact injury
C. Plane III frontal impact injury
D. Plane I lateral impact injury
E. Plane II lateral impact injury

34. Which one of the following statement is incorrect about septal haematoma?

A. It is usually unilateral occurring on the side of injury
B. Undrained haematomas may lead to septal perforation or fibrosis
C. Organised haematoma may result in thickening of cartilage
D. Septal haematoma is treated by incising mucoperichondrium on one side only
E. Both surgical and antibiotic therapy should be given

35. Closed reduction of nasal fracture is indicated in unilateral depressed nasal pyramid fracture. Which instrument is required for reduction of the septal fracture?

A. Walsham forceps
B. Asch forceps
C. Kilner forceps
D. Rowe's disimpaction forceps
E. Septal hook forceps

36. Which one of the following muscle is not attached to the zygoma?

A. Masseter muscle
B. Zygomaticus major muscle
C. Zygomaticus minor muscle
D. Levator labii superioris muscle
E. Medial pterygoid muscle

37. Which one of the following nerves and vessels are responsible for causing ecchymosis of eye in fracture of the zygoma?

A. Zygomaticotemporal nerves and vessels
B. Terminal branches of the facial artery
C. Infraorbital nerve and vessels
D. Supraorbital nerve and vessels
E. Nasociliary nerve and vessels

38. Which of the following nerve often gets damaged in fracture-dislocation of the orbital floor?

A. Zygomatic nerve
B. Infraorbital nerve
C. Lacrimal nerve
D. Supraorbital nerve
E. All of the above

39. Which one of the following statement is incorrect regarding the zygoma?

A. Part of it may be pneumatized with air cells connecting it to the maxillary sinus

B. Zygomaticofacial foramen is a weak area in the zygoma

C. The coronal incision allows exposure of the entire zygomatic arch and roof of the glenoid fossa for arch reconstruction

D. The Mayer view is the best view for evaluation of the zygoma

E. The lateral blepharoplasty incision may be used for zygomatic fracture reduction

40. What causes ipsilateral epistaxis in zygomatic fractures?

A. Injury to the eye

B. Injury to the nose

C. Injury to the maxilla

D. Injury to the conjunctiva

E. Injury to the infraorbital artery

41. Which is the single best plain X-ray view to evaluate fracture of the zygoma?

A. PA view

B. Waters view

C. Lateral view skull

D. Occipitomental view

E. Mento-occipital view

42. The blow-in fracture of the orbit may be observed in which of the following fractures of the zygoma?

A. Arch fracture

B. Laterally displaced fracture

C. Medially displaced fracture

D. Hairline fracture

E. Unrotated body fracture

43. The zygomaticofrontal suture is a key landmark to the diagnosis and treatment of fractures of the zygoma. It is located at which one of the following level?

A. At the level of the lateral canthus

B. Above the level of the lateral canthus

C. Below the level of the lateral canthus

D. Lateral to the lateral canthus

44. Which one of the following approaches should be selected for treating an isolated fracture displacement of the zygomaticomaxillary buttress?

A. Coronal approach

B. Dingman approach

C. Frontozygomatic approach

D. Endoscopic approach

E. Intraoral approach

45. Which of the following is useful for the management of compound comminuted fractures of the zygoma?

A. Reduction of zygomatic arch fracture

B. Reduction of frontozygomatic disjunction

C. Reduction of inferior orbital rim disjunction / fractures

D. Reduction of maxillary – buttress fracture

E. All of the above

46. Which one of the following should be selected to manage a depressed fracture of the zygomatic arch?

A. Gillies approach

B. Facelift approach

C. Coronal approach

D. Intraoral approach

E. Endoscopic approach

47. Which of the following causes diplopia in zygomatic fractures?

A. Eyelid abnormalities

B. Globe abnormalities

C. Muscular abnormalities

D. Neurological abnormalities

E. All of the above

48. Which one of the following part of the mandible is directly implicated in causing restricted mouth opening in zygomatic fractures?

A. Ramus

B. Condyle

C. Coronoid

D. Body

E. Alveolar part

49. All of the following are complications of untreated maxilla fractures except which one of the following?

A. Chronic sinusitis

B. Oroantral fistula

C. Hypoplasia

D. Malunion

E. Nonunion

50. A transverse fracture of the maxilla above the apices of the teeth is called which one of the following?

A. LeFort I fracture

B. LeFort II fracture

C. LeFort III fracture

D. Apical fracture

E. LeFort IV fracture

51. A pyramidal fracture of the maxilla and the nasal bone is called which one of the following?

A. LeFort I fracture
B. LeFort II fracture
C. LeFort III fracture
D. Apical fracture
E. LeFort IV fracture

52. A fracture that disconnects the maxilla, zygoma and nasal bones from the frontal bone is called which one of the following?

A. LeFort III fracture
B. LeFort II fracture
C. LeFort I fracture
D. Apical fracture
E. LeFort IV fracture

53. LeFort who proposed the widely accepted classification of midfacial fractures was which one of the following?

A. Plastic surgeon
B. Oral and maxillofacial surgeon
C. Orthopedic surgeon
D. ENT surgeon
E. General surgeon

54. Maxillary fractures may present all of the following clinical features except which one of the following?

A. Unilateral ecchymosis
B. Facial edema
C. Malocclusion
D. Epistaxis
E. Facial deformity

55. Panfacial fractures are those fractures involving which one of the following bones?

A. Frontal
B. Maxilla
C. Mandible
D. All of the above
E. Any of the above

56. Which of the following is the suitable method of repair of dural tears in patients with fractures of the frontal region?

A. Direct suturing
B. Patch of temporalis fascia
C. Patch of fascia lata
D. Patch of pericranium
E. All of the above

57. Foramina of Breschet is located in which one of the following bone?

A. Maxilla
B. Ethmoid
C. Sphenoid
D. Frontal
E. Temporal

58. The bony orbit is conical or pyramidal in shape. It is formed by seven bones. Name the smallest bone of the orbit:

A. Frontal bone
B. Zygoma
C. Maxilla
D. Lacrimal bone
E. Ethmoid

59. The depth of the bony orbit is more than its height or breadth. The correct depth of the orbit is which one of the following?

A. 35 mm
B. 40 mm
C. 45 mm
D. 50 mm
E. 55 mm

60. The superior and inferior rectus muscles of the eye move the eye ball in which of the following axis of movement?

A. Anteroposterior
B. Vertical
C. Transverse
D. Horizontal
E. All of the above

61. Which one of the following muscle is in intimate relationship to the floor of the orbit?

A. Inferior oblique
B. Inferior rectus
C. Superior rectus
D. Superior oblique
E. Lateral rectus

62. Which one of the following bone gets easily fractured in the orbit?

A. Frontal
B. Zygoma
C. Orbital plate of maxilla
D. Lacrimal bone
E. Sphenoid

63. Enopthalmos in blow-out fractures of the orbit needs treatment in the form of reconstruction of the orbital floor. The location of the optic foramen behind the inferior orbital rim is which one of the following?

A. 20-25 mm
B. 30-35 mm
C. 40-45 mm
D. 50-55 mm
E. 60-65 mm

64. The superior orbital fissure is triangular in shape. It is bounded above by the lesser wing, below by the greater wing of the sphenoid and medially by the body of the sphenoid. It is bounded laterally by which one of the following?

A. Zygomatic bone
B. Frontal bone
C. Palatine bone
D. Temporal bone
E. Sphenoid bone

65. The etiological factors responsible for diplopia in orbital injuries are the following except:

A. Muscle incarceration
B. Muscle contusion / Haematoma
C. Herniation of orbital contents through the fracture site
D. Fracture and dislocation of zygomatic bone
E. Fracture of nasal bone

66. Which one of the following statements about superior oblique muscle is not correct?

A. Arises from the sphenoid bone above the optic canal
B. Passes through the trochlea
C. Lies deep to the superior rectus before getting inserted
D. Insertion into the superolateral part of posterior quadrant of the eyeball
E. Contraction of the muscle will produce extortion of the eye

67. Medial orbital blowout fractures would manifest all of the given clinical signs except which one of the following?

A. Enophthalmos
B. Narrowing of the palpebral fissures
C. Subcutaneous and / or orbital emphysema
D. Squint
E. Epistaxis

68. Lamina papyracea is a smooth plate of bone which encloses which one of the following?

A. Sphenoid bone
B. Lacrimal bone
C. Ethmoid bone
D. Orbit
E. Optic foramen

69. Which one of the following muscle underlies the inferior orbital nerve as it travels down?

A. Levator anguli oris
B. Zygomaticus major
C. Zygomaticus minor
D. Risorius
E. Buccinator

70. Which one of the following statements about inferior oblique muscle is not correct?

A. Arises from the orbital surface of maxilla lateral to the nasolacrimal groove
B. Passes laterally between the inferior rectus and orbital floor and then between the eyeball and lateral rectus
C. Is inserted into the inferolateral part of the posterior quadrant between inferior and lateral recti
D. Supplied by the oculomotor nerve
E. Contraction of the muscle will produce intortion of the eye

71. Which one of the following muscle is most likely to get incarcerated in ocular injuries to produce diplopia?

A. Superior rectus
B. Medial rectus
C. Inferior rectus
D. Superior oblique
E. Lateral rectus

72. Downward displacement of the lateral canthus of the eye suggests involvement of which of the following?

A. Fracture of the frontal process of the zygoma
B. Fracture of the zygomatic process of the frontal bone
C. Fracture of the orbital plate of the zygoma bone
D. Fracture of the zygomaticomaxillary buttress
E. All of the above

73. The superior meatus is the shortest and the shallowest of the three meatuses of the nose. Which one of the following opens into superior meatus?

A. Anterior ethmoidal cells
B. Middle ethmoidal cells
C. Posterior ethmoidal cells
D. Nasolacrimal duct

74. The frontal sinus drains into the nose through the nasofrontal ducts which open in the:

A. Superior meatus
B. Middle meatus
C. Inferior meatus
D. Oropharynx
E. Nasopharynx

75. The middle meatus receives the opening of which one of the following except:

A. Anterior and middle ethmoidal sinuses
B. Frontal sinus (frontonasal duct)
C. Maxillary sinus
D. Nasolacrimal duct

76. The inferior meatus receives the opening of which one of the following?

A. Frontal sinus
B. Nasolacrimal duct
C. Anterior ethmoidal sinus
D. Middle ethmoidal sinus

77. The superior meatus receives the opening of how many ducts and sinuses?

A. One
B. Two
C. Three
D. Four

78. The middle meatus receives the opening of how many ducts and sinuses?

A. One
B. Two
C. Three
D. Four
E. Five

79. The inferior meatus receives the opening of how many structures?

A. One
B. Two
C. Three
D. Four
E. Five

80. The opening of which one of the following paranasal sinus does not allow dependent drainage?

A. Frontal
B. Ethmoidal
C. Sphenoidal
D. Maxillary

81. The blow-out fractures may be categorized into all of the following types based on the type of orbital reconstruction except which one of the following?

A. Trap door
B. Single hinge
C. Double hinge
D. Punched out
E. Comminuted

82. Which one of the following is not a feature of nasoethmoid fracture?

A. Flattened nose
B. Loss of dorsal nasal prominence
C. Lip / columella angle becomes obtuse
D. Hypotelorism due to fracture of the nasal bone

83. The "double ring sign" in nasoethmoidal-orbital injuries is useful for the diagnosis of which one of the following ?

A. Presence of fracture of the cribriform plate
B. Fracture of the orbit
C. Acute extradural haematoma
D. CSF rhinorrhea
E. Herniation of the brain

84. The medial canthal ligament is attached to all of the following except:

A. Frontal process of maxilla
B. Anterior lacrimal crest
C. Posterior lacrimal crest
D. Nasal bones
E. Lacrimal fossa

85. Which one of the following is not true about retrobulbar hematoma?

A. Globe proptosis is present
B. Red, congested eye is present
C. Edematous conjunctiva is present
D. Diagnosis can be confirmed by CT scan
E. Treatment is by drainage

86. Optic nerve injury can be clinically diagnosed by testing the pupillary reaction to light. Which one of the following is diagnostic for an optic nerve injury to the right side?

A. The right pupil contracts on exposure to light flashed by a torch
B. The right pupil does not react
C. The right pupil dilates when torch light is flashed after flashing it on the left side
D. The left pupil contracts on exposure to light

87. The optic foramen is an opening for the passage of the optic nerve and the ophthalmic artery. It is which one of the following?

A. Circular in shape
B. Ovoid in shape
C. Vertically ovoid in shape
D. Horizontally ovoid in shape

88. The muscles supplied by the oculomotor nerve are the following except:

A. Levator palpebrae
B. Superior rectus
C. Inferior rectus
D. Inferior oblique
E. Superior oblique

89. The strongest bone of the face is which one of the following?

A. Frontal bone
B. Mandible
C. Nasal
D. Zygoma
E. Maxilla

90. Frontal lobe injuries produce confusion, coma and personality changes. All of the following cranial nerves may be involved in these injuries except:

A. Cranial nerve III
B. Cranial nerve IV
C. Cranial nerve V
D. Cranial nerve VI
E. Cranial nerve VII

91. Causalgia is characterized by the following except:

A. Burning pain following history of injury to a nerve or its branches
B. Cold, clammy, sweaty skin
C. Hot, dry and scaly skin
D. Atrophy of skin appendages
E. Atrophy of bones, joints and muscle in late cases

92. The relative proportions of the face change markedly during the period of postnatal growth. The ratio of cranium to face size at birth is which one of the following?

A. 2:1
B. 4:1
C. 6:1
D. 8:1
E. 10:1

93. The lip to trachea distance is an important consideration for pediatric intubation. What is the lip to trachea distance at one year of age?

A. 7 cm
B. 10 cm
C. 14-15 cm
D. 15-20 cm

94. Birth injuries result from prolonged labor with difficult passage through the birth canal. Which one of the following muscle is vulnerable to injury during a breech delivery with lateral hyperextension?

A. Shoulder abductor muscles
B. Sternocleidomastoid muscle
C. Trapezius muscle
D. Pectoralis major muscle
E. Platysma

95. Which one of the following bones of the face is more likely to fracture in children below the age of 5 years?

A. Condyle of mandible
B. Neck of the mandible
C. Symphysis of mandible
D. Ramus of mandible
E. Parasymphyseal region of mandible

96. The coronal incision is the workhorse for craniofacial surgery. All of the following are the drawbacks of this incision except:

A. Blood loss
B. Injury to frontal branch of the facial nerve
C. Loss of sensation posterior to the incision
D. Alopecia due to scarring
E. Wide exposure of frontal and orbital region

97. Which one of the following is a favorable position for endoscopic treatment of subcondylar fractures?

A. Lateral override
B. Medial override
C. Anteroposterior override
D. Vertical override
E. All of the above

98. Endoscopic reduction of condylar fractures is indicated in which one of the following clinical situation?

A. Intracapsular fractures
B. Comminuted fractures
C. Medial override of proximal fragment
D. Lateral override of proximal fragment

99. Which one of the following is an absolute contraindication to endoscopic reduction and rigid fixation of mandible condyle fractures?

A. Child younger than 12 years
B. Comminuted fracture
C. Intercondylar fracture
D. Medial override of the proximal fragment

100. The shape of the condyle of the mandible is:

A. Elliptical
B. Ovoid
C. Round
D. Oblong

101. All of the following muscles help in protrusion of the mandible except:

A. Lateral pterygoid
B. Geniohyoid
C. Medial pterygoid
D. Temporalis
E. Masseter

102. TMJ arthroscopy enables the surgeon to perform endoscopic joint examination, biopsy and lavage. What is the preferred approach and point of entry for the temporomandibular joint arthroscopy?

A. Along a line from the tragus to the tip of nose
B. Along a line from the tragus to angle of mouth
C. Along a line from the tragus to the lateral canthus
D. Along a line from the tragus to menton
E. Along a line from the tragus to the pogonion

103. Extra-articular TMJ ankylosis may be due to which one of the following?

A. External trauma
B. Infection
C. Juvenile rheumatoid arthritis
D. Enlargement of muscles of mastication

104. Which one of the following is the procedure of choice for treatment of ankylosis of the jaw?

A. Condylectomy
B. Gap arthroplasty
C. Interpositional arthroplasty
D. Costochondral arthroplasty

105. The average thickness of the cranial vault is 7 mm. The thickest bone in the vault is which one of the following?

A. Frontal
B. Temporal
C. Parietal
D. Occipital

106. The average thickness of the cranial vault is 7 mm. The thinnest bone in the vault is which one of the following?

A. Frontal
B. Temporal
C. Parietal
D. Occipital

107. Which one of the following should be used for large cranioplasty defects?

A. Calvarial bone
B. Split rib graft
C. Iliac crest
D. Tibia

108. Which one of the following bone donor sites is relatively painless?

A. Calvarium
B. Rib
C. Iliac crest
D. Tibia

109. Hydroxyapatite is a common alloplastic material which is used for cranioplasty. It is obtained from which one of the following?

A. Sea fish
B. Marine algae
C. Marine coral
D. Jelly fish
E. Sea weeds

110. Microvascular free flap reconstruction of acquired cranial deformities is useful after tumour removal. Which one of the following free flaps provides a long vascular pedicle for reconstruction and also provides a pliable tissue which can adapt to any type of three dimensional wound requirement?

A. Rectus abdominis myocutaneous flap
B. Latissimus dorsi flap
C. Radial artery forearm flap
D. Pectoralis major flap
E. Omental flap

111. Which is the best modality for treating small cranial defects in children younger than 2 years?

A. Calvarial bone graft
B. Split rib graft
C. Tibial graft
D. Heal by themselves
E. Alloplastic material

112. The preferred area for obtaining cranial grafts is from which one of the following?

A. Frontal bone
B. Right parietal bone in right handed patients
C. Right parietal bone in left handed patients
D. Left parietal bone in left handed patients
E. Any of the above

113. A patient with a full thickness cranial defect located near the frontal sinus should preferably be managed with which one of the following?

A. Norian bone cement
B. Hydroxyapatite cement
C. Acrylic mould
D. Calvarial graft

114. Which one of the following flap is suitable and reliable for closing a hemimaxillary palatal defect?

A. Forehead flap
B. Deltopectoral flap
C. Pectoralis major flap
D. Temporalis flap
E. Facial artery musculomucosal flap

115. Displaced traumatic fractures of the zygoma would produce a deformity which would clinically manifest the following features except:

A. Loss of prominence of the cheek
B. Step deformity in the infraorbital margin
C. Displaced zygomatic-maxillary buttress
D. Deformity of fronto-zygomatic region
E. Upward slanting of the lateral canthus

116. Enophthalmos in traumatic injuries is commonly due to herniation of the orbital contents through which of the following?

A. Orbital floor
B. Posterior limit
C. Lateral wall
D. Superior wall
E. All of the above

117. The scalp extends from the supraorbital margin to the superior nuchal line. It has five layers and is supplied by five arteries. It is supplied by all of the following arteries except:

A. Supraorbital artery
B. Facial artery
C. Superficial temporal
D. Postauricular
E. Occipital

118. The scalp has a rich vascular plexus of arteries which are interconnected with each other so that replantation of the entire scalp based on a single donor vessel can be done. What is the common mode of spread of scalp neoplasms ?

A. Local spread
B. Lymphatic spread
C. Vascular spread
D. All of the above

119. The crane principle is commonly used for restoration of defects in which one of the following situation?

A. Avulsive skin loss
B. Muscle defect
C. Bone defect
D. Nerve defect
E. Tendon defect

120. The scalp of an adult has about 1,40,000 hairs. The rate of growth of these hairs is which one of the following?

A. 1 mm per day
B. Less than 1 mm per day
C. More than 1 mm per day
D. More than 2 mm per day

121. The hair has three phases of normal growth. Laser therapy is effective in which one of the following?

A. Anagen
B. Catagen
C. Telogen
D. Catagen and telogen

122. Male pattern baldness has been classified by Norwood (1975) into seven types. Which one of the following type is not suitable for hair transplantation?

A. Type I
B. Type III
C. Type V
D. Type VI
E. Type VII

123. Many techniques have been described for hair transplantation. Which one of the following technique gives the best result in terms of aesthetics and natural look following surgery?

A. Punch grafts
B. Temporo-parietal occipital strip grafts
C. Macro-hair transplantation
D. Follicular hair transplantation
E. Tissue expansion

124. Which one of the following techniques for hair transplantation give rise to the "doll's hair" look?

A. Punch grafts
B. Temporo-parietal occipital strip grafts
C. Macro-hair transplantation
D. Follicular hair transplantation
E. Tissue expansion

125. The modern technique of follicular grafts has revolutionised hair transplantation. What is the fate of the transplanted hairs?

A. Do not fall off
B. Fall off after some time
C. Fall off but regrowth takes place later after 10-12 weeks
D. The transplanted hairs multiply in numbers to cover the adjacent bald areas of the scalp
E. The transplanted hairs stimulate adjacent hair follicles to increase the overall growth of hairs

126. Which one of the following is the best method for auricular reconstruction?

A. Maternal ear cartilage
B. Silastic implants
C. Autogenous diced cartilage
D. Autogenous cartilage framework

127. The ear is supplied by the following nerves. Which one of these is responsible for creating a cough reflex when attempt is made to clear the wax from the external auditory canal?

A. Great auricular nerve
B. Lesser occipital nerve
C. Auriculotemporal nerve
D. Vagus nerve

128. The cartilaginous frame work is the foundation of auricular reconstruction. Which one of the following techniques uses the maximum amount of rib cartilage in framework design?

A. Tanzer
B. Brent
C. Nagata
D. Spina

129. Many techniques have been described for the repair of split ear lobe using different types of flaps. The use of interpositional conchal cartilage graft in the ear lobe to prevent recurrence was described by which one of the following?

A. Tanzer
B. Brent
C. Nagata
D. Spina
E. Agarwal

130. Cauliflower ear is common in which one of the following?

A. Mountain climbers
B. Newborn children
C. Pugilists
D. Postburn chondritis
E. Benign tumours of the ear

131. The superior auriculocephalic sulcus is an important aesthetic feature of the ear. It is absent in which one of the following condition?

A. Cauliflower ear
B. Constricted ear
C. Cryptotia
D. Chondritis of the ear
E. Prominent ear

132. Prominent ear is due to failure of antihelix to fold leading to widening of the conchoscaphal angle. The range of this angle in prominent ears is near to which one of the following?

A. 30 degrees
B. 60 degrees
C. 90 degrees
D. 150 degrees

133. Worthen flap for closure of lateral forehead defect is which one of the following?

A. Local flap
B. Advancement flap
C. Rotation flap
D. Bilobed flap
E. V-Y advancement flap

134. Reconstruction of partial eyebrow defects can be accomplished using a variety of options. Which one of the following options is least justifiable?

A. Transverse advancement flap
B. V-Y advancement flap
C. Double Z rhombic flap
D. Contralateral eyebrow
E. Pedicled scalp flap

135. Which one of the following method is suitable for reconstructing eyelid defects which are less than 25% of the upper eyelid?

A. Lateral canthotomy with primary closure
B. Mustarde method
C. Nasojugal flap of Tessier
D. Forehead flap
E. Tenzel flap

136. Which one of the following method is suitable for reconstructing total eyelid defect of both the lids?

A. Lateral canthotomy with primary closure
B. Mustarde method
C. Nasojugal flap of Tessier
D. Forehead flap
E. Tenzel flap

137. Which one of the following method is suitable for reconstructing eyelid defects which are less than 25% of the lower eyelid?

A. Lateral canthotomy with primary closure
B. Mustarde method
C. Nasojugal flap of Tessier
D. Forehead flap
E. Tenzel flap

138. In patients with facial paralysis, lid closure can be achieved using gold weights. Gold weight is used therapeutically in which one of the following ways?

A. Taping it to lower midportion of the upper lid
B. Inserting below the skin
C. Inserting above the orbicularis oculi
D. Inserting below the orbicularis oculi
E. Sutured to tarsal plate

139. A child with cyanosis who improves on crying is probably suffering from which one of the following?

A. Atrial septal defect
B. Ventricular septal defect
C. Patent ductus arteriosus
D. Choanal atresia
E. Fallot's tetrology

140. Barking cough is a feature of which one of the following condition?

A. Unilateral paralysis of vocal cords
B. Total paralysis of vocal cords
C. Subglottic stenosis
D. Laryngeal cleft
E. Laryngeal cyst

141. Adult sleep apnea is characterised by all of the following except:

A. Stoppage of breathing for more than 10 seconds at a time
B. Five episodes of apnoea in an hour
C. Irregularities of pulse
D. Right ventricular hypertrophy on echocardiography
E. Left ventricular hypertrophy on echocardiography

142. Sleep apnoea is diagnosed when the number of apnoeas occurring in the night are which one of the following?

A. More than 15 each lasting more than 5 seconds
B. More than 15 each lasting more than 10 seconds
C. More than 30 each lasting more than 5 seconds
D. More than 30 each lasting more than 10 seconds
E. More than 40 each lasting more than 5 seconds

143. Which one of the following is most successful medical treatment for sleep apnea?

A. Reduction of weight
B. Breathing exercises
C. Continuous positive airway pressure (CPAP)
D. Bilevel positive airway pressure (BPAP)
E. Nasopharyngeal intubation

144. The gold standard for surgical treatment of sleep apnea is which one of the following?

A. Adenotonsillectomy
B. Uvulopalatopharyngoplasty
C. Tongue advancement
D. Tongue reduction
E. Tracheostomy

145. The natural elasticity of the upper and lower lips allows defects to a certain limit to be closed primarily without needing extra tissue. Defects of which ofthe following size are amenable to primary closure?

A. Up to 10%
B. Up to 20%
C. Up to 30%
D. Up to 40%
E. Up to 50%

146. Which one of the following is the flap of choice for central full thickness defects of the upper lip?

A. Gillies fan flap
B. Abbe flap
C. Estlander flap
D. Karapandzic flap
E. Schuchardt procedure

147. Which one of the following is the flap of choice for reconstructing lower lip defects of upto two thirds of the lower lip?

A. Gillies fan flap
B. Abbe flap
C. Estlander flap
D. Karapandzic flap
E. Schuchardt procedure

148. Witch's chin deformity is characterised by which one of the following?

A. Prominent chin
B. Double chin
C. Bifid chin
D. Prominent submental crease
E. Accumulation of subcutaneous fat in the chin

149. The Limberg flap is used for which type of defect?

A. Square defect
B. Rectangular defect
C. Circular defect
D. Rhomboidal defect
E. Elliptical defect

150. For smile reconstruction in a case of facial palsy, which one of the following muscle flap would be suitable as a one stage facial reanimation procedure?

A. Pectoralis major flap
B. Latissimus dorsi flap
C. Palmaris longus
D. Radial artery forearm flap
E. Omental transfer

151. Infraorbital anaesthesia in case of maxillofacial injuries is due to fracture of which one of the following surfaces of the maxilla?

A. Anterior
B. Infratemporal
C. Orbital
D. Nasal

152. Which one of the following muscle of facial expression is unpaired?

A. Levator labii superioris alaequae nasi
B. Orbicularis oris
C. Nasalis
D. Buccinator
E. Risorius

153. The 'Mobius syndrome' is characterized by which one of the following?

A. Right side facial palsy
B. Left side facial palsy
C. Bilateral facial palsy
D. Microgenia
E. Cleft lip

154. The face consists of several paired and one unpaired muscle, the orbicularis oris. The number of paired muscles is which one of the following?

A. 13
B. 15
C. 17
D. 19
E. 21

155. Lagophthalmos in cases of facial paralysis can be managed by which of the following?

A. Lateral tarsorrhaphy
B. Gold weight in upper eyelid
C. Temporalis sling
D. Spring
E. All of the above

156. Lower eyelid ectropion can be corrected by which of the following?

A. Tendon sling
B. Lateral canthoplasty
C. Lid shortening
D. Temporalis sling
E. All of the above

157. Balancing of the upper lip in cases of facial paralysis can be done by which of the following?

A. Static slings
B. Rhytidectomy and mucosal excisions
C. Microneurovascular muscle transplantation
D. Temporalis and masseter muscles
E. All of the above

158. Pocketing of the food in the buccal sulcus is caused by paralysis of which one of the following muscle?

A. Mylohyoid
B. Genioglossus
C. Buccinator
D. Digastric
E. Risorius

159. Name the muscle which lies in the Passavant's ridge:

A. Palatopharyngeal
B. Glossopharyngeal
C. Buccopharyngeal
D. Palatoglossus
E. Genioglossus

160. In cases of bilateral facial nerve palsy with the absence of seventh nerve input, the microneurovascular anastomosis can be done alternatively by using which nerve of the face?

A. 11th nerve
B. 12th nerve
C. 5th nerve
D. 6th nerve
E. 7th nerve

161. The parotid gland secretions are carried by the Stensen's duct. It opens in the oral cavity in the upper buccal sulcus at which one of the following location?

A. Opposite the first molar
B. Opposite the second molar
C. Opposite the third molar
D. Opposite the root of the canine
E. Opposite the root of the premolar

162. The pectoralis major myocutaneous flap is supplied by the thoracoacromial artery which leaves the subclavian artery near the middle of the clavicle. The pectoral branch of the thoracoacromial artery lies on which one of the following landmark?

A. A line joining the midpoint of the clavicle with xiphisternum
B. A line joining the tip of the shoulder with the xiphisternum
C. A line joining the tip of the shoulder with the nipple
D. A line joining the midpoint of the clavicle with the nipple
E. A vertical line along the midpoint of the clavicle

163. Microvascular surgery has revolutionised the management of head and neck cancer. Which one of the following free flaps skin paddle is relatively insensate?

A. Radial artery forearm flap
B. Pectoralis major myocutaneous flap
C. Latissimus dorsi flap
D. Anterolateral thigh flap
E. Rectus abdominis myocutaneous flap

164. The free lateral thigh flap is a versatile flap for head and neck reconstruction based on the profunda femoris artery. It is based on which one of the following perforator?

A. First perforator
B. Second perforator
C. Third perforator
D. Fourth perforator
E. Fifth perforator

165. Which one of the following is an indication for using nonvascularized method of mandibular reconstruction?

A. Defects resulting from treatment of mandibular fracture nonunions
B. Large defects
C. Defects of the central segment of the mandible (anterior defects)
D. Composite defects of bone and soft tissue
E. Defects of mandible with scarring

166. Which one of the following free flaps is suitable for mandibular reconstruction in terms of amount of usable length of bone and its adaptability?

A. Ilium on deep circumflex artery
B. Radius on radial artery forearm flap
C. Fibula on peroneal artery
D. Scapula on circumflex scapular artery
E. Second metatarsal

167. Which one of the following free flaps is suitable for mandibular reconstruction in terms of offering the maximum thickness and height of bone?

A. Ilium on deep circumflex artery
B. Radius on radial artery forearm flap
C. Fibula on peroneal artery
D. Scapula on circumflex scapular artery
E. Second metatarsal

168. The size of the bone graft that can be safely taken from the radial forearm donor site is which one of the following?

A. 5 cm
B. 10 cm of bone length with 40% of its circumference
C. 15 cm with 50% of its circumference
D. 20 cm with 40% of its circumference
E. 25 cm with 40% of its circumference

169. Which one of the following nerve is likely to get damaged following harvest of iliac crest graft?

A. Superior epigastric
B. Circumflex iliac
C. Lateral femoral cutaneous
D. Popliteal
E. Sciatic

170. Which one of the following flaps could be used for pharyngo-esophageal reconstruction?

A. Radial forearm flap
B. Deltopectoral flap
C. Pectoralis major myocutaneous flap
D. Jejunal flap
E. All of the above

171. Which one of the following is suitable for total esophageal reconstruction?

A. Gastric pull up
B. Jejunal flap
C. Colonic transfer
D. Pectoralis major myocutaneous flap
E. Radial forearm flap

172. Which one of the following condition is associated with torticollis?

A. Inaccurate visual field
B. Compensatory strabismus
C. Positional plagiocephaly
D. Malocclusion
E. All of the above

173. The platsyma flap for coverage of the lower face is based on which one of the following vessel?

A. Superior thyroid artery
B. Submental artery
C. Suprasternal artery
D. Occipital artery
E. Transverse cervical artery

174. Which one of the following is suitable for repair of radionecrotic defects of the nape of the neck?

A. Deltopectoral flap
B. Pectoralis major myocutaneous flap
C. Latissimus dorsi flap
D. Trapezius musculocutaneous flap
E. Lateral arm flap

175. The trapezius muscle flap for coverage of head and neck defects is based on which one of the following vessels?

A. Intercostal artery
B. Submental artery
C. Suprasternal artery
D. Occipital artery
E. Transverse cervical artery

176. Which one of the following laser modality is helpful in the treatment of the type of vascular malformation shown in the following photograph?

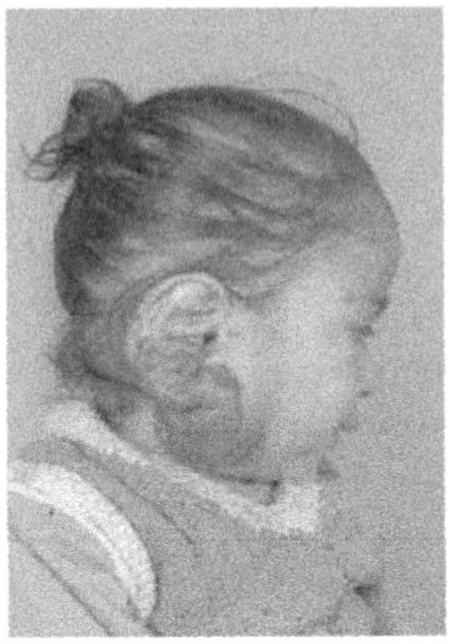

A. Argon-pumped tunable dye
B. Erbium: YAG
C. KTP
D. Pulsed dye
E. Q-switched ruby

177. A 12-year-old boy has persistent ptosis of the right eyelid eight months after undergoing resection for a massive fronto-orbital fibrous dysplasia. On current examination, no levator function is noted in the eyelid and lateral movement of the eyelid is minimal. Which one of the following interventions is the mostappropriate next step in management?

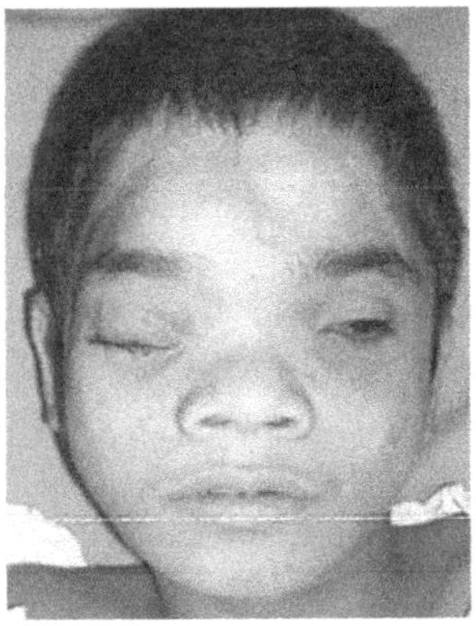

A. Lysis of adhesions
B. Kuhnt-Szymanowski procedure
C. Fasanella-Servat procedure
D. Suspension to the frontalis muscle with fascia lata grafting
E. Advancement of the levator muscle

ANSWERS, EXPLANATIONS AND REFERENCES

1. The correct response is C.

The Langer's lines run parallel to the main fiber bundles in the reticular layer of the dermis and are thought to originate from the ultrastructural organisation of the dermis. These are not clinically seen. If multiple holes are created in the skin, the holes acquire an elliptical shape along the lines of least tension in the area. These lines of least tension are called 'Langer's lines'.

Wrinkles are caused by mechanical forces from underlying muscle fibres and are therefore orientated perpendicular to the direction of the contraction.

Reference:

1. *Gibson T. Karl Langer (1819-1887) and his lines. Br J Plast Surg 1978; 31: 1.*
2. *Langers K. On the anatomy and physiology of the skin.III. The elasticity of the cutis by Professor K Langer, presented at the meeting of 27th November 1861. Br J Plast Surg 1978; 31: 185.*

2. The correct response is B.

The Arnold nerve provides sensation to the external auditory meatus and portions of the concha. Its fibres travel with the auricular branch of the vagus nerve.

Reference:

Wildsmith JA, Strichartz GR. Local anaesthetic drugs- an historical perspective. Br J Anaesth 1984;56:937.

3. The correct response is B.

The Erb's point located along the posterior border of the sternocleidomastoid muscle is useful to block the transverse cervical nerve. The great auricular nerve lies about 1 cm above this point and can be blocked by injecting the local anaesthetic in this location.

Reference:

1. *Wildsmith JA, Strichartz GR. Local anaesthetic drugs- an historical perspective. Br J Anaesth 1984; 56: 937.*
2. *Friedman PM, Mafong EA, Friedman ES et al. Topical anaesthetics update: EMLA and beyond. Dermatol Surg 2001;27:1019.*

4. The correct response is D.

The most common plane of avulsion of scalp is at the level of the loose areolar tissue below the aponeurosis. The deepest layer i.e. pericranium is firmly fixed to the underlying bone.

Reference:

1. *Hussain K, Wijetunge DB, Grubnic S et al. A comprehensive analysis of craniofacial trauma. J Trauma 1994; 36: 34.*
2. *Tolhurst DE, Carstens MH, Greco RJ et al. The surgical anatomy of the scalp. Plast Reconstr Surg 1991; 87: 603.*

5. The correct response is D.

Local anaesthetics are acidic and hence are painful on injection. The pain of injection can be decreased by buffering with sodium bicarbonate. Lidocaine 1% solution can be buffered with 8.4% sodium bicarbonate. Once the solution is buffered, its shelf life is significantly reduced.

The other methods listed do not reduce the pain on injection. Addition of epinephrine causes vasoconstriction, reduces bleeding and increases duration of action of the anaesthetic.

Reference:

1. *Wildsmith JA, Strichartz GR. Local anaesthetic drugs- an historical perspective. Br J Anaesth 1984; 56: 937.*
2. *Chen BK, Eichenfield LF. Pediatric anaesthesia in dermatologic surgery: when hand-holding is not enough. Dermatol Surg 2001; 27: 1010.*

6. The correct response is A.

The parotid duct is vulnerable to injury in lacerations of the face. It lies on the middle third of a line between tragus and middle of upper lip. The other options are incorrect.

The parotid duct travels adjacent to the buccal branches of the facial nerve. If the nerve is paralysed by any injury, then there are high chances of injury to the duct as well.

Reference:

1. *Shah JP, Shah JP. Head and Neck Surgery and Oncology. 3rd ed. Edinburgh, UK: Mosby; 2003: 732.*
2. *Gosain AK, Matloub HS. Surgical management of the facial nerve in craniofacial trauma and long-standing facial paralysis: cadaver study and clinical presentations. J Craniomaxillary Trauma 1999; 5: 29.*

7. The correct response is B.

The infraorbital nerve supplies the lower eyelid. Infratrochlear, branch of nasociliary supplies the upper eyelid.

Reference:

1. *Tyers A, Collin J. Colour Atlas of Ophthalmic Plastic Surgery. New York, Churchill Livingstone, 1995.*
2. *Standring S. Gray's Anatomy. The anatomical basis of clinical practice. 39th ed. Elsevier, Churchill Livingstone, 2005:684.*

8. The correct response is D.

Pseudomonas aeruginosa is the most common offending organism for suppurative chondritis. It is often associated with Staph aureus and Proteus.

Reference:

Dowling JA, Foley FD, Moncrief JA. Chondritis in the burned ear. Plast Reconstr Surg 1968; 42: 115.

9. The correct response is D.

A ring block around the ear will anaesthetise the entire ear except the portion of the concha and the external auditory canal as these are supplied by the Arnold nerve. Arnold's nerve (auricular branch of vagus) travels along the ear canal and hence escapes the ring block. Additional local injection will be required to block this nerve.

Reference:

1. *Shah JP, Shah JP. Head and Neck Surgery and Oncology. 3rd ed. Edinburgh, UK: Mosby; 2003: 732.*
2. *Krugman ME. Management of auricular hematomas with suction assisted lipectomy apparatus. Otolaryngol Head Neck Surg 1989; 101: 504.*

10. The correct response is A.

The great auricular nerve supplies the ear lobule. It is a branch of cervical plexus i.e. second and third cervical. It also supplies the lower part of the ear and skin over the parotid gland.

Reference:

Standring S. Gray's Anatomy. The anatomical basis of clinical practice. 39th ed. Elsevier, Churchill Livingstone, 2005: 515.

11. The correct response is C.

The auriculotemporal nerve supplies the tragus and the concha. It is a branch of the mandibular division of the trigeminal.

Reference:

Standring S. Gray's Anatomy. The anatomical basis of clinical practice. 39th ed. Elsevier, Churchill Livingstone, 2005: 515.

12. The correct response is A.

The complex anatomy of the periorbital region requires extensive quantities of skin to be replaced while correcting contractures. It is also important to do overcorrection to compensate for graft contraction. Full thickness skin may not be available in such large quantities, hence split skin graft is the choice of procedure. Local flaps and free flaps are usually not required. Forehead flap is also unsuitable as it lies in the zone of injury.

Reference:

1. *Achauer BM. Reconstructing the burned face. Clin Plast Surg 1992; 19: 623.*
2. *Jonsson CE, Dalsgaard CJ. Early excision and skin grafting of selected burns of the face and neck. Plast Reconstr Surg 1991; 88: 83.*

13. The correct response is B.

The complex anatomy of the periorbital region requires extensive quantities of skin to be replaced while correcting contractures. It is also important to do overcorrection to compensate for graft contraction. Full thickness skin may not be available in such large quantities, hence split skin graft is the choice of procedure. A thicker split thickness skin graft is preferred over a thin split thickness graft. The postauricular graft may not be available in sufficient quantity for resurfacing. There is no entity like a thick postauricular graft as the thickness of a full thickness graft remains the same.

Forehead flap is also unsuitable as it usually lies in the zone of injury and provides thick skin cover which is unsuitable for resurfacing.

Reference:

1. *Achauer BM. Reconstructing the burned face. Clin Plast Surg 1992; 19: 623.*
2. *Jonsson CE, Dalsgaard CJ. Early excision and skin grafting of selected burns of the face and neck. Plast Reconstr Surg 1991; 88: 83.*

14. The correct response is A.

Medial canthal webbing is common after postburn facial scarring. The procedure of choice for large web is excision of all scar tissue followed by resurfacing with full thickness graft. This is because that no amount of Z plasty or V-M plasty would be able to provide enough skin.

Z plasty is indicated for those webs which are limited to a ridge only. The V-M plasty and double opposing Z plasty are good for mild to moderate deformities.

Reference:

1. *Achauer BM. Reconstructing the burned face. Clin Plast Surg 1992; 19: 623.*
2. *Converse JM, McCarthy JG, Dobrkovsky M et al. Facial burns. In Converse JM, ed: Reconstructive Plastic Surgery. Philadelphia, WB Saunders, 1977: 1628.*

15. The correct response is C.

The best technique for reconstruction of the philtral dimple is that described by Schmid using the triangular fossa of the ear. The cartilage provides the necessary definition for restoration of the philtral dimple and contour of the philtrum.

A full thickness graft is the next best method but does not provide the same quality of contours which can be obtained by placing the cartilage graft. Split thickness graft again does not provide good contour and Abbe flap is unsuitable if the lower lip is also scarred.

Reference:

1. *Achauer BM. Reconstructing the burned face. Clin Plast Surg 1992; 19: 623.*
2. *Schmid E. The use of auricular cartilage and composite grafts in reconstruction of the upper lip with special reference to reconstruction of the philtrum. In Broadbent TR, ed: Transactions of the Third International Congress of Plastic Surgery. Amsterdam, Excerpta Medica, 1964: 306.*

16. The correct response is E.

All of the above options are correct for neck webbing. Neck webbing can occur after release and grafting of post burn neck contracture at the lateral aspect of the neck where the anterior grafts meet posterior unburned skin or at the edge of a graft. They can be prevented by using darts / Z plasties at time of original grafting. The treatment of neck webbing lies in using Z plasty or VY plasties under local or general anaesthesia.

Reference:

1. *Achauer BM. Reconstructing the burned face. Clin Plast Surg 1992; 19: 623.*
2. *Converse JM, McCarthy JG, Dobrkovsky M et al. Facial burns. In Converse JM, ed. Reconstructive Plastic Surgery. Philadelphia, WB Saunders, 1977: 1628.*

17. The correct response is C.

Life-threatening haemorrhage is defined by the loss of more than 3 units of blood or a haematocrit below 29%. Lacerations and crush injuries of the facial region may result in significant haemorrhage that may be life-threatening.

Reference:

1. *Bynoe RP, Kerwin AJ, Parker HH. Maxillofacial injuries and life-threatening hemorrhage: treatment with transcatheter arterial embolization. J Trauma 2003; 55: 74.*
2. *Yang WG, Tsai TR, Hung CC, Tung TC. Life threatening bleeding in a facial fracture. Ann Plast Surg 2001; 46: 159.*

18. The correct response is A.

The Glasgow Coma Scale (GCS) is useful for evaluating patients with head injuries. The scale relates to patient's level of consciousness, eye opening response and ability to speak and move extremities in prognostic grade. A higher scale indicates good prognosis whereas a GCS of 3 and fixed dilated pupils indicate no reasonable chance of survival.

Reference:

1. *Lieberman JD, Pasquale MD, Garcia R, Cipolle MD. Use of admission Glasgow Coma Scale score, pupil size, and pupil reactivity to determine outcome for trauma patients. J Trauma 2003; 55: 437.*
2. *MacLeod JB, Lynn M, McKenney MG. Early coagulopathy predicts mortality in trauma. J Trauma 2003; 55: 39.*

19. The correct response is D.

The Glasgow Coma Scale (GCS) is useful for evaluating patients with head injuries. The scale relates to patient's level of consciousness, eye opening response and ability to speak and move extremities in prognostic grade. The confused verbal response will be assigned a score of 4 in the scale. The other responses would be assigned the following score - No response (1), Incomprehensible sound (2), Inappropriate words (3) and fully oriented (5).

Reference:

1. *Lieberman JD, Pasquale MD, Garcia R, Cipolle MD. Use of admission Glasgow Coma Scale score, pupil size, and pupil reactivity to determine outcome for trauma patients. J Trauma 2003; 55:4 37.*
2. *MacLeod JB, Lynn M, McKenney MG. Early coagulopathy predicts mortality in trauma. J Trauma 2003; 55: 39.*

3

20. The correct response is D.

The spontaneous eye opening is assigned score of 4. The other scores in respect of eye response are as follows: No eye response (1) Eye opening response to painful stimuli (2) Eye opening to verbal request would be assigned (3) points.

Reference:

1. *Lieberman JD, Pasquale MD, Garcia R, Cipolle MD. Use of admission Glasgow Coma Scale score, pupil size, and pupil reactivity to determine outcome for trauma patients. J Trauma 2003; 55: 437.*
2. *MacLeod JB, Lynn M, McKenney MG. Early coagulopathy predicts mortality in trauma. J Trauma 2003; 55: 39.*

21. The correct response is D.

The Glasgow Coma Scale (GCS) is useful for evaluating patients with head injuries. A patient who obeys commands and moves his body according to the given instructions would be assigned 6 score in the best motor response category. If the patient is able to localize the pain, he would be assigned score of 5, withdrawal from pain is score of 4, abnormal flexion is score of 3, abnormal extension is score of 2 and no movements is score of 1.

Reference:

1. *Lieberman JD, Pasquale MD, Garcia R, Cipolle MD. Use of admission Glasgow Coma Scale score, pupil size, and pupil reactivity to determine outcome for trauma patients. J Trauma 2003; 55: 437.*
2. *MacLeod JB, Lynn M, McKenney MG. Early coagulopathy predicts mortality in trauma. J Trauma 2003; 55: 39.*

22. The correct response is B.

A combination of subconjunctival haemorrhage, palpebral ecchymosis and swelling around the eye are indications of fracture of the zygoma. Bilateral haematomas suggest a LeFort, nasoethmoid or anterior cranial fossa fracture.

Reference:

1. *Lim LH, Lam LK, Moore H et al. Associated injuries in facial fratures: a review of 839 patients. Plast Surg 1993; 46: 635.*
2. *Dingman RO, Natvig P. Surgery of facial Fractures. Philadelphia, WB Saunders, 1964.*

23. The correct response is C.

The pupil on the injured side would dilate when light is flashed on the intact side. The pupillary response of dilatation on the injured side is due to Marcus Gunn phenomenon. The afferent impulses can travel upwards from the normal side and produce consensual dilatation of the pupil on the injured side. The afferent reflexes fail to travel up from the injured side and the pupil fails to constrict on the injured side, when light is flashed. It however dilates on the injured side when light is flashed on the normal side.

Reference:

1. *Barton FE, Berry WL. Evaluation of the acutely injured orbit. In Aston SJ, Hornblass A, Meltzer MA, Rees TD, eds: Third International Symposium of Plastic and Reconstructive Surgery of the Eye and Adenexa. Baltimore, Williams and Wilkins, 1982: 34.*
2. *Dingman RO, Natvig P. Surgery of facial Fractures. Philadelphia, WB Saunders, 1964.*

24. The correct response is D.

Computed tomographic scan is indispensable for the evaluation of a patient with facial fractures. Both the axial and coronal views along with the three dimensional reconstruction provide an unparalleled picture of the bony structures as well as soft tissue derangements.

Mayer view is a specific radiograph for visualizing the temporomandibular joint and external auditory canal. Panoramic films are helpful in defining location and displacement of mandibular fractures. Colour doppler has limited and specific role in the management of facial fractures.

Reference:

1. *Kreipke DLK, Moss JJ, Franco JM et al. Computed tomography in facial trauma. Am J Roentgenol 1984; 142: 1041.*
2. *Kreipke DLK, Noyek AM, Cooper PW. CT in facial trauma. J Otolaryngol 1983; 12: 2.*

25. The correct response is B.

The neck of the mandible is the weakest area. It is most likely to get fractured and out of all the fractures, the maximum numbers of fractures occur in the region of the neck of the mandible (36%).

Reference:

1. *Kruger GO. Textbook of Oral Maxillofacial Surgery, 6th ed. St. Louis, CV Mosby, 1984.*
2. *Dingman RO, Natvig P. Surgery of facial Fractures. Philadelphia, WB Saunders, 1964.*

26. The correct response is D.

The compression plate osteosynthesis concept was developed for extremity fracture treatment but is to be used with caution in the craniofacial skeleton. It is correct that the compression of the bone ends conceptually speeds fracture healing but compression of craniofacial fracture may result in malunion due to undesirable movement of well reduced fractures. Hence non-compressive fixation is recommended for craniofacial fractures.

Reference:

1. *Dingman RO, Natvig P. Surgery of facial Fractures. Philadelphia, WB Saunders, 1964.*
2. *Spiessl B. New concepts in Maxillofacial Bone Surgery. New York, Springer Verlag, 1976.*

27. The correct response is C.

The distance between the two threads of a screw used for osteosynthesis is known as pitch of the screw. A cutting flute is seen in the inferior end of the screw.

Reference:

1. *Spiessl B. New concepts in Maxillofacial Bone Surgery. New York, Springer Verlag, 1976.*
2. *Assael LA. Craniofacial fractures. In Prein J, ed: Manual of Internal Fixation in the Craniofacial Skeleton: Techniques as Recommended by the AO/ASIF Group. New York, Springer Verlag, 1997:120.*

28. The correct response is A.

Primary bone grafting is routinely used in management of facial fractures. These grafts help in maintaining the contour and projection of the bone in areas of severe comminution. The nasal skeleton, orbital walls and rims and the frontal bone are areas where primary bone grafting has been successful. It is not usually indicated in the mandible as there is a significant incidence of infection.

Reference:

1. *Gruss JS, Mackinnon SE, Kasel E et al. The role of primary bone grafting in complex craniomaxillofacial trauma. Plast Reconstr Surg 1985;75: 17.*
2. *Gruss JS. Complex craniofacial trauma:evolution of management: a trauma unit's experience. J Trauma 1990; 30: 377.*

29. The correct response is C.

The rib graft is the easiest to contour out of the options given. It is good for recontouring to internal orbital shapes. The marrow may be curetted out of a split rib to make a very thin nasal onlay graft. The calvarial is the most difficult to contour. MMCA is not an autogenous material.

Reference:

1. *Gruss JS, Mackinnon SE, Kasel E et al. The role of primary bone grafting in complex craniomaxillofacial trauma. Plast Reconstr Surg 1985;75: 17.*
2. *Gruss JS. Complex craniofacial trauma: evolution of management: a trauma unit's experience. J Trauma 1990; 30:377.*

30. The correct response is A.

The calvarial is the most difficult to contour. The rib graft is the easiest to contour out of the options given. It is good for recontouring to internal orbital shapes. The marrow may be curetted out of a split rib to make a very thin nasal onlay graft. MMCA is not an autogenous material.

Reference:

1. *Gruss JS, Mackinnon SE, Kasel E et al. The role of primary bone grafting in complex craniomaxillofacial trauma. Plast Reconstr Surg 1985;75: 17.*
2. *Gruss JS. Complex craniofacial trauma: evolution of management: a trauma unit's experience. J Trauma 1990; 30:377.*

31. The correct response is D.

Deviation of chin to the opposite side on opening the mouth is not a feature of subcondylar fracture. The rest are correct signs of this type of fracture.

Reference:

1. *Hovinga J, Boering G, Stegenga B. long-term results of non-surgical management of condylar fractures in children. J Oral Maxillofac Surg 1999; 28: 429.*
2. *Norholt SE, Krishanan V, Sinder-Pederson S, Jensen I. Pediatric condylar fractures: a long term follow up of 55 patients. J Oral Maxillofac Surg 1993; 51: 1302.*

32. The correct response is B.

The most common form of condylar head dislocation is medial and anterior with the condylar head fractured at the neck. This is due to the pull of the lateral pterygoid on the condyle. Other dislocations have also been recorded.

Reference:

1. *Assael L. Open versus closed reduction of adult mandibular condyle fractures: an alternative interpretation of the evidence. J Oral Maxillofac Surg 2003; 61: 1333.*
2. *Ellis E III, McFadden D, Simon P et al. Surgical complications with open treatment of mandibular condylar process fractures. J Oral Maxillofac Surg 2000; 58: 950.*

33. The correct response is B.

Nasal fractures can be divided into lateral impact and frontal impact injuries. Lateral impact injuries are unilateral while frontal impact injuries are bilateral. A patient with fractures involving lower half of both the nasal bones with telescoping of the septum is classifiable into plane II frontal impact injury. Plane I injury involves the distal ends of the nasal bones while plane III injuries are truly nasoethmoidal orbital fractures.

Reference:

1. *Stranc MF, Robertson LA. Classification of injuries to the nasal skeleton. Ann Plast Surg 1979; 2: 468.*
2. *Stranc MF. Primary treatment of nasoethmoid injuries with increased intercanthal distance. Br J Plast Surg 1970; 23: 8.*

34. The correct response is A.

Septal haematomas are often bilateral as fractures of the cartilaginous septum permit the passage of blood from one side to the other. Undrained haematomas may lead to septal perforation or fibrosis. Organised haematoma may result in thickening of cartilage. Septal haematoma is treated by incising mucoperichondrium on one side only as incision on both sides may lead to a septal perforation.

Reference:

1. *Stranc MF, Robertson LA. Classification of injuries to the nasal skeleton. Ann Plast Surg 1979; 2: 468.*
2. *Stranc MF. Primary treatment of nasoethmoid injuries with increased intercanthal distance. Br J Plast Surg 1970; 23: 8.*

35. The correct response is B.

The Asch forceps is the instrument of choice for reduction of a septal fracture. The Walsham forceps is useful for nasal fracture reduction, specifically in performing upward and outward displacement followed by repositioning of the fragments. Rowe's forceps is used for LeFort I osteotomy.

Reference:

1. *Verwoerd CDA. Present day treatment of nasal fractures: closed versus open reduction. Facial Plast Surg 1992; 8: 220.*
2. *Stranc MF. Primary treatment of nasoethmoid injuries with increased intercanthal distance. Br J Plast Surg 1970; 23: 8.*

36. The correct response is E.

The medial pterygoid is not attached to the zygoma. It is attached to the ramus and angle of the mandible.

Reference:

1. *Shah JP, Shah JP. Head and Neck Surgery and Oncology. 3rd ed. Edinburgh, UK: Mosby; 2003: 732.*
2. *Standring S. Gray's Anatomy. The anatomical basis of clinical practice. 39th ed. Elsevier, Churchill Livingstone, 2005: 515.*

37. The correct response is A.

The zygomatico-temporal and zygomaticofacial vessels pass through the foramen in the bone. Fracture and displacement of zygoma causes damage to these fine vessels, which causes ecchymosis of the eye. These vessels are branches of the lacrimal artery, which is a branch of the ophthalmic artery from the internal carotid artery system. The other options are incorrect.

Reference:

1. *Sungeil P, Lindquist C. Paresthesia of the infraorbital nerve following fracture of the zygomatic complex. Int J Oral Maxillofac Surg 1987; 16: 363.*
2. *Standring S. Gray's Anatomy. The anatomical basis of clinical practice. 39th ed. Elsevier, Churchill Livingstone, 2005: 478.*

38. The correct response is B.

The infraorbital nerve travels obliquely from lateral to medial across the floor of the orbit. In the posterior portion of the orbit, the nerve is in a groove while in the anterior portion of the orbit, it is located in a canal. Both of these locations constitute a weak portion of the bone hence the nerve is often compressed in fractures involving the orbital floor. The other options are incorrect.

Reference:

1. *Hwang K, Shu MS, Lee S, Chung IH. Cutaneous distribution of the infraorbital nerve. J Craniofac Surg 2004; 15: 3.*
2. *Hwang K, Shu MS, Lee S, Chung H. Zygomaticotemporal nerve passage in the temporal area. J Craniofac Surg 2004; 15: 209.*

39. The correct response is D.

The Mayer view is good for visualizing the temporomandibular joint and is not preferred for zygoma radiography. The rest of the options are all true. The zygoma forms the upper outer part of the maxillary antrum and hence may be pneumatised with air cells. Zygomaticofacial foramen is a weak area in the zygoma. The coronal incision allows exposure of the entire zygomatic arch and roof of the glenoid fossa for arch reconstruction. The lateral blepharoplasty incision may be used for zygomatic fracture reduction in the area of the zygomaticofrontal suture.

Reference:

1. *Barclay TL. Four hundred malar-zygomatic fractures. Transactions of the International Society of Plastic Surgeons, Second Congress. Edinburgh, EandS Livingstone, 1960: 259.*
2. *Dingman RO, Alling CC. Open reduction and internal wire fixation of maxillofacial fractures. J Oral Surg 1954; 12: 140.*

40. The correct response is D.

The lateral and superior walls of the maxillary sinuses are involved in fractures of the zygoma. It is injury to the maxillary antral lining, which is responsible for unilateral epistaxis in most of the cases.

Reference:

1. *Barclay TL. Four hundred malar-zygomatic fractures. Transactions of the International Society of Plastic Surgeons, Second Congress. Edinburgh, EandS Livingstone, 1960: 259.*
2. *Harison DH. Nasal injuries: their pathogenesis and treatment. Br J Plast Surg 1979; 32: 57.*

41. The correct response is B.

The Waters view is the single best plain film to demonstrate depression and malalignment of the zygoma at its buttresses, depression of the orbital floor and for information about the sutures related to the zygoma.

Reference:

1. *Hollier L, Thornton J, Pazmino P, Stal S. The management of orbitozygomatic fractures. Plast Reconstr Surg 2003; 111: 2386.*
2. *Dingman RO, Alling CC. Open reduction and internal wire fixation of maxillofacial fractures. J Oral Surg 1954; 12: 140.*

42. The correct response is C.

Medially displaced zygoma fractures may narrow the volume of the orbit and lead to exophthalmos. These are the so called blow-in fractures. The other categories would not produce this type of fracture.

Reference:

1. *Gruss JS, Mackinnon SE, Kasel E et al. The role of primary bone grafting in complex craniomaxillofacial trauma. Plast Reconstr Surg 1985; 75: 17.*
2. *Gruss JS. Complex craniofacial trauma:evolution of management: a trauma unit's experience. J Trauma 1990; 30: 377.*

43. The correct response is B.

The zygomaticofrontal suture is a key landmark to the diagnosis and treatment of fractures of the zygoma. It is located about 8-10 mm above the level of the lateral canthus.

Reference:

1. *Hollier L, Thornton J, Pazmino P, Stal S. The management of orbitozygomatic fractures. Plast Reconstr Surg 2003; 111: 2386.*
2. *Anastassou GE, Van Damme PA. Evaluation of the anatomical position of the lateral canthal ligament: clinical application and guidelines. J Craniofac Surg 1996; 7: 429.*

44. The correct response is E.

The upper buccal sulcus approach or the intraoral approach is preferred for treating fracture displacements of the zygomaticomaxillary buttress without any associated injuries like arch fractures. This approach allows good exposure and an elevator can be used through the anterior wall of the fractured maxillary sinus to elevate the body of the zygoma before performing plate osteosynthesis of the fracture. Dingman approach is good for arch fractures, and coronal approach is used for those where exposure of the entire zygomatic arch is required. Endoscopic approach is used for assisting the repair of zygomatic fractures by defining the orbital floor defect.

Reference:

1. *Hollier L, Thornton J, Pazmino P, Stal S. The management of orbitozygomatic fractures. Plast Reconstr Surg 2003; 111: 2386.*
2. *Mayer M, Manson PN. Rigid fixation in facial fractures. Philadelphia, JB Lippincott, 1991. Problems in Plastic Surgery.*

45. The correct response is E.

All of the above measures would be required to manage compound comminuted fractures of the zygoma. Reduction should first be done by drilling holes in the fractured ends, which should be held by wires initially. After the zygoma has been reduced in position, plate and screws should be used for final fixation as required.

Reference:

1. *Hollier L, Thornton J, Pazmino P, Stal S. The management of orbitozygomatic fractures. Plast Reconstr Surg 2003; 111: 2386.*
2. *Mayer M, Manson PN. Rigid fixation in facial fractures. Philadelphia, JB Lippincott, 1991. Problems in Plastic Surgery.*

46. The correct response is A.

The Gillies approach (closed reduction) is suitable for depressed fractures of the zygomatic arch. In this, the elevator can be taken behind the zygomatic arch, which can be easily reduced. The temporalis fascia is attached to its upper border from one end to the other. The face lift approach can also be used, if plating is required, to be done. The other approaches do not provide this convenience and ease with the closed approach.

Reference:

1. *Hollier L, Thornton J, Pazmino P, Stal S. The management of orbitozygomatic fractures. Plast Reconstr Surg 2003; 111: 2386.*
2. *Perino KE, Zide MF, Kinnebrew MC. Late treatment of malunited malar fracture. J Oral Maxillofac Surg 1980; 42: 20.*

47. The correct response is C.

The diplopia is due to muscular abnormalities caused by displacement of lateral canthus downwards which affects the lateral rectus muscle, causing imbalance in the muscular mechanism.

Reference:

1. *Perino KE, Zide MF, Kinnebrew MC. Late treatment of malunited malar fracture. J Oral Maxillofac Surg 1980; 42: 20.*
2. *Hollier L, Thornton J, Pazmino P, Stal S. The management of orbitozygomatic fractures. Plast Reconstr Surg 2003; 111: 2386.*

48. The correct response is C.

The coronoid process is in intimate relationship to the body of the zygoma. The coronoid process and the undersurface of the zygoma are about 1 cm away from each other. Any lateral displacements of the body of the zygoma impinge on the condyle and lead to difficulty in mouth opening.

Reference:

1. *Perino KE, Zide MF, Kinnebrew MC. Late treatment of malunited malar fracture. J Oral Maxillofac Surg 1980; 42: 20.*
2. *Hollier L, Thornton J, Pazmino P, Stal S. The management of orbitozygomatic fractures. Plast Reconstr Surg 2003; 111: 2386.*

49. The correct response is C.

Maxillary hypoplasia is not a known complication of untreated maxilla fractures.

Reference:

1. *Dingman RO, Alling CC. Open reduction and internal wire fixation of maxillofacial fractures. J Oral Surg 1954; 12: 140.*
2. *Stajcic Z. The buccal fat pad in the closure of oro-antral communications. J Craniomaxillofac Surg 1992; 20: 193.*

50. The correct response is A.

A transverse fracture of the maxilla above the apices of the teeth is called LeFort I fracture. It courses above the apices of teeth, sectioning the entire alveolar process, vault of the palate and inferior ends of the pterygoid processes. This is also known as Guerin fracture. This fracture is almost always bilateral.

Reference:

1. *Manson PN. Some thoughts on the classification and treatment of LeFort fractures. Ann Plast Surg 1986; 17: 356.*
2. *Mayer M, Manson PN. Rigid fixation in facial fractures. Philadelphia, JB Lippincott, 1991. Problems in Plastic Surgery.*

51. The correct response is B.

A pyramidal fracture of the maxilla and the nasal bone is called LeFort II fracture. The fracture line extends above the level of apices of teeth laterally and posteriorly in the zygomaticomaxillary buttress and extends through the pterygoid plates in the same fashion. Fracture lines travel medially and superiorly to pass through the medial portion of the inferior orbital rim and extend across the nose to separate a pyramid shaped central maxillary segment.

Reference:

1. *Manson PN. Some thoughts on the classification and treatment of LeFort fractures. Ann Plast Surg 1986; 17: 356.*
2. *Mayer M, Manson PN. Rigid fixation in facial fractures. Philadelphia, JB Lippincott, 1991. Problems in Plastic Surgery.*

52. The correct response is A.

A fracture that disconnects the maxilla, zygoma and nasal bones from the frontal bone is called LeFort III fracture or craniofacial disjunction. The fracture extends through the zygomaticofrontal suture and the nasal frontal suture and across the floor of the orbits to effectively separate all midfacial structures from the cranium.

Reference:

1. *Rowe NL, Killey HC. Fractures of the facial skeleton, 2nd ed, Baltimore, Williams and Wilkins, 1968.*
2. *Manson PN. Some thoughts on the classification and treatment of LeFort fractures. Ann Plast Surg 1986; 17: 356.*

53. The correct response is C.

LeFort was a French orthopedic surgeon. He proposed a classification based on fractures produced experimentally in the skulls around 1900. The fractures of maxilla were classified as LeFort I, II and III.

Reference:

1. *Rowe NL, Killey HC. Fractures of the facial skeleton, 2nd ed, Baltimore, Williams and Wilkins, 1968.*
2. *Manson PN. Some thoughts on the classification and treatment of Le Fort fractures. Ann Plast Surg 1986; 17: 356.*

54. The correct response is A.

Maxillary fractures usually produce a bilateral rather than an unilateral ecchymosis. The rest of the options are correct. Facial oedema depends upon the severity of fracture.

Reference:

1. *Rowe NL, Killey HC. Fractures of the facial skeleton, 2nd ed, Baltimore, Williams and Wilkins, 1968.*
2. *Manson PN. Some thoughts on the classification and treatment of LeFort fractures. Ann Plast Surg 1986; 17: 356.*

55. The correct response is D.

All of the above. Conceptually, panfacial fractures involve all the three areas of the face including frontal bone, midface and the mandible.

Reference:

Manson P, Clark N, Robertson B, Crawley W. Comprehensive management of pan facial fractures. J Craniomaxillofac Trauma 1995; 11: 43.

56. The correct response is E.

All of the above mentioned methods are suitable for repair of dura and its tears. Dural patch of temporalis, fascia lata or pericranium can be used for repair of dura. Direct suturing may also be done for minor tears.

Reference:

1. *Manson P, Clark N, Robertson B, Crawley W. Comprehensive management of pan facial fractures. J Craniomaxillofac Trauma 1995; 11: 43.*
2. *Rohrich R, Shewmake K. Evolving concepts of craniomaxillofacial trauma management. Clin Plast Surg 1992; 19: 1.*

57. The correct response is D.

The foramina of Breschet are located in the frontal sinus. The mucosa of the sinus follows the veins present there in. When the sinus is planned to be closed, the mucosa needs to be stripped thoroughly down into the nasal frontal duct.

Reference:

Donald PJ. The tenacity of frontal sinus mucosa. Otolaryngol Head Neck Surg 1979; 87: 557.

58. The correct response is D.

The lacrimal bone is the smallest bone of the orbit.

Reference:

1. *Manson PN, Illif N. Surgical anatomy of the orbit: In Marsh J ed: Current Therapy in Plastic and Reconstructive Surgery. Philadelphia, BC Decker, 1989: 117.*
2. *Standring S. Gray's Anatomy. The anatomical basis of clinical practice. 39th ed. Elsevier, Churchill Livingstone, 2005: 688.*

59. The correct response is C.

The correct depth of the orbit is 45 mm. The height of the eye, i.e. vertical dimension is 35 mm and breadth of the eye, i.e. horizontal dimension is 40 mm. Minor variations can be present from one person to another.

Reference:

1. *Manson PN, Illif N. Surgical anatomy of the orbit: In Marsh J ed: Current Therapy in Plastic and Reconstructive Surgery. Philadelphia, BC Decker, 1989: 117.*
2. *Standring S. Gray's Anatomy. The anatomical basis of clinical practice. 39th ed. Elsevier, Churchill Livingstone, 2005: 688.*

60. The correct response is C.

The superior and the inferior rectus move the eye on its transverse axis. The medial and the lateral rectus move the eye on its vertical axis. The superior and the inferior oblique move the eye on the antero-posterior axis to produce intorsion and extorsion of the eye.

Reference:

1. *Manson PN, Illif N. Surgical anatomy of the orbit: In Marsh J ed: Current Therapy in Plastic and Reconstructive Surgery. Philadelphia, BC Decker, 1989: 117.*
2. *Standring S. Gray's Anatomy. The anatomical basis of clinical practice. 39th ed. Elsevier, Churchill Livingstone, 2005: 688.*

61. The correct response is A.

The inferior oblique is close to the floor of the orbit. It passes laterally between the inferior rectus and the floor of the orbit.

Reference:

1. *Manson PN, Illif N. Surgical anatomy of the orbit: In Marsh J ed: Current Therapy in Plastic and Reconstructive Surgery. Philadelphia , BC Decker, 1989: 117.*
2. *Standring S. Gray's Anatomy. The anatomical basis of clinical practice. 39th ed. Elsevier, Churchill Livingstone, 2005: 688.*

62. The correct response is C.

The orbital plate of maxilla is present in the floor of the orbit and is thin and therefore the one that gets easily fractured in orbital fractures. In addition to it, the ethmoids are also prone to fracture easily.

Reference:

1. *Catone GA, Morrissette MP, Carlson ER. Retrospective analysis of untreated orbital blowout fractures. J Oral Maxillofac Surg 1998; 46: 1033.*
2. *Manson PN, Illif N. Surgical anatomy of the orbit: In Marsh J ed: Current Therapy in Plastic and Reconstructive Surgery. Philadelphia, BC Decker, 1989: 117.*

63. The correct response is C.

The optic foramen is located 40-45 mm behind the inferior orbital rim. This is important when performing inferior orbital dissection. The position of instruments in floor dissection can be checked by putting the Freer elevator into the maxillary sinus and feeling the back of sinus which is located 5-10 mm in front and 10 mm below the optic foramen.

Reference:

1. *Catone GA, Morrissette MP, Carlson ER. Retrospective analysis of untreated orbital blowout fractures. J Oral Maxillofac Surg 1998; 46: 1033.*
2. *Manson PN, Illif N. Surgical anatomy of the orbit: In Marsh J ed: Current Therapy in Plastic and Reconstructive Surgery. Philadelphia , BC Decker, 1989: 117.*

64. The correct response is B.

The lateral boundary of the superior orbital fissure is formed by the "frontal bone", between the greater and lesser wings.

Reference:

1. *Catone GA, Morrissette MP, Carlson ER. Retrospective analysis of untreated orbital blowout fractures. J Oral Maxillofac Surg 1998; 46: 1033.*
2. *Manson PN, Illif N. Surgical anatomy of the orbit: In Marsh J ed: Current Therapy in Plastic and Surgery. Philadelphia , BC Decker, 1989: 117.*

65. The correct response is E.

Fracture of the nasal bone is an unlikely cause for diplopia. The rest of the factors listed are correct. The 12 muscles of both the sides act in tandem and not individually. Any disturbance in the functioning and alignment of these muscles will produce diplopia.

Reference:

1. *Mathog RH, Archer KF, Nesi F. Post-traumatic enophthalmos and diplopia. Otolaryngol Head Neck Surg 1989; 94: 69.*
2. *Lyon DB, Newman SA. Evidence of direct damage to extraocular muscles as a cause of diplopia following orbital trauma. Ophthalmic Plast Reconstr Surg 1989; 5: 81.*

66. The correct response is E.

The superior oblique muscle on contraction does not produce extortion. It produces intortion of the eye.

Reference:

1. *Mathog RH, Archer KF, Nesi F. Post-traumatic enophthalmos and diplopia. Otolaryngol Head Neck Surg 1989; 94: 69.*
2. *Lyon DB, Newman SA. Evidence of direct damage to extraocular muscles as a cause of diplopia following orbital trauma. Ophthalmic Plast Reconstr Surg 1989; 5: 81.*

67. The correct response is D.

Squint is not a feature of medial orbital blowout fractures.

Reference:

1. *Mathog RH, Archer KF, Nesi F. Post-traumatic enophthalmos and diplopia. Otolaryngol Head Neck Surg 1989;94:69.*
2. *Prasad SS. Blowout fractures of the medial wall of the orbit. In Bleeker GM, Lyle TK, eds: Proceedings of the Second International Symposium on Orbital Disorders, vol 14. Basel, Karger, 1975.*

68. The correct response is C.

Lamina papyracea is a smooth plate of bone which encloses the ethmoid cells and forms a large part of the medial wall of the orbit. It is vulnerable to fracture as it is papery thin in structure.

Reference:

1. *Prasad SS. Blowout fractures of the medial wall of the orbit. In Bleeker GM, Lyle TK, eds: Proceedings of the Second International Symposium on Orbital Disorders, vol 14. Basel, Karger, 1975.*
2. *Jones E, Evans JN. "Blowout" fractures of the orbit: an investigation into their anatomical basis. J Laryngol Otol 1967; 81: 1109.*

3

69. The correct response is A.

The muscle which underlies the inferior orbital nerve is 'Levator anguli oris'. The inferior orbital nerve is protected by a muscle in front of it and a muscle behind it.

Reference:

1. *Manson PN, Illif N. Surgical anatomy of the orbit: In Marsh J ed: Current Therapy in Plastic and Reconstructive Surgery. Philadelphia , BC Decker, 1989: 117.*
2. *Rowe NL, Killey HC. Fractures of the facial skeleton, 2nd ed, Baltimore, Williams and Wilkins, 1968.*

70. The correct response is E.

The muscle on contraction does not produce intortion. It produces extortion of the eye.

Reference:

Manson PN, Illif N. Surgical anatomy of the orbit: In Marsh J ed: Current Therapy in Plastic and Reconstructive Surgery. Philadelphia, BC Decker, 1989: 117.

71. The correct response is C.

The inferior rectus muscle is the one to be incarcerated in ocular injuries.

The procedure to diagnose incarceration is called "Forced duction test." The local anaesthesia is instilled in the eye. Once the effect is obtained the patient is made to lie in a preoperative room or in the operating room. The inferior rectus muscle is held about 1 cm behind the limbus by a forceps and the eyeball is rotated up and down. If it can be easily done, the muscle is not incarcerated.

Reference:

1. *Manson PN, Illif N. Surgical anatomy of the orbit: In Marsh J ed: Current Therapy in Plastic and Reconstructive Surgery. Philadelphia , BC Decker, 1989: 117.*
2. *Kakibuchi M, Fukazawa K, Fukuda K. Combination of transconjuctival and endonasal- transantral approach in the repair of blowout fractures involving the orbital floor. Br J Plast Surg 2004; 57: 37.*

72. The correct response is A.

Downward displacement of the lateral canthus of the eye suggests involvement of the frontal process of the zygoma. The lateral canthal ligament is attached to the frontal process of the zygoma at the Whitnall's tubercle. Frontozygomatic disjunction or fracture would produce downward displacement of the zygoma and this would result in downward displacement of the lateral canthus of the eye.

Reference:

1. *Manson PN, Illif N. Surgical anatomy of the orbit: In Marsh J ed: Current Therapy in Plastic and Reconstructive Surgery. Philadelphia , BC Decker, 1989: 117.*
2. *Hammer B, Kunz C, Schramm A, et al. Repair of complex orbital fractures: technical problems, state-of-the art solutions and future prospective [review]. Ann Acad Med Singapore 1999; 28: 687.*

73. The correct response is C.

The posterior ethmoidal cells and the sphenoidal sinus open into the superior meatus. The anterior and middle ethmoidal sinuses open into the middle meatus.

Reference:

Standring S. Gray's Anatomy. The anatomical basis of clinical practice. 39th ed. Elsevier, Churchill Livingstone, 2005: 570.

74. The correct response is B.

The frontal sinus drains into the nose through the nasofrontal ducts which open and drain into the middle meatus of the nose. The anterior and middle ethmoidal sinuses also drain into the middle meatus. Canulation of the frontal sinus is also done through the middle meatus.

Reference:

1. *Manson PN, Illif N. Surgical anatomy of the orbit: In Marsh J ed: Current Therapy in Plastic and Reconstructive Surgery. Philadelphia , BC Decker 1989. 117.*
2. *Hammer B, Kunz C, Schramm A, et al. Repair of complex orbital fractures: technical problems, state-of-the art solutions and future prospective [review]. Ann Acad Med Singapore 1999; 28: 687.*

75. The correct response is D.

The nasolacrimal duct opens into the inferior meatus and all the structures including anterior / middle ethmoidal sinus, frontal and maxillary sinuses open in the middle meatus.

Reference:

1. *Manson PN, Illif N. Surgical anatomy of the orbit: In Marsh J ed: Current Therapy in Plastic and Reconstructive Surgery. Philadelphia, BC Decker, 1989: 117.*
2. *Hammer B, Kunz C, Schramm A, et al. Repair of complex orbital fractures: technical problems, state-of-the art solutions and future prospective [review]. Ann Acad Med Singapore 1999; 28: 687.*

76. The correct response is B.

The nasolacrimal duct is the one that opens into the inferior meatus and helps in the discharge of tears.

Reference:

1. *Manson PN, Illif N. Surgical anatomy of the orbit: In Marsh J ed: Current Therapy in Plastic and Reconstructive Surgery. Philadelphia, BC Decker 1989: 117.*
2. *Hammer B, Kunz C, Schramm A, et al: Repair of complex orbital fractures: technical problems, state-of-the art solutions and future prospective [review]. AnnAcad Med Singapore 1999;28:687.*

77. The correct response is B.

The superior meatus receives opening of two structures viz. posterior ethmoidal and sphenoidal sinus.

Reference:

1. *Manson PN, Illif N. Surgical anatomy of the orbit and In Marsh J ed: Current Therapy in Plastic and Reconstructive Surgery. Philadelphia, BC Decker, 1989: 117.*
2. *Hammer B, Kunz C, Schramm A, et al. Repair of complex orbital fractures: technical problems, state-of-the art solutions and future prospective [review]. Ann Acad Med Singapore 1999; 28: 687.*

78. The correct response is D.

The middle meatus receives openings of total of four structures. It receives the openings of 3 sinuses and one duct i.e. anterior and middle ethmoidal sinuses, maxillary sinus and the frontonasal duct from frontal sinus.

Reference:

Manson PN, Illif N. Surgical anatomy of the orbit: In Marsh J ed: Current Therapy in Plastic and Reconstructive Surgery. Philadelphia, BC Decker, 1989: 117.

79. The correct response is A.

The inferior meatus of the nose receives the opening of the nasolacrimal duct only.

Reference:

Manson PN, Illif N. Surgical anatomy of the orbit: In Marsh J ed: Current Therapy in Plastic and Reconstructive Surgery. Philadelphia, BC Decker, 1989: 117.

80. The correct response is D.

The opening of the maxillary sinus is high above its floor and is poorly placed for natural drainage in the sitting or standing posture. It will however allow drainage during the sleeping position on the side.

Reference:

Manson PN, Illif N. Surgical anatomy of the orbit: In Marsh J ed: Current Therapy in Plastic and Reconstructive Surgery. Philadelphia , BC Decker, 1989: 117.

81. The correct response is E.

Burm has categorized blow-out fractures into the types as trap door, single hinge, double hinge and punched out. Comminuted type is not described. The basis of this classification bears relevance to the type of orbital reconstruction that would be required in these fractures.

Reference:

1. *Burm JS, Chung CH, Oh SJ. Pure orbital blow-out fracture: new concepts and the importance of the medial orbital wall. Plast Reconstr Surg 1999; 103: 1439.*
2. *Burm JS, Oh SJ. Direct local approach through a W-shaped incision in moderate or severe blow-out fractures of the medial orbital wall. Plast Reconstr Surg 2001; 107: 920.*

82. The correct response is D.

Hypotelorism does not usually occur in nasoethmoid fracture. On the contrary hypertelorism may occur due to traumatic telecanthus. The other features are correct. The root of the nose gets pushed in and the dorsum of the nose may also lose its prominence. The nose may also get telescoped. The septum gets depressed, fractured and may develop hematomas.

Reference:

Paskert JP, Manson PN. The bimanual examination for assessing instability in nasoethmoid orbital fractures. Plast Reconstr Surg 1989; 83: 165.

83. The correct response is D.

The double ring sign in nasoethmoidal-orbital injuries is useful for the diagnosis of CSF rhinorrhea. A small amount of nasal drainage is placed on a paper towel. The blood component produces a ring while the CSF migrates out and produces another ring outside. This double ring sign is diagnostic of CSF leak.

Reference:

Bell R, Dierks E, Homer L, Potter B. Management of cerebrospinal fluid leak associated with craniomaxillofacial trauma. J Oral Maxillofac Surg 2004; 62: 676.

84. The correct response is E.

The medial canthal ligament is attached to all the listed structures except the lacrimal fossa. It forms a roof for the lacrimal sac. It has a three dimensional triangular attachment around the lacrimal sac to provide necessary protection.

Reference:

1. *Manson PN, Illif N. Surgical anatomy of the orbit: In Marsh J ed: Current Therapy in Plastic and Reconstructive Surgery. Philadelphia, BC Decker, 1989: 117.*
2. *Anderson RL.The medial canthal tendon branches out. Arch Ophthalmol 1977; 95: 2051.*

85. The correct response is E.

All of the above features may be present in retrobulbar haematoma. It is not usually possible to drain the haematoma because they are diffuse in nature.

Reference:

MacKinnon CA, David DJ, Cooter RD. Blindness and severe visual impairment in facial fractures: an 11 year review. Br J Plast Surg 2002; 55: 1.

86. The correct response is C.

The right pupil dilates when torch light is flashed after flashing it on the left side. The pupillary dilatation on exposure to light indicates that the afferent impulses are not being carried by the optic nerve. This phenomenon is called "Marcus Gunn pupillary phenomenon", when pupil on the normal side contracts and the affected side dilates.

Reference:

Anderson RL, Panje WR, Gross CE. Optic nerve blindness following blunt forehead trauma. Ophthalmology 1992; 89: 445.

87. The correct response is C.

The optic foramen is vertically ovoid in shape measuring 6 mm x 5 mm. The ophthalmic artery lies below the optic nerve. The optic foramen is the anterior opening of the optic canal which is about 1 cm in length. The dural sheath is firmly attached to the canal. The ophthalmic vein leaves the eye through the superior oblique fissure.

Reference:

1. *Anderson RL, Panje WR, Gross CE. Optic nerve blindness following blunt forehead trauma. Ophthalmology 1992; 89: 445.*
2. *Manson PN, Illif N. Surgical anatomy of the orbit: In Marsh J ed: Current Therapy in Plastic and Reconstructive Surgery. Philadelphia, BC Decker 1989: 117.*

88. The correct response is E.

Oculomotor nerve does not supply the superior oblique muscle, which is supplied by the trochlear nerve.

Reference:

1. *Anderson RL, Panje WR, Gross CE. Optic nerve blindness following blunt forehead trauma. Ophthalmology 1992; 89: 445.*
2. *Manson PN, Illif N. Surgical anatomy of the orbit: In Marsh J ed: Current Therapy in Plastic and Reconstructive Surgery. Philadelphia , BC Decker, 1989: 117.*

89. The correct response is A.

The frontal bone is the strongest bone of the face requiring 150 g per square inch of force for the production of fracture. This is due to the dense structure of the frontal bone.

Reference:

Swearingen JJ. Tolerances of the human face to crash impact. Report from the office of Aviation Medicine, Federal Aviation Agency, July 1965.

90. The correct response is E.

All of the cranial nerves (III, IV,V,VI) may be involved in frontal lobe injuries if extension of the fracture occurs to the superior orbital fissure. Cranial nerve VII is usually not involved in these injuries.

Reference:

1. *Anderson RL, Panje WR, Gross CE. Optic nerve blindness following blunt forehead trauma. Ophthalmology 1992; 89: 445.*
2. *Manson PN, Illif N. Surgical anatomy of the orbit: In Marsh J ed: Current Therapy in Plastic and Reconstructive Surgery. Philadelphia , BC Decker, 1989: 117.*

91. The correct response is C.

Hot, dry and scaly skin is not a feature of causalgia. The cause for causalgia is not known. The rest of the features are true for causalgia.

Reference:

Crockford DA. Post-traumatic facial pain. In Converse JM, ed: Reconstructive Plastic Surgery, 2nd ed. Philadelphia, WB Saunders, 1977: 741.

92. The correct response is D.

The proportions of the face change markedly during the period of postnatal growth. The ratio of cranium to face size at birth is 8:1, but falls to 4:1 by 5 years of age and reaches 2:1 in the adult.

Reference:

Enlow DH. Handbook of Facial Growth, 2nd ed. Philadelphia, WB Saunders, 1982.

93. The correct response is B.

The lip to trachea distance is an important consideration for pediatric intubation. This distance at one year of age is 10-11 cm.

Reference:

1. *Dufresne CR, Manson PN. Pediatric facial trauma in MaCarthy JG, ed: Plastic Surgery. Philadelphia, WB Saunders, 1990: 1142.*
2. *Lebowitz PW, Newberg LA, Gillette MT et al. Clinical anaesthesia procedures of the Massachusetts General Hospital, Boston, Little Brown, 1982.*

94. The correct response is B.

In breech delivery the neck has a chance to get extended and may get laterally pulled, resulting in injury to the sternocleidomastoid muscle with resultant tear, haematoma and subsequently fibrosis producing torticollis.

Reference:

Roemer FJ. Relation of torticollis to breach delivery. Am J Obstet Gynecol 1954; 68: 1146.

95. The correct response is A.

The condyle of the mandible is more likely to get fractured because of its vascular and trabecular pattern. The neck is small and resilient however after the age of 5 years, the fractures of the neck are more likely because of the neck getting longer and more slender.

Reference:

Lee CY, McCullon C III, Blaustein DI, Mohammadi H. Sequelae of unrecognized, untreated mandibular condylar fractures in the pediatric patient. Ann Dent 1993; 52: 5.

3

96. The correct response is E.

The coronal incision provides wide exposure of frontal and orbital region which is an advantage with this incision. The rest can be considered drawbacks to the coronal incision.

Reference:

Gerbino G, Roccia F, Benech A, Caldarelli C. Analysis of 158 frontal sinus fractures: current surgical management and complications. J Craniomaxillofac Surg 2000; 28: 133.

97. The correct response is A.

The lateral override is a favourable position for endoscopic treatment of subcondylar fractures. In this position, the lateral (proximal fragment) surface of the condylar fracture can be seen easily. In the medial override, the condylar portion, i.e. the proximal fragment lies medial to the ascending ramus.

Reference:

1. *Lindahl L. Condylar fractures of the mandible. IV. Function of the masticatory system. Int J Oral Surg 1977;6: 195-203.*
2. *Lee C, Mueller RV, Lee K, et al. Endoscopic subcondylar fracture repair: functional, aesthetic, and radiographic outcomes. Plast Reconstr Surg 1998; 102: 1434.*

98. The correct response is D.

In lateral override the endoscopic reduction is easy and hence is indicated.

Reference:

1. *Lindahl L. Condylar fractures of the mandible. IV. Function of the masticatory system. Int J Oral Surg 1977;6:195-203.*
2. *Lee C, Mueller RV, Lee K, et al. Endoscopic subcondylar fracture repair: functional, aesthetic, and radiographic outcomes. Plast Reconstr Surg 1998; 102: 1434.*

99. The correct response is C

An intercondylar fracture is an absolute contraindication to endoscopic treatment because these are located within the joint capsule and are thus not amenable to endoscopic repair. The proximal fragment will not afford sufficient room to accommodate at least two screws of the 2.0 plate. The rest are relative contraindications.

Reference:

1. *Haug RH, Assael LA. Outcomes of open versus closed treatment of mandibular subcondylar fractures. J Oral Maxillofac Surg 2001; 59: 370.*
2. *Lee C, Mueller RV, Lee K, et al. Endoscopic subcondylar fracture repair: functional, aesthetic, and radiographic outcomes. Plast Reconstr Surg 1998; 102: 1434.*

100. The correct response is A.

The shape of the condyle is elliptical measuring from 20 mm medial to lateral and 10 mm in anteroposterior.

Reference:

Zide BM. The temporomandibular joint. In McCarthy JG, ed: Plastic Surgery. Philadelphia, WB Saunders, 1990: 1475-1513.

101. The correct response is B.

Geniohyoid does not protrude the mandible. The rest help in elevating or protruding the mandible. The lateral pterygoid muscle has two heads; the transverse head gets attached to the meniscus and stabilizes it during the movement, the inferior head, i.e. oblique portion of the lateral pterygoid is attached to the neck of the condyle and helps to protrude it by acting together with the muscle of the other side.

Reference:

Zide BM. The temporomandibular joint. In McCarthy JG, ed: Plastic Surgery. Philadelphia, WB Saunders, 1990: 1475-1513.

102. The correct response is C.

The measured landmarks for entry to the TMJ have been established. The point of entry is along a line from the tragus to the lateral canthus. The site is 10 mm anterior to the tragus and 2 mm inferior to the line. Use of these landmarks will help prevent complications involving the temporal branch of the facial nerve and the auriculotemporal branch of the trigeminal nerve.

Reference:

1. *McCain JP, Sanders B, Koslin MG et al. Temporomandibular joint arthroscopy. J Oral Maxillofac Surg 1992; 50: 926.*
2. *Holmlund A, Hellsing G. Arthroscopy of the temporomandibular joint. Int J Oral Surg 1985; 14: 169.*

103. The correct response is D.

Extra-articular TMJ ankylosis can be due to enlargement of muscles of mastication, facial nerve or the coronoid process. The common causes of intra-articular ankylosis are trauma, infection and juvenile rheumatoid arthritis.

Reference:

Freedus M, Zitoc W, Doyle P. Principles of treatment for temporomandibular joint ankylosis. J Oral Surg 1975; 33: 757.

104. The correct response is D.

The best results for treatment of ankylosis of the jaw are obtained by the use of costo-chondral arthroplasty. The costochondral graft harvested from the rib is the optimal approach to reconstruction and is the preferred technique. A gap arthroplasty involves removal of bone but leaves a gap and is thus prone to recurrence of ankylosis. Condylectomy alone is not favoured.

Reference:

1. *Munro IR, Chen YR, Park BY. Simultaneous total correction of temporomandibular joint ankylosis and facial asymmetry. Plast Reconstr Surg 1986; 77: 517.*
2. *Gallagher DM, Wolford LM. Comparison of Silastic and Proplast implants in the temporomandibular joint after condylectomy for osteoarthritis. J Oral Maxillofac Surg 1982; 40: 627.*

105. The correct response is D.

The average thickness of skull vault is about 7 mm but has considerable variations and it reduces in the elderly. The thickest bone is occipital and the thinnest is the temporal bone.

Reference:

1. *Pensler J, McCarthy JG. The calvarial donor site: an anatomic study in cadavers. Plast Reconstr Surg 1985; 75: 648.*
2. *Tessier P. Dysostoses cranio-faciales. Transactions of the Fourth International Congress of Plastic and Reconstructive Surgery, Rome, 1967, Amsterdam, Excerpta Medica, 1969.*

106. The correct response is B.

The average thickness of skull vault is about 7 mm but has considerable variations and it reduces in the elderly. The thickest bone is occipital and the thinnest is the temporal bone.

Reference:

1. *Pensler J, McCarthy JG. The calvarial donor site: an anatomic study in cadavers. Plast Reconstr Surg 1985; 75: 648.*
2. *Tessier P. Dysostoses cranio-faciales. Transactions of the Fourth International Congress of Plastic and Reconstructive Surgery, Rome, 1967, Amsterdam, Excerpta Medica, 1969.*

107. The correct response is B.

Split rib grafts are useful when large defects are to be reconstructed. Calvarial bone although lies in the same surgical field is a good source of bone but the amount of bone is limited. The split ribs are usually fitted into a shelf made in the adjacent intact skull and plates can be used for fixation.

Reference:

1. *Munro IR, Guyuron B. Split-rib cranioplasty. Ann Plast Surg 1981;7:341.*
2. *Manson PN, Ruas E, Iliff N et al. Single eyelid incision for exposure of the zygomatic bone and orbital reconstruction. Plast Reconstr Surg 1987; 79: 120.*

108. The correct response is A.

The calvarial bone graft site has the advantage of being painless. All other bone graft sites are painful. The calvarial bone graft site however may have complications such as dural tear with bleeding, CSF leak and meningitis.

Reference:

1. *Pensler J, McCarthy JG. The calvarial donor site: an anatomic study in cadavers. Plast Reconstr Surg 1985; 75: 648.*
2. *Kline RM Jr, Wolfe SA. Complications associated with the harvesting of cranial bone grafts. Plast Reconstr Surg 1995; 95: 5.*

109. The correct response is C.

Hydroxyapatite is a common alloplastic material which is used for cranioplasty. It can either be manufactured synthetically or formed by chemically converting the naturally occurring porous calcium carbonate skeleton of marine coral.

Reference:

1. *Constantino PD, Friedman CD, Jones K et al. Experimental hydroxyapatite cement cranioplasty. Plast Reconstr Surg 1992; 90: 174.*
2. *Burstein FD, Cohen SR, Hudgins R et al. The use of hydroxyapatite cement in secondary craniofacial reconstruction. Plast Reconstr Surg 1999; 104: 1270.*

110. The correct response is E.

The omental free flap fits the bill. It has rich, interconnecting vascular network which allows it to conform to almost any three dimensional wound requirement and provides both coverage and dead space obliteration. This flap also has an extremely long vascular pedicle that can easily reach the neck vessels for purpose of microvascular anastomosis.

Reference:

1. *Barrow DL, Nahai F, Tindall GT. The use of the greater omentum vascularised free flaps for neurosurgical disorders requiring reconstruction. J Neurosurg 1984; 60: 305.*
2. *Thomson JG, Restifo RJ. Microsurgery for cranial base tumours. Clin Plast Surg 1995; 22: 563.*

111. The correct response is D.

Cranial bone defects in children younger than 2 years or so heal by themselves and do not require bone grafting. The bone grafts are useful in later age groups. Alloplastic materials are not preferred for children and if necessary are reserved for use in resurfacing minor surface irregularities.

Reference:

Wolfe SA. Cranial defects. In Wolfe SA, Berkowitz S. Plastic Surgery of the facial skeleton. Boston, Little Brown, 1989: 692.

112. The correct response is C.

The preferred area for obtaining cranial grafts is from the right parietal bone in left handed patients. The parietal bone is the thickest having good width of the diploe and in right handed patients the left hemisphere is dominant hence the contralateral parietal bone should be chosen depending upon the hand dominance.

Reference:

Pensler J, McCarthy JG. The calvarial donor site: an anatomic study in cadavers. Plast Reconstr Surg 1985; 75: 648.

113. The correct response is D.

Cranial defects can be managed using either autogenous bone or alloplastic materials. Defects that are small and are away from the frontal sinus can be treated with alloplastic materials, however for defects near the frontal sinus, autogenous bone is the preferred method of treatment.

Reference:

Wolfe SA, Johnson P. Frontal sinus injuries: primary care and management of late complications. Plast Reconstr Surg 1988; 82: 781.

114. The correct response is D.

The temporalis flap is a reliable and suitable pedicled flap for closing hemimaxillary type of palatal defects. The temporalis muscle needs to be mobilised well and the zygomatic arch may also require removal to facilitate tension free entry of this muscle to fill up the defect. Forehead flap, deltopectoral flap and pectoralis major flaps are not the flaps of choice for such defects. The facial artery musculomucosal flap is good for small defects of the palate.

Reference:

Wolfe SA. Use of temporalis muscle for closure of palatal defects. Presented at 66th Annual meeting of American Association of Plastic Surgeons, Nashville, Tenn, May 3-6, 1987.

115. The correct response is E.

Upward slanting of the lateral canthus would not be seen in zygomatic fractures. On the contrary if lateral canthal detachment occurs then the slanting occurs in the downward direction.

Reference:

Wolfe SA. Application of craniofacial surgical precepts in orbital reconstruction following trauma and tumor removal. J Maxillofac Surg 1982;10:212.

116. The correct response is A.

Enophthalmos occurs commonly due to the herniation of orbital contents through the inferior wall and also the medial wall. Treatment includes reconstruction of the continuity of the wall along with repositing back the displaced structures.

Reference:

1. *Wolfe SA. Posttraumatic orbital deformities. In Wolfe SA, Berkowitz S: Plastic Surgery of the Facial Skeleton. Boston, Little, Brown, 1989: 572-624.*
2. *Wolfe SA. Correction of a lower eyelid deformity caused by multiple extrusions of alloplastic orbital floor implants. Plast Reconstr Surg 1981; 68: 429.*

117. The correct response is B.

The scalp is not supplied by the facial artery. It is supplied by supraorbital and supratrochlear arteries which are terminal branches of the internal carotid artery on the anterior side and the forehead. The superficial temporal, postauricular and occipital artery are branches of external carotid artery and supply the lateral and posterior aspects of the scalp.

Reference:

Tremolada C, Candiani P, Signorini M, et al. The surgical anatomy of the subcutaneous facial system of the scalp. Ann Plast Surg 1994; 32: 8-14.

118. The correct response is A.

The scalp has a rich vascular plexus of arteries which are interconnected with each other so that replantation of the entire scalp based on a single donor vessel can be done. The lymphatic network of the scalp is unique in that there are no lymph nodes and therefore no barriers to lymphatic flow. Skin cancers of the scalp tend to spread by local extension rather than through lymphatic or vascular channels.

Reference:

1. *Tremolada C, Candiani P, Signorini M, et al. The surgical anatomy of the subcutaneous facial system of the scalp. Ann Plast Surg 1994; 32: 8-14.*
2. *Minor LB, Panje WR. Malignant neoplasms of the scalp. Etiology, resection and reconstruction. Otolaryngol Clin North Am 1993; 26: 279-293.*

119. The correct response is A

The crane principle can be used for treating avulsive skin losses. A local flap needs to be transferred onto the defect. Several weeks later the flap is elevated leaving behind a cuff of tissue over the defect which can be resurfaced by a graft. The flap can be put back to its original place. The other options are not indications for using the crane principle.

Reference:

1. *Millard DR. The crane principle for the transport of subcutaneous tissue. Plast Reconstr Surg 1969; 43: 451-462.*
2. *Terkonda RP, Sykes JM. Concepts in scalp and forehead reconstruction. Otolaryngol Clin North Am 1997; 30: 519-539.*

120. The correct response is B.

The growth of a normal hair on the scalp is less than 1 mm per day. It is about 0.35 mm per day, which means that hair would grow by about 1 cm in a month's time. This rate however can be affected by age, nutrition, pregnancy and environmental factors.

Reference:

Sawaya ME. Regulation of the human hair cycle. Curr Probl Dermatol 2001; 13: 206-210.

121. The correct response is A.

The laser therapy is effective in the anagen phase which is the growth phase of the hair cycle.

Reference:

Courtois M, Loussouarn G, Hourseau C, et al. Hair cycle and alopecia. Skin Pharmacol 1994; 7:84-89.

122. The correct response is E.

Type VII is unsuitable for hair transplantation because only a frill of hairs are present which are inadequate to serve as donor hairs for transplantation. The other categories are as follows: Type I-Mild frontal recession;Type II- Fronto-temporal recession reaching upto the coronal plane;Type III- Vertex-Fronto-temporal recession and balding of the vertex;Type IV-Type III + vertex balding;Type V- Fronto - temporal recession and vertex balding are still separate. There is a bridge of hairs in between. Type VI- Bridge of hairs between frontal region and vertex is lost;Type VII-Frontal, vertex and occipital baldness. Only a frill of hairs is presents in the occipital region which extends from one ear to the other.

Reference:

Norwood OT. Male pattern baldness: classification and incidence. South Med J 1975; 68: 1359-1365.

123. The correct response is D.

The follicular hair transplantation is the current state of the art technique for hair transplantation which gives the best results. Temporo-parietal occipital strip grafts and the rest of the techniques have donor site morbidity. Tissue expansion is a multistaged procedure.

Reference:

Unger WP. The history of hair transplantation. Dermatol Surg 2000; 26: 181-189.

124. The correct response is A.

The punch graft technique gives rise to the "doll's hair" look which is often obvious in the frontal hairline.

The follicular hair transplantation is the current state of the art technique for hair transplantation which gives the best results. Temporo-parietal occipital strip grafts and the rest of the techniques have donor site morbidity. Tissue expansion is a multistaged procedure.

Reference:

1. *Unger WP. The history of hair transplantation. Dermatol Surg 2000; 26: 181-189.*
2. *Stough D, Whitworth JM. Methodology of follicular unit hair transplantation. Dermatol Clin 1999; 17: 297-306.*

125. The correct response is C.

The transplanted hairs do fall off and then regrowth takes place after about 10-12 weeks of initial transplantation. The other options are incorrect. The transplanted hairs do not multiply and they also do not stimulate the adjacent hair follicles into growing more hairs.

Reference:

1. *Unger WP. The history of hair transplantation. Dermatol Surg 2000; 26: 181-189.*
2. *Stough D, Whitworth JM. Methodology of follicular unit hair transplantation. Dermatol Clin 1999; 17: 297-306.*

126. The correct response is D.

The best results for auricular reconstruction can only be produced by autogenous costal cartilage framework. Maternal cartilage resorbs in due course of time. Silastic ears run a high risk of extrusion. Diced cartilage does not give good results because of the overgrowth of fibrous tissue around the diced cartilage graft moulds and transferring these moulds from their donor site to the ear as free grafts also does not give the desired shape and contours.

Reference:

Brent B. Auricular repair with autogenous rib cartilage grafts: two decades of experience with 600 cases. Plast Reconstr Surg 1992; 90: 355.

127. The correct response is D.

The cough reflex is produced by the sensory impulses which are carried by auricular branches of the vagus nerve. The afferents so carried are responsible for producing this reflex.

Reference:

Standring S. Gray's Anatomy. The anatomical basis of clinical practice. 39th ed. Elsevier, Churchill Livingstone, 2005: 674.

128. The correct response is C.

The Nagata technique uses the maximum amount of costal cartilage in the design of framework as compared to the other existing techniques of ear reconstruction.

Reference:

Nagata S. Modification of the stages in total reconstruction of the auricle. Plast Reconstr Surg 1994; 93: 221.

129. The correct response is E.

Agarwal described the use of interpositional conchal cartilage graft in the ear lobe to prevent recurrence. The conchal cartilage graft also allows simultaneous reperforation of the ear lobe in the same sitting.

Reference:

Agarwal R, Chandra R. A new technique for repair of acquired split-ear-lobe deformity: the free conchal cartilage sandwich graft. J Plast Recon Aesth Surg. 2010; 63, 499-505.

130. The correct response is C.

The cauliflower ear is common in pugilists and it occurs due to direct blow to the ear causing a haemorrhage. The blood collects between the perichondrium and the cartilage producing a clot that organises and distorts the ear.

Reference:

Tanzer RC. Total reconstruction of the external ear. Plast Reconstr Surg 1959; 23: 1.

131. The correct response is C.

Cryptotia is a congenital deformity in which the upper pole of the ear cartilage is buried beneath the scalp. The superior auriculocephalic sulcus is hence absent but can be demonstrated by gentle finger pressure.

It is present in the rest of the conditions.

Constricted ear is characterised by deformity of helical and scaphal hooding due to tight encircling helix.

Reference:

1. *Matsumoto K. The characteristics of cryptotia and its therapy. Jpn J Plast Reconstr Surg 1977; 20: 563.*
2. *Ohmori S, Matsumoto K. Treatment of cryptotia, using Teflon string. Plast Reconstr Surg 1972; 49-33.*

132. The correct response is D.

Prominent ear deformity is due to failure of antihelix to fold leading to a widened conchoscaphal angle as much as 150 degrees. The normal values are 90 degrees.

Reference:

1. *McDowell AJ. Goals in otoplasty for protruding ears. Plast Reconstr Surg 1968; 42: 189.*
2. *Straith RE. Correction of the protruding ear. Plast Reconstr Surg 1959; 24: 277.*

133. The correct response is C.

Worthen flap is a large rotation flap which extends across the width of the forehead to close a lateral forehead or suprabrow defect. The rest of the options are incorrect.

Reference:

Worthen EF. Repair of forehead defects by rotation of local flaps. Plast Reconstr Surg 1976; 57: 204-206.

134. The correct response is D.

Reconstruction of partial eyebrow defects can be accomplished using local flaps. The transverse advancement flap, V-Y advancement flap, double Z rhombic flap and pedicled scalp flap are all viable and justifiable options. The use of contralateral eyebrow is rarely justified for partial eyebrow defects due to donor site deformity.

Reference:

1. *McConnell CM, Neale HW. Eyebrow reconstruction in the burn patient. J Trauma 1977; 17: 362-366.*
2. *Kasai K, Ogawa Y. Partial eyebrow reconstruction using subcutaneous pedicle flaps to preserve the natural hair direction. Ann Plast Surg 1990; 24: 117-125.*

135. The correct response is A.

Reconstruction of eyelid defects of less than 25% of the upper eyelid, can be done using a lateral canthotomy which allows satisfactory closure of the eyelid. For defects greater than this the options listed from B to E are reasonable and justifiable.

Reference:

Mustarde JC. Reconstruction of the upper lid. In Mustarde JC: Repair and Reconstruction in the Orbital Region, 3rd ed. Edinburgh, Churchill Livingstone 1991: 191-327.

136. The correct response is D.

The forehead flap is the only option that can be used for resurfacing total eyelid defects of both the lids. Lateral canthotomy is good for closing defects less than 25% of the lid. Mustarde, Tessier's flap and Tenzel flap are good for closing defects more than 25% of the lid but these cannot cover total defects of both the lids.

Reference:

Mustarde JC. Reconstruction of the upper lid. In Mustarde JC: Repair and Reconstruction in the Orbital Region, 3rd ed. Edinburgh, Churchill Livingstone 1991: 191-327.

137. The correct response is A.

Reconstruction of eyelid defects of less than 25% of the lower eyelid, can be done using a lateral canthotomy which allows satisfactory closure of the eyelid. For defects greater than this the options listed from B to E are reasonable and justifiable.

Reference:

Mustarde JC. Reconstruction of the upper lid. In Mustarde JC: Repair and Reconstruction in the Orbital Region, 3rd ed. Edinburgh, Churchill Livingstone 1991: 191-327.

138. The correct response is E.

The use of gold weight is a time honoured and effective method for treating poor lid closure in patients with facial palsy. Commercially available gold weights come in 5 gm to 15 gm sizes and the best way is to suture the gold weight to the midportion of the tarsal plate.

Reference:

Jobe R. Lid loading with gold for upper lid paralysis. Plast Reconstr Surg 2000; 106: 735-736.

139. The correct response is D.

The classical presentation of the patient with bilateral choanal atresia is with cyanosis that is improved on crying. This indicates a nasal obstruction and crying facilitates augmented air entry by the mouth and improves the cyanosis. Cyanosis caused by other conditions does not improve with crying.

Reference:

1. *Tellier AL, Cormier-Daire V, Abadie V, et al. CHARGE syndrome: report of 47 cases and review. Am J Med Genet 1998; 76: 402-409.*
2. *Keller JL, Kacker A. Choanal atresia, CHARGE association, and congenital nasal stenosis. Otolaryngol Clin North Am 2000; 33: 1343-1351.*

140. The correct response is C.

Barking cough is a characteristic feature of subglottic stenosis. It is a congenital anomaly in which there is a deformed and diminutive cricoid cartilage. The patient has difficulty in inspiration and a characteristic barking sound is produced on coughing.

It is not observed in other disease conditions listed in the options.

Reference:

Milczuk HA, Smith JD, Everts EC. Congenital laryngeal webs: surgical management and clinical embryology. Int J Pediatr Otolaryngol 2000; 52(1): 1-9.

141. The correct response is E.

Left ventricular hypertrophy is not a feature of sleep apnea. It is the right ventricular hypertrophy which develops in patients of sleep apnea due to poor oxygenation, increased pulmonary artery pressure which subsequently leads to right ventricular hypertrophy.

Reference:

Wlaker RP. Snoring and obstructive sleep apnea. In Bailey BJ, Calhoun KH, Derkay CS, et al eds: Head and Neck Surgery-Otolryngology, vol 1, 3rd ed. Philadelphia, Lippincott Williams and Wilkins, 2001: 579-597.

142. The correct response is D.

Sleep apnoea is diagnosed when there are more than 30 apnoeas per night with each of these apnoea lasting for more than 10 seconds and accompanied by a cardiac arrhythmia.

Reference:

1. *Walker RP. Snoring and obstructive sleep apnea. In Bailey BJ, Calhoun KH, Derkay CS, et al, eds: Head and Neck Surgery-Otolryngology, vol 1, 3rd ed. Philadelphia, Lippincott Williams and Wilkins, 2001: 579-597.*
2. *Meoli AL, Casey KR, Clark RW et al. Hypopnoea in sleep disordered breathing in adults.Sleep 2001; 24: 469-470.*

143. The correct response is D.

BPAP or bilevel positive airway pressure has been the most successful medical modality for the management of sleep apnoea and has taken over the usefulness of CPAP. The patient wears a mask strapped to the face and appropriate airway pressure is determined which holds the hypopharynx open and relieves obstructed breathing.

Reference:

1. *Walker RP. Snoring and obstructive sleep apnea. In Bailey BJ, Calhoun KH, Derkay CS, et al, eds: Head and Neck Surgery- Otolaryngology, vol 1, 3rd ed. Philadelphia, Lippincott Williams and Wilkins, 2001: 579-597.*
2. *Meoli AL, Casey KR, Clark RW et al. Hypopnoea in sleep disordered breathing in adults. Sleep 2001; 24: 469-470.*

144. The correct response is E.

The aim of surgical treatment of sleep apnoea is to correct the anatomic obstruction. All the procedures listed help to achieve this aim to a certain extent but the gold standard for treatment of sleep apnoea is tracheostomy.

Reference:

1. *Walker RP. Snoring and obstructive sleep apnea. In Bailey BJ, Calhoun KH, Derkay CS, et al, eds: Head and Neck Surgery-Otolryngology, vol 1, 3rd ed. Philadelphia, Lippincott Williams and Wilkins, 2001: 579-597.*
2. *Fujita S, Conway W, Zorick F, et al. Surgical correction of anatomic abnormalities in obstructive sleep apnea syndrome: uvulopalatopharyngoplasty. Otolaryngol Head Neck Surg 1981; 89: 923.*

145. The correct response is C.

Defects of up to 30% of the upper or lower lip can be closed primarily. This is possible due to the elasticity of the lip. Defects more than 30% size require additional tissue from the normal lip to reconstruct the deformity.

Reference:

1. *Constantinis J, Federspiel P, Iro H. Functional and aesthetic objectives in the lip reconstruction. Facial Plast Surg 1999; 15: 337.*
2. *Lesavoy MA. Lip deformities and their reconstruction. In Lesavoy MA, ed: Reconstruction of the Head and Neck. Baltimore, Williams and Wilkins, 1981: 95.*

146. The correct response is B.

The Abbe flap from the lower lip based on the labial artery is the flap of choice for central upper lip defects. Estlander flap is a transposition flap from the upper lip and is used for defects of the lateral lower lip. Gillies fan flap is an extension of the Estlander flap and is for upper lip defects. Schuchardt procedure is used for reconstruction of the labiomental region.

Reference:

1. *Karapandzic M. Reconstruction of lip defects by local arterial flaps. Br J Plast Surg 1974; 27: 93.*
2. *Abbe RA. A new plastic operation for the relief of deformity due to double harelip. The classic reprint. Plast Reconstr Surg 1968; 42: 481.*

147. The correct response is E.

The Schuchardt procedure is used for reconstruction of the labiomental region for defects of upto two thirds of the lower lip. The Abbe flap from the lower lip based on the labial artery is the flap of choice for central upper lip defects. Estlander flap is a transposition flap from the upper lip and is used for defects of the lateral lower lip. Gillies fan flap is an extension of the Estlander flap and is for upper lip defects.

Reference:

1. *Karapandzic M. Reconstruction of lip defects by local arterial flaps. Br J Plast Surg 1974; 27:93.*
2. *Abbe RA. A new plastic operation for the relief of deformity due to double harelip. The classic reprint. Plast Reconstr Surg 1968; 42: 481.*

148. The correct response is D.

The witch's chin is characterised by ptosis of the premental soft tissues, a prominent submental crease and often a loss of chin projection. The other options listed are not seen in this deformity. Repair is by use of anteriorly based de-epithelialized triangular flaps buried posteriorly in a subcutaneous pocket.

Reference:

Lesavoy ML, Creasman C, Schwartz RJ. A technique for correcting witch's chin deformity. Plast Reconstr Surg 1996; 97: 842.

149. The correct response is D.

The Limberg flap is suitable for use in rhomboidal defects with a small angle of about 60°. A number of Limberg flaps can be fashioned around a defect and the best flap is chosen depending upon the presence of skin laxity around the defect.

Reference:

Mullin WR. Surgery of the forehead and cheek regions. In Lesavoy MA, ed: Reconstruction of the Head and Neck. Baltimore, Williams and Wilkins, 1981: 29.

150. The correct response is B.

The latissimus dorsi muscle flap with the thoracodorsal nerve and vessels can be used to treat such cases. The nerve is taken to the other side of the face through the upper lip and anastomosed to branches of the facial nerve. The vessels are anastomosed to branches of the facial artery on the same side. The muscle, an average of 3 cm × 8 cm is taken from the latissimus dorsi.

Reference:

Harii K, Asato H, Yoshimura K, et al. One-stage transfer of the latissimus dorsi muscle for reanimation of paralysed face: a new alternative. Plast Reconstr Surg 1998; 102: 942.

151. The correct response is C.

The infraorbital nerve traverses through the floor of the orbit to emerge through the infraorbital foramen. Fracture of the floor of the orbit and the infraorbital margin is likely to damage the infraorbital nerve and cause anaesthesia in its distribution.

Reference:

Standring S. Gray's Anatomy. The anatomical basis of clinical practice. 39th ed. Elsevier, Churchill Livingstone, 2005: 478.

152. The correct response is B.

The orbicularis oris is the only unpaired muscle of facial expression. There are a total of 17 paired muscles in the human face which work in synergy to produce the various facial expressions.

Reference:

McLaughlin CR. Surgical support in permanent facial paralysis. Plast Reconstr Surg 1953; 11: 302.

153. The correct response is C.

The 'Mobius syndrome' is characterised by bilateral facial palsy which is congenital. The rest of the options are incorrect.

Reference:

Falco NA, Eriksson E. Facial nerve palsy in the newborn: incidence and outcome. Plast Reconstr Surg 1990; 85:1.

154. The correct response is C.

The numbers of paired muscles are seventeen (17). In all, there are thirty five (35) in the face for various movements and expressions of the face. The names of the facial muscles according to the facial regions are - Forehead (3): Frontalis, procerus, corrugator supercilli; Nose (3): Dilator nares, compressor nares, depressor nasii; Eyes (1): Orbicularis oculi;Lips (3): Levator labii superioris, alaequae nasii and levator anguli oris. Mouth (2) paired: Zygomaticus minor and zygomaticus major, orbicularis oris (unpaired); Cheek (2): Risorius and buccinator. Lower lip (3) Depressor anguli oris, depressor labii inferioris and mentalis.

Reference:

McLaughlin CR. Surgical support in permanent facial paralysis. Plast Reconstr Surg 1953; 11: 302.

155. The correct response is E.

All of the above measures are helpful in the management of lagophthalmos.

Reference:

Salimbeni G: Eyelid reanimation in facial paralysis by temporalis muscle transfer. Operative Techniques Plast Reconstr Surg 1999; 6: 159.

156. The correct response is E.

All of the above are useful in the management of lower eyelid ectropion.

Reference:

Jelk GW, Glat PM, Jelks EB, et al. Evolution of the lateral canthoplasty: technique and indications. Plast Reconstr Surg 1997; 100: 1396.

157. The correct response is E.

All of the above modalities are useful in the reanimation of the upper lip in facial paralysis. Temporalis and masseter muscles can be used with the help of tendon or facial slings to balance the upper lip and elevate the commissure up in cases of facial paralysis with good results. Microneurovascular anastomosis gives good results in expert hands. Use of static slings is not very helpful. Rhytidectomy only partially helps in the treatment of facial palsy.

Reference:

Terzis JK, Kalantarian B. Microsurgical strategies in 74 patients for restoration of dynamic depressor muscle mechanism. Plast Reconstr Surg 2000; 105: 1917.

158. The correct response is C.

The paralysis of the buccinator causes pocketing of the food in the buccal sulcus. It also expels air from the oral cavity like a trumpeteer. The buccinator muscle arises from the:

1. Alveolar processes of maxilla and mandible
2. Pterygomandibular raphe
3. Pterygoid hamulus

It gets inserted into the orbicularis oris. It gets its nerve supply from the lower buccal branches of the facial nerve.

Reference:

Standring S. Gray's Anatomy. The anatomical basis of clinical practice. 39th ed. Elsevier, Churchill Livingstone, 2005: 505.

159. The correct response is A.

Palatopharyngeal muscle fibres of superior constrictor lie in the Passavant's ridge. The superior constrictor has four parts, i.e. pterygopharyngeal, buccopharyngeal, mylopharyngeal and glossopharyngeal. It arises from-

1 Pterygoid hamulus
2. Medial pterygoid plate
3. Pterygomandibular raphe
4. Mylohyoid line
5. Side of tongue
6. Palatine aponeurosis

The Passavant's ridge becomes more prominent in cases of cleft palate.

Reference:

Standring S. Gray's Anatomy. The anatomical basis of clinical practice. 39th ed. Elsevier, Churchill Livingstone, 2005: 628.

160. The correct response is C.

The nerve to the masseter which is a branch of the 5th nerve is normal in patients with bilateral facial nerve paralysis. It runs on the undersurface of the muscle and enters this surface of the muscle belly approximately 2 cm below the zygomatic arch. The other options are incorrect.

Reference:

Zuker RM, Goldberg CS, Manktelow RT. Facial animation in children with Moebius syndrome after segmental gracilis muscle transplant. Plast Reconstr Surg 2000; 106: 1.

161. The correct response is B.

The Stensen's duct opens opposite the second molar tooth in the upper buccal sulcus. The other options are incorrect.

Reference:

Stringer SP. Flaps and grafts for reconstruction. In Million RR, Cassisi NJ, eds: Management of Head and Neck Cancer: A Multidisciplinary approach, 2nd ed. Philadelphia, JB Lippincott, 1994: 157.

162. The correct response is B.

The thoracoacromial artery descends down between the pectoralis major and minor muscles and then enters the under surface of the pectoralis major muscle. Its pectoral branch lies along a line joining the tip of the shoulder with the xiphisternum.

Reference:

Ariyan S. Further experiences with the pectoralis major myocutaneous flap for the immediate repair of defects from excisions of head and neck cancer. Plast Reconstr Surg 1979; 64: 605.

163. The correct response is E.

The rectus abdominis myocutaneous flap does not carry its nerve supply with it. The muscle atrophies in due course of time (3-6 months). Thus sensory neurotisation of the skin paddle is difficult due to the muscle's multisegmental innervation.

Reference:

Evans GR. The rectus abdominis flap. In Evans GR, ed: Operative Plastic Surgery. New York, McGraw-Hill, 2000: 362.

164. The correct response is C.

The lateral thigh flap is a fasciocutaneous flap based on the third perforator of the profunda femoris artery. The axis of this flap lies along a line drawn from the greater trochanter to the lateral condyle of the femur. This line corresponds to the lateral intermuscular septum. The calibre of this vessel ranges from 1.5 to 2.5 mm.

Reference:

1. *Baek SM. Two new cutaneous free flaps: the medial and lateral thigh flaps. Plast Reconstr Surg 1983; 71: 354.*
2. *Hayden RE. Lateral thigh flap. Otolaryngol Clin North Am 1994; 27: 1171.*

165. The correct response is A.

The improvement in microvascular techniques has opened innumerable possibilities and success for vascularized mandibular reconstruction, however the indications of nonvascularised mandibular reconstruction include small defects including the ramus or the body of the mandible, bone-only defects, defects not requiring soft tissue reconstruction and defects resulting from treatment of mandibular fracture nonunions.

Reference:

1. *Eppley BL. Nonvascularised methods of mandible reconstruction. Operative Techniques Plast Reconstr Surg 1996; 3: 226.*
2. *Duncan MJ, Manktelow RT, Zuker RM et al. Mandibular reconstruction in the irradiated patient: the role of osteocutaneous free tissue transfer. Plast Reconstr Surg 1985; 76: 829.*

166. The correct response is C.

The fibula will provide good amount of bone about 20-25 cm for mandibular reconstruction, for lateral and /or central defects. It has a segmental blood supply. It can be osteotomised and can be bent to conform to the shape of the mandible.

Reference:

Hidalgo DA. Free flap mandibular reconstruction. Clin Plast Surg 1994; 21: 25.

167. The correct response is A.

The use of the ilium on deep circumflex iliac artery provides bone of maximum thickness and height and is second only to the fibula in the amount of usable length. This flap accommodates osseointegrated implants easily and the intrinsic shape of the ilium resembles that of the hemi-mandible.

Reference:

Taylor GI, Townsend P, Corlett R. Superiority of the deep circumflex iliac vessels as the supply for free groin flaps. Plast Reconstr Surg 1979; 64: 745.

168. The correct response is B.

The radial forearm donor site allows about 10 cm of bone length with 40% of its circumference. The thickness of bone is limited to one cortex because at least 60% of its circumference must remain intact to prevent postoperative fracture.

Reference:

1. *Soutar D, SchekerL, Tanner N et al. The radial forearm flap: a versatile method for intraoral reconstruction. Br J Plast Surg 1983; 36: 1.*
2. *Mathes SJ, Nahai F. Reconstructive Surgery: principles, anatomy, and technique. New York, Churchill Livingstone, 1997: 658, 659.*

169. The correct response is C.

The lateral femoral cutaneous nerve is the one most likely to be damaged especially during harvest of large portions of the iliac crest graft.

Reference:

1. *Shpitzer T, Neligan P et al. The free iliac crest and fibula flaps in vascularised oromandibular reconstruction: comparison and long-term evaluation. Head Neck 1999; 21: 639.*
2. *Mathes SJ, Nahai F. Reconstructive Surgery: principles, anatomy, and technique. New York, Churchill Livingstone, 1997: 658, 659.*

170. The correct response is E.

All of the above flaps can be used for pharyngo-esophageal reconstruction. Each of these have their own advantages and disadvantages which should be weighed when choosing an appropriate flap for a given defect.

Reference:

1. *Fabian RL. Pectoralis major myocutaneous flap reconstruction of the laryngopharynx and cervical esophagus. Laryngoscope 1988; 98: 1227.*
2. *Mathes SJ, Nahai F. Reconstructive Surgery: principles, anatomy, and technique. New York, Churchill Livingstone, 1997: 658, 659.*

171. The correct response is C.

Colonic transfer has been used for pharyngo-esophageal reconstruction when total esophagectomy has been performed. The ideal method of transposition is through the posterior mediastinum but substernal and even subcutaneous routes have been described.

Reference:

1. *Schusterman MA, Shestak K, deVries EJ et al. Reconstruction of the cervical esophagus: free jejunal transfer versus gastric pull-up. Plast Reconstr Surg 1990; 85: 16.*
2. *Mathes SJ, Nahai F. Reconstructive Surgery: principles, anatomy, and technique. New York, Churchill Livingstone, 1997: 658, 659.*

172. The correct response is E.

All of the above findings may be present in torticollis. A tilted head may cause field disturbances along with deformation of the cranium and jaws. A double Z-plasty at the upper and the lower end of the muscle gives very good and desirable results.

Reference:

Cheng JC, Au AW. Infantile torticollis: a review of 624 cases. J Pediatr Orthop 1994; 14: 802.

173. The correct response is B.

The Platysma flap is based on the submental artery as the dominant pedicle and the suprasternal artery as the minor pedicle. It is useful for defects of the lower face, anterior neck and for intraoral reconstruction.

Reference:

1. *Mathes SJ, Nahai F. Reconstructive Surgery: principles, anatomy and technique. New York, Churchill Livingstone, 1997: 658, 659.*
2. *Hurwitz DJ, Rabson JA, Futrell JW. The anatomic basis for the platsyma skin flap. Plast Reconstr Surg 1983; 72: 302.*

174. The correct response is D.

The trapezius musculocutaneous flap can be easily rotated to cover the defects of the nape of the neck.

Reference:

1. *Mathes SJ, Nahai F. Reconstructive Surgery: principles, anatomy and technique. New York, Churchill Livingstone, 1997: 658, 659.*
2. *Ugurlu K, Ozcelik D, Huthut I, et al. Extended vertical trapezius myocutaneous flap in head and neck reconstruction as a salvage procedure. Plast Reconstr Surg 2004; 114: 339.*

175. The correct response is E.

The vertical trapezius flap for head and neck reconstruction is based on the transverse cervical artery as its dominant blood supply. The minor pedicle consists of branches of occipital artery and the intercostal arteries.

Reference:

1. *Mathes SJ, Nahai F. Reconstructive Surgery: principles, anatomy and technique. New York, Churchill Livingstone, 1997: 658, 659.*
2. *Panje W. Myocutaneous trapezius flap. Head Neck Surg 1980; 2: 206.*

176. The correct response is D.

The pulsed dye laser is specifically designed for vascular lesions with a wavelength of 585 nm. It provides selective photothermolysis without unwanted thermal damage and can be used in patients with light and dark skin tones. The target chromophore for this capillary malformation is oxyhemoglobin in the ectatic vessels within the dermis. The three primary absorption peaks are 418 nm, 542 nm, and 577 nm.

The KTP laser has a wavelength of 532 nm. It does work well with telangiectasias however it has decreased tissue penetration and is not as effective as the pulsed-dye laser in treatment of vascular malformations. The erbium:YAG (2490-nm) and Q-switched ruby (694-nm) lasers are not targeting the oxyhemoglobin chromophore and are used in other cutaneous applications.The argon-pumped tunable dye laser can be used to treat capillary malformations. However, it causes nonspecific thermal damage with higher incidences of hypertrophic scarring, textural changes, and dyspigmentation.

References:

1. *Achauer BM. Lasers in plastic surgery: current practice. Plast Reconstr Surg. 1997; 99: 1442-1450.*
2. *Lam SM. Practical considerations in the treatment of capillary vascular malformations or port wine stains. Facial Plast Surg. 2004; 20: 71-76.*

177. The correct response is D.

The ptosis is best managed by a frontalis suspension procedure. It is generally agreed that the fascia lata is the material of choice for the sling. Alloplastic materials, such as silicone slings, can also be used but have a risk of extrusion and infection. The advantage of alloplastic sling reconstruction is that there are no risks to the donor site.

The Fasanella-Servat procedure involves excision of a portion of the conjunctiva, tarsus, orbital septum, levator aponeurosis, and Müller muscle. It can be used in cases of mild ptosis (1-2 mm). Levator function must be present. The Kuhnt-Szymanowski procedure is used to correct lower eyelid ectropion. It involves a wedge excision of the lower eyelid.

Levator advancement surgery could possibly be used in this case if, during exploration of the eyelid, the levator was noted to be present and not compromised by scar. However, in this case the levator mechanism was likely excised in the process of debriding the wound tract and inflammatory tissue. Therefore, in light of the degree of ptosis, the noted limited elevation of the upper eyelid, and the mechanism of injury, frontalis suspension is a better choice for ptosis repair in this patient.

Reference:

1. *Finsterer J. Ptosis: causes, presentation, and management. Aesthetic Plast Surg. 2003; 27: 193-204.*
2. *Iliff JW, Pacheco EM. Ptosis surgery. In: Tasman W, Jaeger EA, eds. Duane's Clinical Ophthalmology. Philadelphia: Lippincott Williams and Wilkins; 2001: 1-18.*

4

CRANIOFACIAL AND CLEFT

QUESTIONS

1. **The face develops from the five branchial arches during the fourth to eighth weeks of development. The maxilla and mandible develop from which one of the following arches?**
   A. First branchial arch
   B. Second branchial arch
   C. Third branchial arch
   D. Fourth branchial arch
   E. Fifth branchial arch

2. **The neurocranium is composed of two parts, cartilaginous neurocranium and the membranous neurocranium. Which one of the following bones is a part of the cartilaginous neurocranium?**
   A. Petrous temporal bone
   B. Frontal bone
   C. Squamosal bone
   D. Parietal bone
   E. Occipital bone

3. **The neurocranium is composed of two parts, cartilaginous neurocranium and the membranous neurocranium. Which one of the following bones is a part of the membranous neurocranium?**
   A. Sphenoid
   B. Ethmoid bone
   C. Squamosal bone
   D. Petrous temporal
   E. Base of occipital bone

4. **Which one of the following bones is a part of the viscerocranium?**
   A. Petrous temporal bone
   B. Frontal bone
   C. Maxilla
   D. Parietal bone
   E. Occipital bone

5. **Tessier classified craniofacial clefts bearing numbers zero to fourteen. This classification has been based on which one of the following reference point?**
   A. Ear
   B. Nose
   C. Orbit
   D. Mouth
   E. A line joining the lateral canthus of the eye to the tragus of ear

6. **Which one of the following Tessier cleft is the most laterally placed on the face?**
   A. Number 6 cleft
   B. Number 7 cleft
   C. Number 8 cleft
   D. Number 9 cleft
   E. Number 10 cleft

7. **The most common craniofacial cleft also known as otomandibular dysostosis is which one of the following?**
   A. Number 6 cleft
   B. Number 7 cleft
   C. Number 8 cleft
   D. Number 9 cleft
   E. Number 10 cleft

8. Treacher Collins syndrome characterised by clefting in the maxillozygomatic, temporozygomatic and frontozygomatic regions is a combined manifestation of which one of the following clefts?

A. Number 5, 6 and 7 clefts
B. Number 6, 7 and 8 clefts
C. Number 7, 8 and 9 clefts
D. Number 8, 9, 10 and 11 clefts
E. Number 9, 10, 11 and 12 clefts

9. Orbital hypertelorism is commonly associated with facial clefting. Which one of the following cranial clefts may be associated with hypotelorism?

A. Number 10 cleft
B. Number 11 cleft
C. Number 12 cleft
D. Number 13 cleft
E. Number 14 cleft

10. Tessier cleft number 30 is a cleft affecting the:

A. Nose
B. Upper lip
C. Lower lip
D. Lateral canthus
E. Oral commissure

11. Which one of the following is the cleft that passes through the Cupid's bow and alar cartilage dome resembling the common cleft lip?

A. Number 0 cleft
B. Number 1 cleft
C. Number 2 cleft
D. Number 3 cleft
E. Number 4 cleft

12. The secondary palate consists of which one of the following structure?

A. Premaxilla
B. Incisor teeth
C. Uvula
D. Anterior septum
E. Soft tissues of the lip

13. The Kernahan's striped 'Y' classification is based on which one of the following key landmarks?

A. Nasal septum
B. Incisor teeth
C. Incisive foramen
D. Septal angle
E. Anterior nasal spine

14. Which one of the following muscle forms a sling that suspends the palate from the cranial base and is a critical muscle involved in velopharyngeal closure?

A. Tensor veli palatini
B. Levator veli palatini
C. Palatopharyngeus
D. Superior constrictor
E. Palatoglossus

15. Serous otitis media in patients with cleft palate is primarily due to dysfunction of which one of the following muscle causing loss of ability to dilate the Eustachian tube?

A. Tensor veli palatini
B. Levator veli palatini
C. Palatopharyngeus
D. Superior constrictor
E. Palatoglossus

16. The function of musculus uvulae is which one of the following?

A. No active function. Has passive role in maintaining the bulk of the palate
B. Elevation of the velum
C. Forms the cleft muscle of Veau along with fibres of the levator
D. Closure of the Eustachian tube
E. Contributes to the Passavant's ridge

17. Which one of the following muscles forms the anterior pretonsillar sphincter and helps to propel the food?

A. Tensor veli palatini
B. Levator veli palatini
C. Palatopharyngeus
D. Superior constrictor
E. Palatoglossus

18. The tensor veli palatini dilates the Eustachian tube and helps in milking the tube of its contents. This action is achieved by pull on the tube in which of the following direction?

A. Inferiorly, laterally and posteriorly
B. Superiorly, laterally and anteriorly
C. Inferiorly, laterally and anteriorly
D. Superiorly, laterally and posteriorly
E. Inferiorly, medially and posteriorly

19. Which one of the following muscle is the main component of the Passavant's ridge?

A. Tensor veli palatini
B. Levator veli palatini
C. Palatopharyngeus
D. Superior constrictor
E. Palatoglossus

20. Which one of the following modality is suitable as a diagnostic tool to evaluate the velopharynx before surgery in patients with occult submucous clefts?

A. Clinical examination
B. Nasoendoscopy
C. Fluoroscopy
D. MRI
E. Contrast enhanced computed tomography

21. Which one of the following velopharyngeal muscles is innervated by the mandibular nerve?

A. Tensor veli palatini
B. Levator veli palatini
C. Palatopharyngeus
D. Superior constrictor
E. Palatoglossus

22. The incisive foramen is located in the anterior part of the palate. Which one of the following structure passes through it?

A. Greater palatine nerve
B. Nasopalatine nerve
C. Lesser palatine nerve
D. Alveolar nerve
E. Nasopalatine artery

23. The greater palatine foramen is present in which one of the following bones?

A. Maxilla
B. Palatine bone
C. Vomer
D. Sphenoid
E. Pterygoid

24. The lesser palatine foramina are present in which one of the following bones?

A. Maxilla
B. Palatine bone
C. Vomer
D. Sphenoid
E. Pterygoid

25. Which one of the following muscles does not participate in velopharyngeal function during speech production?

A. Tensor veli palatini
B. Levator veli palatini
C. Palatopharyngeus
D. Superior constrictor
E. Palatoglossus

26. Fracturing the hook of pterygoid hamulus during palatoplasty produces which one of the following changes?

A. Converts the tensor veli palatini into levator veli palatini
B. Allows the tendon of the tensor palatini to slip and roll out of the groove
C. No change in the functioning of the tensor veli palatini
D. Tendon hooking around the hamulus gets relaxed
E. Increases the tension on the tensor veli palatini

27. Many classifications have been proposed for clefts taking into consideration various themes. Which one of the following classification systems is based on the evaluation of cephalometric radiographs?

A. Davis and Ritchie
B. Veau
C. Pruzansky
D. Kernahan and Stark
E. Spina

28. Many classifications have been proposed for clefts taking into consideration various themes. Which one of the following classification systems is based on the anatomic structures involved?

A. Davis and Ritchie
B. Veau
C. LAHSHAL
D. Kernahan and Stark
E. Spina

29. Many classifications have been proposed for clefts taking into consideration various themes. Which one of the following classification systems is based on codes and symbolic representation?

A. Davis and Ritchie
B. Veau
C. Villar-Sancho
D. Kernahan and Stark
E. Spina

30. The palatal aponeurosis is formed by which one of the following muscle?
A. Tensor veli palatini
B. Levator veli palatini
C. Palatopharyngeus
D. Superior constrictor
E. Palatoglossus

31. The tensor veli palatini muscle takes origin from which one of the following cranial bones?
A. Maxilla
B. Palatine bone
C. Vomer
D. Sphenoid
E. Pterygoid

32. The levator veli palatini muscle takes origin from which one of the following bones?
A. Maxilla
B. Palatine bone
C. Vomer
D. Sphenoid
E. Temporal

33. Which one of the following muscles is the only intrinsic muscle of the palate?
A. Tensor veli palatini
B. Levator veli palatini
C. Musculus uvulae
D. Superior constrictor
E. Palatoglossus

34. The palatoglossus muscle forms which one of the following?
A. The anterior pillar of the tonsil
B. The posterior pillar of the tonsil
C. Both the pillars of the tonsil
D. Passavant's ridge
E. Uvula

35. The palatopharyngeus muscle forms which one of the following?
A. Anterior pillar of the tonsil
B. Posterior pillar of the tonsil
C. Both the pillars of tonsils
D. Passavant's ridge
E. Uvula

36. Which one of the following craniosynostoses has the highest familial occurrence?
A. Coronal B. Sagittal
C. Metopic D. Lambdoid

37. Which of the following are the features of Apert's syndrome?
A. Brachycephaly
B. Midface hypoplasia
C. Complex syndactyly
D. Hydrocephalus
E. All of the above

38. The degree of hypertelorism is based on the intercanthal distance. A distance of 30-34 mm would be classified into which one of the following category?
A. First degree
B. Second degree
C. Third degree
D. Fourth degree

39. An encephalocoele is a herniation of which of the following through a defect in the cranium?
A. Dura
B. CSF
C. Brain tissue
D. All of the above

40. Malformations in the frontonasal region tend to follow a similar anatomic path to present in the prenasal space between the skin and nasal cartilages. The starting point of these malformations is which one of the following?
A. Between the orbits at the nasal root
B. Between the frontal and ethmoid bones
C. Evagination of dura through foramen cecum
D. Evagination of dura through a medial orbital defect
E. Dural evagination between the frontal process of maxilla and nasal bone

41. Which one of the following is the commonest syndrome associated with cleft lip and palate?
A. Stickler syndrome
B. Robin sequence
C. Van der Woude syndrome
D. Velocardiofacial syndrome
E. DiGeorge syndrome

42. Cleft palate is associated with a variety of syndromes. Which one of the following is associated with bilateral paramedian lower lip pits?
A. Stickler syndrome
B. Robin sequence
C. Van der Woude syndrome
D. Velocardiofacial syndrome
E. DiGeorge syndrome

43. **Cleft palate is associated with a variety of syndromes. Which one of the following is associated with medial displacement of the carotid artery into the pharynx which must be considered while planning pharyngeal flap surgery?**
   A. Stickler syndrome
   B. Robin sequence
   C. Van der Woude syndrome
   D. Velocardiofacial syndrome
   E. Saethre-Chotzen syndrome

44. **Which one of the following is a characteristic distinguishing feature of Goldenhar syndrome?**
   A. Mandible hypoplasia
   B. Maxillary canting
   C. Epibulbar dermoid
   D. Lack of pneumatisation of mastoid air cells
   E. Hypoplasia of zygoma

45. **The deformity in craniofacial microsomia is related to which of the following?**
   A. Ear
   B. Mandible
   C. Maxilla
   D. Pterygoid process of sphenoid bone
   E. All of the above

46. **Which one of the following is true regarding the jaw opening in a case of craniofacial microsomia?**
   A. Jaw does not deviate on opening
   B. Jaw deviates to the affected side
   C. Jaw deviates to the normal side
   D. Clicking of jaw is present on the affected side
   E. Jaw movements are painful on the affected side

47. **Which of the following may be present in craniofacial microsomia in addition to the characteristic findings observed in the ear, mandible and maxilla?**
   A. Facial nerve palsy
   B. Soft tissue hypoplasia
   C. Zygomatic hypoplasia
   D. Temporal bone hypoplasia
   E. All of the above

48. **'Boat head' shape of the skull is found in which one of the following craniosynostoses?**
   A. Trigonocephaly
   B. Plagiocephaly
   C. Brachycephaly
   D. Scaphocephaly
   E. Acrocephaly

49. **'Tower head' shape of the skull is found in which one of the following craniosynostoses?**
   A. Trigonocephaly
   B. Plagiocephaly
   C. Brachycephaly
   D. Scaphocephaly
   E. Turricephaly

50. **Which one of the following is the commonest nonsyndromic synostoses?**
   A. Sagittal
   B. Unicoronal
   C. Bicoronal
   D. Metopic
   E. Lambdoid

51. **Brow recession would be found in which of the following craniosynostoses?**
   A. Sagittal
   B. Coronal
   C. Lambdoid
   D. Metopic
   E. All of the above

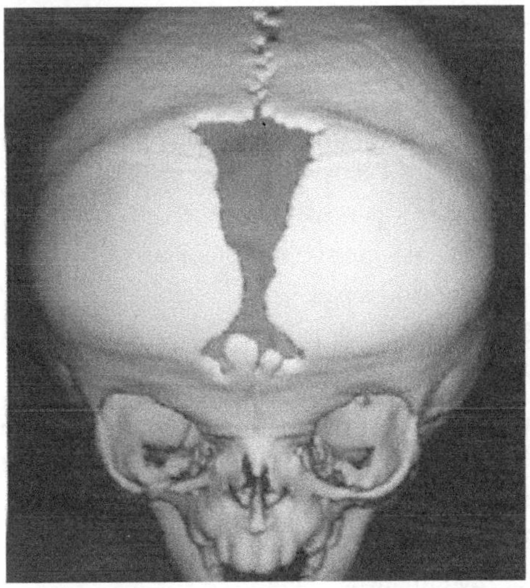

52. **A six month old infant is brought by parents who are concerned with the abnormal shape of the head. The CT scan of the child is shown in the picture. This type of craniosynostoses is consistent with which one of the following head shape?**
   A. Brachycephaly
   B. Turricephaly
   C. Acrocephaly
   D. Trigonocephaly
   E. Plagiocephaly

53. Which of the following craniosynostoses is most common in newborns and is often associated with behavioural impairment?

A. Sagittal
B. Coronal
C. Lambdoid
D. Metopic
E. All of the above

54. Excessive caudal protrusion of one mastoid with minimalization of the other is a pathognomonic clinico-radiologic sign of which of the following craniosynostoses?

A. Sagittal
B. Coronal
C. Lambdoid
D. Metopic
E. All of the above

55. Adhesion cheiloplasty is used for which of the following indication?

A. Wide cleft
B. Complete cleft of primary palate with protruding premaxilla
C. Older children with wide cleft
D. All of the above

56. Which one of the following technique is suitable for staged reconstruction of asymmetric bilateral clefts?

A. Skoog's periosteoplasty
B. Millard's gingivoperiosteoplasty
C. Tennison repair
D. Mohler repair
E. LeMesurier technique

57. Which one of the following muscles is responsible for initiating the smile by raising the upper lip?

A. Levator labii superioris
B. Levator labii superiors alaequae nasi
C. Zygomaticus major
D. Zygomaticus minor
E. Buccinator

58. Peaking of the cleft side of the Cupid's bow is an expression of an undesirable postoperative result. It is due to which of the following?

A. Inadequate rotation of the flap
B. Inadequate horizontalization of the Cupid's bow
C. Scar contraction
D. All of the above
E. None of the above

59. V-Y or Y-V plasty is used to improve upon the postoperative results of cleft lip repair in which of the following situation?

A. Wide nostril by moving the alar base medially
B. Vestibular webbing
C. Centralization of the columella
D. Correction of alar eversion
E. All of the above

60. Vermilion notching following cleft lip repair is due to which of the following?

A. Vermilion deficiency
B. Inadequate muscle repair
C. Dehiscence of muscle repair
D. All of the above

61. The alar web in cleft lip nose deformity consists of which of the following?

A. Skin fold only
B. Alar cartilage
C. Skin fold with alar cartilage
D. Interdomal fat
E. All of the above

62. Which of the following factors is responsible for the protrusion of the premaxilla in bilateral clefts?

A. Unrestrained septal growth
B. Foetal tongue thrust
C. Lack of bony continuity in the maxilla
D. Lack of muscular continuity in the upper lip
E. All of the above

63. Which one of the following method is not advisable for management of the projecting premaxilla in bilateral clefts?

A. Elastic traction
B. Resection and pinning
C. Traction over premaxillary moulds
D. Repair of the lip
E. Pin retained appliances

64. The forked flap used in repair of bilateral clefts takes donor tissue from which of the following structure?

A. Nasal mucosa
B. Buccal mucosa
C. Prolabial skin
D. Prolabial vermilion
E. Columella

65. Which one of the following is the most serious complication following bilateral cleft lip and nose repair in the immediate postoperative period?

A. Wound dehiscence
B. Haemorrhage
C. Airway obstruction
D. Infection
E. Hypertrophic scarring

66. Which one of the following authors has described a cartilage graft to lengthen the short medial crus?

A. Millard
B. Cronin
C. McCarthy
D. Mulliken
E. Noordhoff

67. The anterior nasal spine is poorly formed or absent in which one of the following?

A. Right unilateral cleft lip
B. Left unilateral cleft lip
C. Incomplete cleft lip
D. Microform cleft lip
E. Bilateral cleft lip

68. A notch in the posterior hard palate would be found in which one of the following?

A. Right unilateral cleft lip
B. Left unilateral cleft lip
C. Incomplete cleft lip
D. Submucous cleft palate
E. Complete cleft lip and palate

69. Which one of the following was the first to describe the mucoperiosteal plane of dissection for closure of cleft palate?

A. Dieffenbach
B. von Langenbeck
C. von Graefe
D. van der Woude
E. Kilner

70. The optimal time for repair of cleft palate for children with apparently normal development is which one of the following?

A. At time of birth
B. At time of lip repair between the age 6-9 months
C. 9-12 months
D. School going age between 4-5 years
E. At time of permanent canine eruption between ages 7-8 years

71. Which one of the following method of repair lengthens the palate but leaves large open raw areas on the palate anteriorly?

A. von Langenbeck method
B. Two flap palatoplasty
C. Veau-Wardill-Kilner
D. Intravelar palatoplasty
E. Double opposing Z-Plasty

72. Which one of the following is true regarding Furlow's double opposing Z-plasty?

A. The levator muscle is not dissected
B. The levator muscle is included in the anteriorly based flap
C. The levator muscle is included in the posteriorly based flap
D. Z-plasty is performed on the oral surface
E. The central limb of the Z is placed perpendicular to the cleft margin

73. The vomer flap is commonly used for closure of nasal lining in repair of the cleft palate. Which one of the following structure needs to be incised for raising this flap?

A. Cleft margin
B. Posterior border of hard palate
C. Palatal mucoperiosteum
D. Septum
E. Buccal mucosa

74. Which of the following is a valid reason for alveolar cleft bone grafting?

A. Closure of the fistula
B. Stabilisation of the maxillary arch
C. Support for root of the teeth
D. Provides support for prosthesis
E. All of the above

75. Primary alveolar bone grafting is done at time of:

A. Repair of cleft lip
B. Repair of cleft palate
C. Eruption of first molar
D. Eruption of second molar
E. Before eruption of canine

76. Secondary alveolar bone grafting is done at time of:

A. Repair of cleft lip
B. Repair of cleft palate
C. Before eruption of first molar
D. Before eruption of second molar
E. Before eruption of canine

77. Which one of the following conditions would be more challenging for the orthodontist?

A. Incomplete cleft lip
B. Complete unilateral cleft lip
C. Complete unilateral cleft lip and palate
D. Bilateral incomplete cleft lip
E. Bilateral complete cleft lip and palate

78. Which one of the following is the correct description of teeth relationship in a cleft patient with posterior crossbite in the primary dentition phase?

A. Palatal displacement of the maxillary primary canine
B. Labial displacement of the maxillary primary canine
C. Palatal displacement of the mandibular primary canine
D. Maxillary cleft side primary canine erupts laterally to the lower one
E. All of the above

79. The technique of maxillary distraction using rigid external device requires which of the following steps?

A. Intraoral splint
B. LeFort 1 osteotomy
C. Placement of halo frame
D. Distraction and retention
E. All of the above

80. The perception of inordinate nasal resonance during the production of vowels is which one of the following?

A. Nasal emission
B. Hypernasality
C. Hyponasality
D. Mixed hypernasality and hyponasality
E. Nasal substitution

81. The structures involved in velopharyngeal closure are all of the following except:

A. Soft palate
B. Uvula
C. Posterior pharyngeal wall
D. Lateral pharyngeal wall
E. Hard palate

82. Submucous cleft palate is characterised by a triad of bifid uvula, separation of the soft palate musculature in the midline and which one amongst the following?

A. Cleft lip
B. Cleft alveolus
C. Notch in the bony posterior hard palate
D. Absent anterior nasal spine
E. Palatal fistula

83. Which of the following complications may be seen after posterior pharyngeal flap surgery?

A. Postoperative airway obstruction
B. Bleeding
C. Sleep apnea
D. Death
E. All of the above

84. The greatest criticism of Orticochea's sphincter pharyngoplasty is which one of the following?

A. Bulky flaps
B. Inadequate size of the lateral port
C. Inadequate soft palate closure
D. Low level of inset of flaps
E. Poor speech results

85. Completion of nasal growth determines the timing and extent of surgery in cleft lip rhinoplasty. Nasal growth ceases in girls at which one of the following age?

A. 5-6 years
B. 11-12 years
C. 16-18 years
D. 23-24 years
E. After 30 years

86. The philtrum is an important part of the upper lip and requires careful attention at time of repair of cleft lip. The width of philtrum in a normal adult male at the level of Cupid's bow is which one of the following?

A. 2-4 mm
B. 4-8 mm
C. 8-12 mm
D. 12-16 mm

87. The philtrum is an important part of the upper lip and requires careful attention at time of repair of cleft lip. The width of philtrum in a child at the level of Cupid's bow is which one of the following?

A. 4 mm
B. 6 mm
C. 8 mm
D. 10 mm
E. 12 mm

88. Which of the following statement is true regarding the philtral columns?

A. Philtral columns run parallel from columella to the Cupid's bow

B. Philtral columns gradually narrow as they approach the columella

C. Philtral columns gradually diverge as they approach the columella

D. None of the above

89. Secondary deformities of the cleft lip and palate are common. The 'whistle' deformity refers to which one of the following?

A. Nose

B. Lip

C. Vermilion

D. Buccal mucosa

E. Whistle shaped scar on the lip

90. Secondary deformities of the cleft lip and palate are common. Deficiencies of the labial sulcus are most common after which one of the following?

A. Alveolar bone graft

B. Closure of anterior fistula

C. Unilateral cleft lip repair

D. Bilateral cleft lip repair

E. Abbe flap

91. Which one of the following procedures is suitable for correcting a tight upper lip deformity?

A. Abbe flap

B. Estlander flap

C. Gillies fan flap

D. Karapandzic flap

E. Millard flap

92. Which one of the following is the commonest secondary deformity seen in patients with bilateral cleft lip?

A. Short lip

B. Long lip

C. Tight lip

D. Wide lip

E. Scarred lip

93. Which one of the following statement best describes the caudal septum in unilateral cleft lip nose deformity?

A. It is situated in the midline

B. It is deviated towards the cleft side

C. It is deviated towards the non-cleft side

D. It is deviated towards the non-cleft side while the body of the septum often blocks the cleft side vestibule

E. It is deviated towards the non-cleft side while the body of the septum often blocks the non-cleft side vestibule

94. The septospinal ligament in unilateral cleft lip nose deformity is attached between anterior nasal spine and which one of the following?

A. Vomer

B. Columella

C. Caudal septum

D. Maxilla

E. Septovomerine suture

95. Which one of the following correctly describes the nasal sill in incomplete unilateral cleft lip nose deformity?

A. Not affected

B. Depressed

C. Widened

D. Depressed and widened

E. Absent

96. Which of the following abnormalities in the maxilla may be observed in patients with unilateral cleft lip nose deformity?

A. Short vertical height of maxilla

B. Maxillary arch collapse

C. Absent pyriform margin

D. Maxillary hypoplasia

E. All of the above

97. Grade I hypertelorism according to the Tessier classification will have an interorbital distance of?

A. 25-30 mm

B. 30-34 mm

C. 34-40 mm

D. More than 40 mm

98. Which one of the following is not a feature of orbital hypertelorism?

A. Lateralization of the orbital cavities

B. Inferiorly displaced cribriform plate

C. Expansion of anterior ethmoidal cells

D. Expansion of posterior ethmoidal cells

E. Increased interorbital distance

99. Which of the following is treated by a bipartition procedure?

A. Midline maxillary clefts

B. Translocation of orbits in hypertelorism

C. Inverted V- deformity of maxillary occlusion

D. Double barrel nose

E. All of the above

100. A U-shaped midfacial osteotomy with paramedian bone resection is done in which of the following procedure?

A. Bipartition procedure
B. LeFort III osteotomy
C. LeFort II osteotomy
D. Subcranial osteotomy
E. All of the above

101. Which one of the following characteristic would be present in Tessier number 0 cleft?

A. Nasal septum is intact but deviated
B. Cleft of the nostril
C. Nasal process of maxilla flattened and displaced laterally
D. Cleft of lip
E. Downslanting of the eyes

102. Which one of the following feature is present in Tessier number 1 cleft?

A. Nasal deformity in the middle third of the alar rim
B. Hypoplastic ala
C. Notching in the area of the soft triangle of the nose
D. Direct communication between oral, nasal and orbital cavities
E. Ethmoid sinus may be involved

103. Which one of the following feature is present in Tessier number 2 cleft?

A. Nasal deformity is in the middle third of the alar rim
B. The lacrimal system is disrupted
C. Notching in the area of the soft triangle of the nose
D. Direct communication of the oral, nasal and orbital cavities
E. Anterior maxillary arch is flat
F. Frontal process of maxilla is disrupted

104. Direct communication of the oral, nasal and orbital cavities is found in which one of the following?

A. Tessier no. 1 cleft
B. Tessier no. 2 cleft
C. Tessier no. 3 cleft
D. Tessier no. 4 cleft
E. Tessier no. 5 cleft

105. Direct confluence between the oral cavity, maxillary sinus and orbital cavity exists in which one of the following?

A. Tessier no. 1 cleft
B. Tessier no. 2 cleft
C. Tessier no. 3 cleft
D. Tessier no. 4 cleft
E. Tessier no. 0 cleft

106. A Tessier no. 6 cleft is characterized by which of the following?

A. Antimongoloid slant
B. Hypoplasia of zygoma
C. Soft tissue furrow from angle of mouth to the latral canthus
D. Occlusal tilt
E. All of the above

107. Which one of the following cleft passes through the pterygomaxillary junction?

A. Tessier no. 1 cleft
B. Tessier no. 3 cleft
C. Tessier no. 5 cleft
D. Tessier no. 7 cleft
E. Tessier no. 9 cleft

108. Which one of the following cleft occurs at the frontozygomatic suture?

A. Tessier no. 2 cleft
B. Tessier no. 4 cleft
C. Tessier no. 6 cleft
D. Tessier no. 8 cleft
E. Tessier no. 10 cleft

109. A dermatocoele which is a true lateral commissure coloboma occurs in which one of the following cleft?

A. Tessier no. 2 cleft
B. Tessier no. 4 cleft
C. Tessier no. 6 cleft
D. Tessier no. 8 cleft
E. Tessier no. 10 cleft

110. Changes in the cribriform plate are the hallmark of which one of the following cleft?

A. Tessier no. 7 cleft
B. Tessier no. 11 cleft
C. Tessier no. 12 cleft
D. Tessier no. 13 cleft
E. Tessier no. 14 cleft

111. A Tessier no. 12 cleft is characterised by the following features except:

A. Enlarged frontal sinuses
B. Hypertelorism
C. Midline tuft of hair
D. Widening of the frontal process of maxilla
E. Normal frontonasal angle

112. A paramedian frontal encephalocoele is typically present in which one of the following cleft?

A. Tessier no. 7 cleft
B. Tessier no. 11 cleft
C. Tessier no. 12 cleft
D. Tessier no. 13 cleft
E. Tessier no. 14 cleft

113. A Tessier no. 14 cleft is characterised by which of the following?

A. Hypertelorism
B. Hypotelorism
C. Flattening of glabella
D. Tuft of hair on the forehead
E. All of the above

114. The Tessier no. 30 cleft involves which of the following?

A. Cranium
B. Orbit
C. Upper jaw
D. Lower jaw
E. All of the above

115. Ankyloglossia may be seen in which one of the following cleft?

A. Tessier no. 0 cleft
B. Tessier no. 11 cleft
C. Tessier no. 12 cleft
D. Tessier no. 13 cleft
E. Tessier no. 30 cleft

116. Total absence of the tongue may be seen in which one of the following cleft?

A. Tessier no. 0 cleft
B. Tessier no. 11 cleft
C. Tessier no. 12 cleft
D. Tessier no. 13 cleft
E. Tessier no. 30 cleft

117. Abnormalities of the lateral third of the upper eyelid and eyebrow are hallmarks of which one of the following cleft?

A. Tessier no. 9 cleft
B. Tessier no. 11 cleft
C. Tessier no. 12 cleft
D. Tessier no. 13 cleft
E. Tessier no. 30 cleft

118. The Tessier cleft which is medial to the lower lacrimal punctum is which one of the following?

A. Tessier 1
B. Tessier 2
C. Tessier 3
D. Tessier 7
E. Tessier 8

119. The Tessier cleft which is medial to the medial canthus of the eye with colobomas extending to the root of the eyebrow is which one of the following?

A. Tessier 7
B. Tessier 8
C. Tessier 9
D. Tessier 11
E. Tessier 12

120. Which Tessier cleft may be commonly associated with palsy of the VII nerve?

A. Tessier 7
B. Tessier 8
C. Tessier 9
D. Tessier 11
E. Tessier 12

121. Which one of the following Tessier cleft is associated with clefting along the frontal bone with widening of the olfactory groove?

A. Tessier 10
B. Tessier 11
C. Tessier 12
D. Tessier 13
E. Tessier 14

122. Which one of the following Tessier cleft may be associated with transverse orbital dystopia?

A. Tessier 10
B. Tessier 11
C. Tessier 12
D. Tessier 13
E. Tessier 14

123. The term diprosopus refers to which of the following?

A. Facial bipartition
B. Facial cleft
C. Facial duplication
D. Facial defect
E. Facial agenesis

124. Treacher Collins syndrome results from which one of the following?

A. Exposure to radiation
B. Mutation of gene TCOF1
C. Mutation of T-box gene
D. Deficiency of homeobox gene
E. Deficiency of NADH dehydrogenase

125. The Pi procedure is used to treat which one of the following craniosynostosis?

A. Scaphocephaly
B. Brachycephaly
C. Plagiocephaly
D. Trigonocephaly
E. Multisutural craniosynostosis

126. The Hung Span technique is used to treat which of the following craniosynostosis?

A. Scaphocephaly
B. Brachycephaly
C. Plagiocephaly
D. Trigonocephaly
E. Multisutural craniosynostosis

127. Which one of the following conditions is seen in bilateral coronal craniosynostosis?

A. Scaphocephaly
B. Brachycephaly
C. Plagiocephaly
D. Trigonocephaly
E. Multisutural craniosynostosis

128. Unilateral coronal craniosynostosis would produce which one of the following condition?

A. Scaphocephaly
B. Brachycephaly
C. Plagiocephaly
D. Trigonocephaly
E. Multisutural craniosynostosis

129. The classic "Harlequin sign" in plagiocephaly is seen on which one of the following modality?

A. Clinical examination
B. Radiograph
C. Computed tomogram
D. Doppler examination
E. Magnetic resonance imaging

130. The classic "Harlequin sign" is produced in plagiocephaly due to abnormality in which one of the following bone?

A. Frontal bone
B. Sphenoid bone
C. Parietal bone
D. Occipital bone
E. Temporal bone

131. Which one of the following syndrome is not associated with limb abnormalities?

A. Crouzon syndrome
B. Apert syndrome
C. Pfeiffer syndrome
D. Saethre-Chotzen syndrome
E. Carpenter syndrome

132. The classic "copper beaten" skull is frequently though nonspecifically associated with which one of the following condition?

A. Intracranial infection
B. Intracranial tumour
C. Intracranial hypertension
D. Intracranial vascular malformation
E. Intracranial foreign body (copper)

133. The "Cloverleaf skull" deformity is seen in which one of the following condition?

A. Intracranial infection
B. Intracranial tumour
C. Intracranial hypotension
D. Intracranial vascular malformation
E. Sutural synostosis

134. The "Cloverleaf skull" deformity is treated best by which one of the following modality?

A. Masterly inactivity
B. Conservative measures
C. Ventriculoperitoneal shunting
D. Orthotic cranioplasty
E. Radical craniectomy

135. The bony deformity of the orbit in Treacher Collins syndrome is due to involvement of which one of the following bones?

A. Frontal
B. Maxilla
C. Ethmoid
D. Zygoma
E. Nasal

136. The "Egg shaped" orbit is seen in which one of the following condition?

A. Coronal craniosynostosis
B. Craniofacial microsomia
C. Frontoethmoid meningoencephalocoele
D. Orbital hypertelorism
E. Treacher Collins syndrome

137. A concave antegonial notch with markedly obtuse gonial angle of the mandible is a distinguishing feature of which one of the following condition?

A. Masseteric hypertrophy
B. Craniofacial microsomia
C. Pierre Robin sequence
D. TMJ ankylosis
E. Treacher Collins syndrome

138. Colobomas of the lower eyelid are pathognomonic of which one of the following condition?

A. Masseteric hypertrophy
B. Craniofacial microsomia
C. Pierre Robin sequence
D. TMJ ankylosis
E. Treacher Collins syndrome

139. The triad of Pierre Robin sequence consists of which one of the following?

A. Glossoptosis, micrognathia and cleft palate
B. Glossoptosis, cleft palate and maxillary hypoplasia
C. Glossoptosis, cleft palate and TMJ ankylosis
D. Glossoptosis, micrognathia and airway obstruction
E. Glossoptosis, micrognathia and TMJ ankylosis

140. The triad of glossoptosis, micrognathia and airway obstruction is found in which of the following?

A. Stickler syndrome
B. 22q11 deletion
C. Foetal alcohol syndrome
D. Pierre Robin sequence
E. All of the above

141. Upper airway obstruction is a characteristic feature of Pierre Robin sequence. Which of the following is a potential cause of airway obstruction in this syndrome?

A. Tracheomalacia
B. Acute angulation of the basicranium
C. Lingual anomalies
D. Subglottic anomalies
E. All of the above

142. Which of the following is the characteristic feature of the nose in Treacher Collins syndrome?

A. Obtuse nasofrontal angle
B. Dorsal hump
C. Drooping tip of nose
D. Wide and deep nasal root
E. All of the above

143. The children with Pierre Robin syndrome should be nursed preferably in which of the following position after a feed?

A. Supine
B. Lateral
C. Semiprone
D. Prone
E. Any of the above

144. All patients with Pierre Robin sequence do not need surgery. Which of the following is the physiologic criteria for surgical intervention in Pierre Robin sequence?

A. Respiratory rate > 60/minute
B. $PaO_2 < 65$ mm Hg
C. $PaCO_2 > 60$ mm Hg
D. Weight gain < 100 gm / week
E. All of the above

145. The tongue-lip adhesion procedure is done in patients with which one of the following condition?

A. Unilateral cleft lip
B. Bilateral cleft lip
C. Cleft palate
D. Craniofacial microsomia
E. Pierre Robin sequence

146. Reconstruction of the mandibular ramus, condyle and the glenoid fossa is required in which of the following mandibular deformity?

A. Pruzansky Type I
B. Pruzansky Type IIA
C. Pruzansky Type IIB
D. Pruzansky Type III
E. All of the above

147. Romberg's disease is a progressive hemifacial atrophy. Which of the following etiological factor has been proposed for its pathogenesis?

A. Infection
B. Neuritis
C. Vasculitis
D. Sympathetic dysfunction
E. All of the above

148. Which of the following are the tissue changes in Romberg's disease?

A. Skin fibrosis
B. Fibrosis of blood vessels
C. Fibrosis of synovia
D. Excess collagen deposition
E. All of the above

149. Which one of the following would be the most suitable flap for facial contour correction in Romberg's disease?

A. Omentum
B. Groin flap
C. Superficial inferior epigastric flap
D. Circuflex scapular flap
E. Radial artery forearm flap

150. Which one of the following is unsuitable for correction of facial contour?

A. Liquid silicone
B. Fat graft
C. Dermal graft
D. Implants
E. Free tissue transfer

151. A 20-year-old female presents with a rapidly developing lesion on the nose that is prone to bleeding (photo shown). Which of the following is the most likely diagnosis?

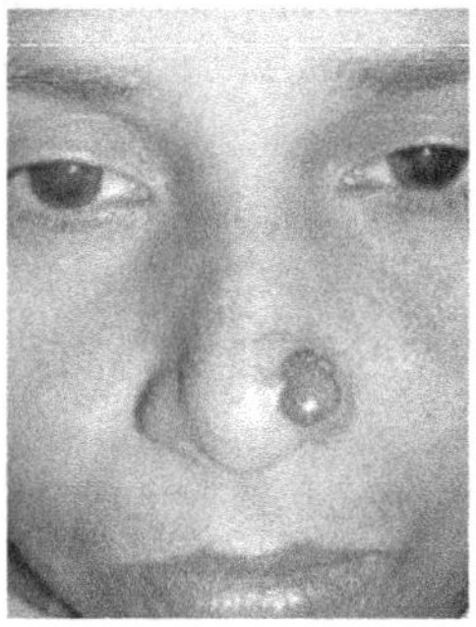

A. Implantation dermoid
B. Mucocele
C. Nevus sebaceus of Jadassohn
D. Pyogenic granuloma
E. Vascular malformation

152. A lady develops this swelling shown in the picture few months after getting her ear pierced by a gun. The diagnosis of this lesion is most likely to be which one of the following?

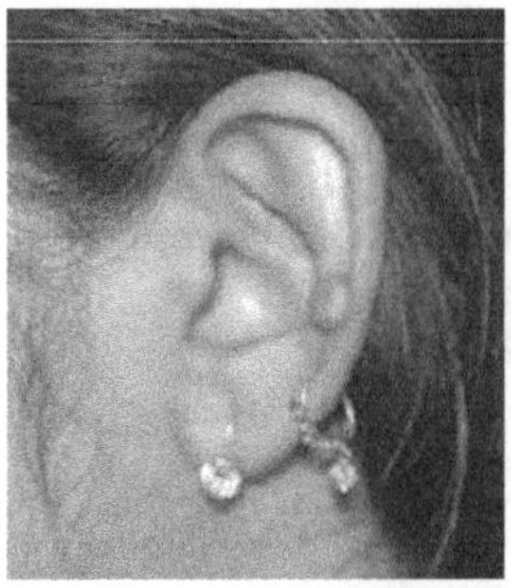

A. Implantation dermoid
B. Mucocele
C. Keloid
D. Pyogenic granuloma
E. Vascular malformation

153. A 20-year-old female presents late for correction of her facial deformity with a deformed ear and retruded chin. In addition she also complains of flattening of cheek bones and slanting eyes. Her lateral view clinical photograph and three dimensional computed tomogram are shown. Which one of the following is the most likely diagnosis for her?

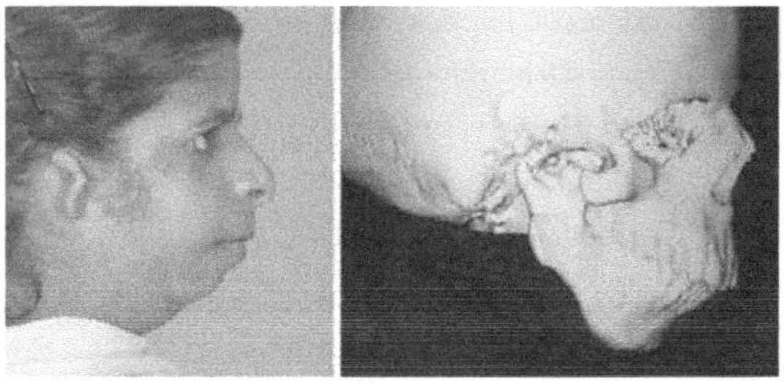

A. Tessier no. 1,2,3 cleft
B. Tessier no. 2,3,4 cleft
C. Tessier no. 3,4,5 cleft
D. Tessier no. 6,7, 8 cleft
E. Pierre Robin syndrome

154. A two week old infant is brought by parents with complaints of difficulty in respiration and feeding. The facial profile shows a marked hypoplasia of mandible with severe degree of retrogenia (picture shown). The clinical diagnosis of this child is consistent with which one of the following diagnosis?

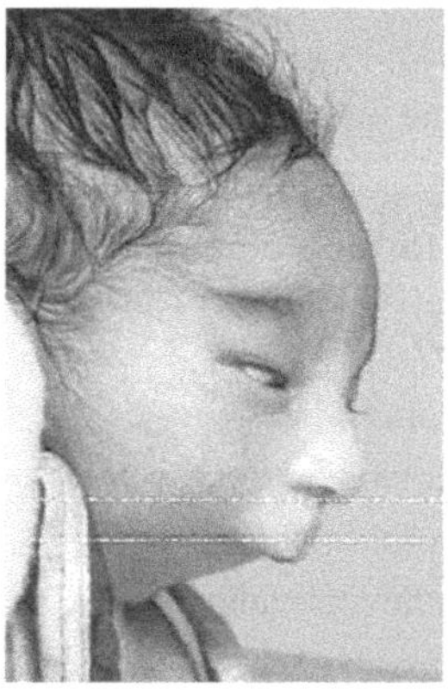

A. Romberg's disease
B. Treacher Collins syndrome
C. Pierre Robin sequence
D. Apert's syndrome
E. Goldenhar syndrome

155. **A 14-year-old boy with bilateral cleft lip and palate deformity underwent repair of bilateral cleft lip at 7 months of age and repair of cleft palate at 12 months of age. He did not return since his last operation for follow up and now has severe facial deformity with maxillary hypoplasia corroborated by cephalometry. He was started on orthodontic treatment, but a 14-mm negative overjet remains (photo shown). Which of the following procedure is most appropriate for him at this stage?**

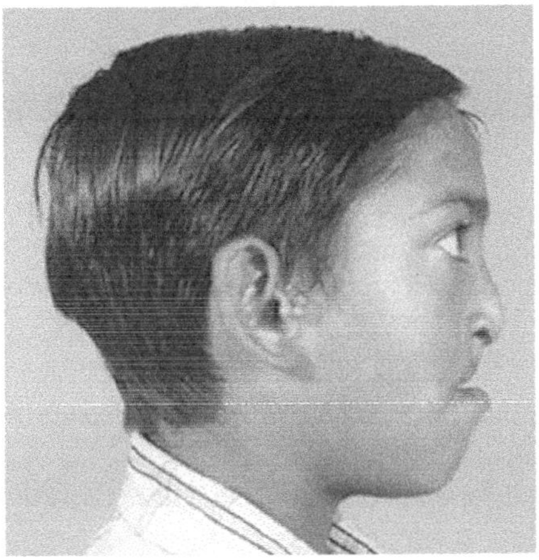

A. LeFort I osteotomy with distraction
B. LeFort I osteotomy with immediate advancement
C. LeFort III osteotomy with distraction
D. LeFort II osteotomy with immediate advancement
E. Face mask therapy

ANSWERS, EXPLANATIONS AND REFERENCES

1. **The correct response is A.**

The maxilla and mandible develop from the first brancial arch. The muscles of facial expression and mastication and other striated muscles in the head and neck are also derived from mesoderm in the first and second arches.

Reference:

1. *Helms JA, Schneider RA. Cranial skeletal biology. Nature 2003; 423: 326-331.*
2. *Moore KL, Persaud TVN. The Developing Human: Clinically Oriented Embryology, 6th ed. Philadephia, WB Saunders, 1998: 220.*

2. **The correct response is A.**

The petrous temporal bone is part of the cartilaginous neurocranium or the chondrocranium and forms the base of the skull. The membranous portion of the neurocranium forms the cranial vault and is composed of seven bones; the paired frontal, squamosal, parietal and portion of the occipital bone.

Reference:

1. *Moore KL, Persaud TVN. The Developing Human: Clinically Oriented Embryology, 6th ed. Philadephia, WB Saunders, 1998; 237-238.*
2. *Jiang X, Jseki S, Maxson RE et al. Tissue origins and interactions in the mammalian skull vault. Dev Biol 2002; 241: 106-116.*

3. **The correct response is C.**

The squamosal bone is not cartilaginous, it is a part of the membranous neurocranium. The membranous portion of the neurocranium forms the cranial vault and is composed of seven bones; the paired frontal, squamosal, parietal and portion of the occipital bone.

Reference:

1. *Moore KL, Persaud TVN. The Developing Human: Clinically Oriented Embryology, 6th ed. Philadelphia, WB Saunders, 1998: 237-238.*
2. *Jiang X, Jseki S, Maxson RE et al. Tissue origins and interactions in the mammalian skull vault. Dev Biol 2002; 241: 106-116.*

4. **The correct response is C.**

The bones of the facial skeleton, including the mandible and the maxilla, compose the viscerocranium. These bones are derived primarily from the cranial neural crest cells of the first branchial arch.

The rest of the bones are derived from the cartilaginous neurocranium.

Reference:

1. *Moore KL, Persaud TVN. The Developing Human: Clinically Oriented Embryology, 6th ed. Philadephia, WB Saunders, 1998: 237-238.*
2. *Jiang X, Jseki S, Maxson RE et al. Tissue origins and interactions in the mammalian skull vault. Dev Biol 2002; 241: 106-116.*

5. **The correct response is C.**

The orbit is the reference point for classification of craniofacial clefts as described by Tessier. The orbit separates the cranial or "northbound" clefts from the facial or "southbound" clefts. All of the craniofacial clefts are formed by the combination of northbound and southbound clefts.

Reference:

Tessier P. Anatomical classification of facial, craniofacial and latero-facial clefts. J Maxillofac Surg 1976; 4: 69.

6. The correct response is B.

The Tessier number 7 cleft is the one that is most laterally placed cleft. It begins at the oral commissure and runs to the preauricular hair line. The skeletal cleft passes through the pterygomaxillary junction. The zygomatic body is severely malformed, hypoplastic and displaced. It is also seen in Treacher Collins syndrome.

Reference:

1. *Tessier P. Anatomical classification of facial, craniofacial and latero-facial clefts. J Maxillofac Surg 1976; 4: 69.*
2. *Gorlin RJ, Jue KL, Jacobsen U et al. Oculoauriculovertebral syndrome. J Pediatr 1963; 63: 991.*

7. The correct response is B.

The number 7 cleft is the most common craniofacial cleft also known as otomandibular dysostosis, craniofacial microsomia, hemifacial microsomia and first and second branchial arch syndrome besides others.

Reference:

1. *Tessier P. Anatomical classification of facial, craniofacial and latero-facial clefts. J Maxillofac Surg 1976; 4: 69.*
2. *Gorlin RJ, Jue KL, Jacobsen U et al. Oculoauriculovertebral syndrome. J Pediatr 1963; 63: 991.*

8. The correct response is B.

Treacher Collins syndrome is a combination of Tessier 6,7 and 8 clefts. Tessier cleft no.6 explains the coloboma of lower eyelid. Tessier cleft no. 7 results in hypoplastic zygoma and hypoplastic masseter muscle besides ear malformations. Cleft no. 8 gives the eyes its antimonogoloid slant due to lack of lateral eye support i.e. hypoplastic zygoma. In a typical case the above involvement is bilateral.

Reference:

1. *Tessier P. Anatomical classification of facial, craniofacial and latero-facial clefts. J Maxillofac Surg 1976; 4: 69.*
2. *Kawamoto HK Jr. The kaleidoscopic world of rare craniofacial clefts: order out of chaos (Tessier classification). Clin Plast Surg 1976; 3: 529.*

9. The correct response is E.

Hypotelorism may be present with an agenesis in a number 14 cleft. A spectrum of holoprosencephalic disorders including cyclopia, ethmocephaly and cebocephaly may also be present. The cranium is typically microcephalic.

Reference:

1. *Tessier P. Anatomical classification of facial, craniofacial and latero-facial clefts. J Maxillofac Surg 1976; 4:69.*
2. *Cohen MM Jr, Jirasek JE, Guzman RT et al. Holoprosencephaly and facial dysmorphia: nosology, aetiology and pathogenesis. Birth defects 1971; 7: 125.*

10. The correct response is C.

Tessier number 30 cleft affects the lower lip and the chin. The anterior third of the tongue may be bifid and attached to the split mandible by a dense fibrous band. Ankyloglossia and total absence of the tongue have also been reported with midline mandibular clefts.

Reference:

1. *Tessier P. Anatomical classification of facial, craniofacial and latero-facial clefts. J Maxillofac Surg 1976; 4: 69.*
2. *Cosman B, Crikelair GF. Midline branchiogenic syndromes. Plast Reconstr Surg 1969; 44: 41.*

11. The correct response is B.

The number 1 cleft is similar to the common cleft lip and passes through the Cupid's bow and alar cartilage dome resembling the common cleft lip. Notching in the area of the soft triangle of the nose is a characteristic feature. The nasal tip and nasal septum deviate away from the cleft.

Reference:

1. *Tessier P. Anatomical classification of facial, craniofacial and latero-facial clefts. J Maxillofac Surg 1976; 4: 69.*
2. *van der Meulen JC, Mazzola R, Vermey-Keers C et al. A morphogenetic classification of craniofacial malformations. Plast Reconstr Surg 1983; 71: 560.*

12. The correct response is C.

The primary palate consists of premaxilla, anterior septum and soft tissues of the lip. The secondary palate consists of the hard palate posterior to the incisive foramen, soft palate and the uvula.

Reference:

1. *Tessier P. Anatomical classification of facial, craniofacial and latero-facial clefts. J Maxillofac Surg 1976; 4: 69.*
2. *Millard R, ed: Cleft Craft, vol 1. Boston, Little Brown, 1977.*

13. The correct response is C.

The Kernahan's striped 'Y' classification is based on the incisive foramen as the key anatomic landmark for easy documentation of the cleft lip and nose deformity. It is one of the most widely followed classification systems for clefts. It has also been modified from time to time by various workers. Elsahy added a triangle for the nasal floor on the top of 'Y'. Millard added another inverted triangle for the nasal deformity on top of the Elsahy's triangle. Smith advocated changes in the numerical system for the anterior and the posterior clefts. Noordhoff advocated a double 'Y' concept using the letter code and number code for easy acceptability.

Reference:

1. *Kernahan DA. The striped Y. A symbolic classification for cleft lips and palates. Plast Reconstr Surg 1971; 47: 469.*
2. *Kernahan DA. On cleft lip and palate classifications. Plast Reconstr Surg 1973; 51: 578.*

14. The correct response is B.

The levator veli palatini is a cylindrical muscle forming a sling that suspends the soft palate from the cranial base. It takes superior attachment to the Eustachian tube and the muscle bundles descend on each side anteriorly and medially towards the soft palate.

Reference:

1. *Huang MH, Lee ST, Rajendran K. Anatomic basis of cleft palate and velopharyngeal surgery: implications from a fresh cadaveric study. Plast Reconstr Surg 1998; 101: 613.*
2. *Seif S, Dellon AL. Anatomic relationships between the human levator and tensor veli palatine and the eustachian tube. Cleft Palate J 1978; 15: 329.*

15. The correct response is B.

The paratubal muscles, particularly the levator veli palatini is responsible for the dilatation function of the Eustachian tube. This is important for adequate drainage of the middle ear. The loss of function in cleft palate is due to the substantial anterior bony insertion on the posterior margin of the hard palate of this muscle.

The other muscles attached to the Eustachian tube are - Tensor palati from the superolateral aspect near the isthmus of the tube and salpingopharyngeus from the posteroinferior aspect of the eustachian tube near the pharyngeal opening.

Reference:

1. *Doyle WJ, Kitajari M, Sando I. The anatomy of the auditory tube and paratubal musculature in a one-month-old cleft palate patient. Cleft Palate J 1983; 20: 218.*
2. *Doyle WJ, Reilly JS, Jardini L. Effect of palatoplasty on the function of the Eustachian tube in children with cleft palate. Cleft Palate J 1986; 23: 63.*
3. *Martin HS, Lee ST, Rajendran K. A fresh cadaveric study of the paratubal muscles: implications for Eustachian tube function in cleft palate. Plast Reconstr Surg 1997; 100: 840.*

16. The correct response is A.

The musculus uvulae is a paired muscle which runs longitudinally in the nasal midline of the velum. Its function consists of a passive space occupying role that prevents attenuation of the midline bulk caused by the lateral traction from the levator during velopharyngeal closure. The other options are incorrect.

Reference:

1. *Doyle WJ, Kitajari M, Sando I. The anatomy of the auditory tube and paratubal musculature in a one-month-old cleft palate patient. Cleft Palate J 1983; 20: 218.*
2. *Doyle WJ, Reilly JS, Jardini L. Effect of palatoplasty on the function of the Eustachian tube in children with cleft palate. Cleft Palate J 1986; 23: 63.*

17. The correct response is E.

The palatoglossus arises from the transverse muscle fibres of the tongue and inserts into the muscles of the soft palate. It functions to narrow the pharyngo-oral isthmus and forms the anterior pretonsillar sphincter and helps to propel the food.

Reference:

1. *Nishio J, Matsuya T, Machida J, Miyazaki T. The motor nerve supply of the velopharyngeal muscles. Cleft Palate J 1976; 13: 20.*
2. *Millard R, ed: Cleft Craft, vol 1. Boston, Little Brown, 1977.*

18. The correct response is C.

The correct action of the tensor veli palatini is to pull the Eustachian tube inferiorly, laterally and anteriorly. This action in concert with the action of levator veli palatini helps to create a pumping action on the contents of the tube leading to its emptying towards the oral side.

Reference:

1. *Ross MA. Functional anatomy of the tensor palatini: its relevance in cleft palate surgery. Arch Otolaryngol 1971; 93:1.*
2. *Rood SR, Doyle WJ. Morphology of tensor veli palatine, tensor tympani and dilator tubae muscles. Ann Otol Rhinol Laryngol 1978; 87: 202.*

19. The correct response is D.

The superior constrictor is the main component of the Passavant's ridge. It causes the anterior displacement of the posterior pharyngeal wall by fibres that meet across the posterior midline.

Reference:

1. *Huang MH, Lee ST, Rajendran K. Anatomic basis of cleft palate and velopharyngeal surgery: implications from a fresh cadaveric study. Plast Reconstr Surg 1998; 101: 613.*
2. *Seif S, Dellon AL. Anatomic relationships between the human levator and tensor veli palatine and the Eustachian tube. Cleft Palate J 1978; 15: 329.*

20. The correct response is D.

MRI offers the best objective imaging modality for evaluating the muscles of the palate, especially the levator veli palatini. This muscle can be clearly seen at its origin at the Eustachian tube with other muscles in the palate. The MRI clearly depicts the anatomy of the velopharynx and hence is considered a suitable modality for preoperative and postoperative evaluation of the velopharynx.

Reference:

1. *Kuehn DP, Ettema ST, Goldwasser MS et al. Magnetic resonance imaging in the evaluation of occult submucous cleft palate. Cleft Palate J 2001; 38: 421.*
2. *Ettema SL, Kuehn DP, Perlman A et al. Magnetic resonance imaging of the levator veli palatini muscle during speech. Cleft Palate J 2002; 39: 130.*

21. The correct response is A.

The tensor veli palatini is different from the rest of the velopharyngeal muscles in having its nerve supply from a branch originating from the mandibular nerve. The rest of the muscles are supplied by branches from the glossopharyngeal and vagus nerves.

Reference:

1. *Broomhead IW. The nerve supply of the muscles of the soft palate. Br J Plast Surg 1951; 4: 1.*
2. *Nishio J, Matsuya T, Machida J, Miyazaki T. The motor nerve supply of the velopharyngeal muscles. Cleft Palate J 1976; 13: 20.*

22. The correct response is B.

The nasopalatine nerve and sphenopalatine artery pass through this foramen which is located in the premaxilla derived portion of the palate.

Reference:

1. *Maue-Dickson W, Dickson DR. Anatomy and physiology related to cleft palate: current research and clinical implications. Plast Reconstr Surg 1980; 65: 83.*
2. *Boorman JG, Freedlander E. Surgical anatomy of the velum and pharynx. In Jackson IT, Sommerlad BC, eds: Recent advances in Plastic Surgery, No. 4. Edinburgh, Churchill Livingstone, 1992: 17.*

23. The correct response is B.

The foramen is present in the palatine bone in its posterolateral portion. It lies medial to the last molar tooth.

Reference:

1. *Maue-Dickson W, Dickson DR. Anatomy and physiology related to cleft palate: current research and clinical implications. Plast Reconstr Surg 1980; 65: 83.*
2. *Boorman JG, Freedlander E. Surgical anatomy of the velum and pharynx. In Jackson IT, Sommerlad BC, eds: Recent advances in Plastic Surgery, No. 4. Edinburgh, Churchill Livingstone, 1992: 17.*

24. The correct response is B.

The lesser palatine foramina are present in the palatine bone posterolateral to the orifice of the greater palatine foramen.

Reference:

1. *Maue-Dickson W, Dickson DR. Anatomy and physiology related to cleft palate: current research and clinical implications. Plast Reconstr Surg 1980; 65: 83.*
2. *Boorman JG, Freedlander E. Surgical anatomy of the velum and pharynx. In Jackson IT, Sommerlad BC, eds: Recent advances in Plastic Surgery, No. 4. Edinburgh, Churchill Livingstone, 1992: 17.*

25. The correct response is D.

The superior constrictor exists below the level of the hard palate and therefore it does not play a role in velopharyngeal function during speech production. It originates from the posterior pharyngeal raphe and courses downward and forward to insert into the pterygoid hamulus, the lateral pterygoid plate, pterygomaxillary ligament, the mandible and the floor of the mouth.

Reference:

1. *Maue-Dickson W, Dickson DR. Anatomy and physiology related to cleft palate: current research and clinical implications. Plast Reconstr Surg 1980; 65: 83.*
2. *Boorman JG, Freedlander E. Surgical anatomy of the velum and pharynx. In Jackson IT, Sommerlad BC, eds: Recent advances in Plastic Surgery, No. 4. Edinburgh, Churchill Livingstone, 1992: 17.*

26. The correct response is D.

The tendon of tensor veli palatini hooking around the pterygoid hamulus gets relaxed following fracture of the hook of the hamulus. This in turn reduces the tension on the palatal stitch line. The tendon does not roll out on its own from the groove. It can however be hooked and rolled out or cut by a knife or scissor.

Reference:

1. *Maue-Dickson W, Dickson DR. Anatomy and physiology related to cleft palate: current research and clinical implications. Plast Reconstr Surg 1980; 65: 83.*
2. *Boorman JG, Freedlander E. Surgical anatomy of the velum and pharynx. In Jackson IT, Sommerlad BC, eds: Recent advances in Plastic Surgery, No. 4. Edinburgh, Churchill Livingstone, 1992: 17.*

27. The correct response is C.

Pruzansky proposed a classification that divided clefts into four general categories; lip only, lip and palate, palate alone and congenital insufficiency of the palate. Within each category, terminology (complete, incomplete) could be used. This was based on the evaluation of cephalometric radiographs and casts of the face and jaws of more than 350 patients. Davis and Ritchie classification and Veau's classification are based on the morphologic characteristics and features. Kernahan and Stark and Spina's classifications are based on embryologic development.

Reference:

1. *Pruzansky S. Description, classification and analysis of unoperated clefts of the lip and palate. Am J Orthod 1953; 39: 590.*
2. *Kernahan DA, Stark RB. A new classification for cleft lip and cleft palate. Plast Reconstr Surg 1958; 22: 435.*

28. The correct response is C.

Kriens proposed the LAHSHAL code to represent clefts of the lip, alveolus and palate based on the anatomic structures involved. This formula is a concise, descriptive code that is amenable to computer data processing.

Davis and Ritchie classification and Veau's classification are based on the morphologic characteristics and features. Kernahan and Stark and Spina's classifications are based on embryologic development.

Reference:

1. *Kriens O. Documentation of cleft lip, alveolus and palate. In Bardach J. Morris HL, eds. Multidisciplinary management of cleft lip and palate. Philadelphia, WB Saunders, 1990: 127.*
2. *Kernahan DA, Stark RB. A new classification for cleft lip and cleft palate. Plast Reconstr Surg 1958; 22: 435.*

29. The correct response is C.

The Villar-Sancho classification uses codes or symbolic representations of Greek words for the defect to be described. K for lip, G for maxillary process, U for hard palate and S for soft palate.

Davis and Ritchie classification and Veau's classification are based on the morphologic characteristics and features. Kernahan and Stark and Spina's classifications are based on embryologic development.

Reference:

1. *Villar-Sancho B. A proposed new international classification of congenital cleft lip and palate. Plast Reconstr Surg 1962; 30: 263.*
2. *Kernahan DA, Stark RB. A new classification for cleft lip and cleft palate. Plast Reconstr Surg 1958; 22: 435.*

30. The correct response is A.

The palatal aponeurosis is formed by the tensor veli palatini after it hooks around the pterygoid hamulus and fans out in the palate. The other muscles do not form the palatal aponeurosis.

Reference:

1. *Maue-Dickson W, Dickson DR. Anatomy and physiology related to cleft palate: current research and clinical implications. Plast Reconstr Surg 1980; 65: 83.*
2. *Boorman JG, Freedlander E. Surgical anatomy of the velum and pharynx. In Jackson IT, Sommerlad BC, eds: Recent advances in Plastic Surgery, No. 4. Edinburgh, Churchill Livingstone, 1992: 17.*

31. The correct response is D.

The tensor veli palatini takes triple origins from a) Scaphoid fossa of the sphenoid bone b) Cartilaginous portion of the Eustachian tubes (posterolateral) and c) Spine of the sphenoid bone. Its fibres travel downwards and inferiorly up to the pterygoid hamulus, where its tendon bends at a right angle and goes on to insert itself along the posterior border of the hard palate and in the midline raphe where it joins the tensor veli palatini muscle of the other side. It almost lies in a horizontal plane, which enables it to tighten the palate and push the bolus downwards. The tendon acting from below helps in opening the Eustachian tube. It is supplied by the mandibular branch of Trigeminal nerve.

Reference:

1. *Maue-Dickson W, Dickson DR. Anatomy and physiology related to cleft palate: current research and clinical implications. Plast Reconstr Surg 1980; 65: 83.*
2. *Boorman JG, Freedlander E. Surgical anatomy of the velum and pharynx. In Jackson IT, Sommerlad BC, eds: Recent advances in Plastic Surgery, No. 4. Edinburgh, Churchill Livingstone, 1992: 17.*

32. The correct response is E.

The levator muscle has a triple origin from a) Petrous portion of temporal bone, b) Cartilaginous portion of the Eustachian tube (posteromedial) and c) Tympanic part of temporal bone. The fibres of the levator travel downwards to form the central portion of the soft palate by merging with the fibres from the other side. The two muscles together form an oblique sling, which on contraction moves and pulls the palate upwards and backwards. Muscle fibres from the palatoglossus and palatopharyngeus intermingle with the fibres of the levator.

Reference:

1. *Dickson DR. Anatomy of the normal velopharyngeal mechanism. Clin Plast Surg 1975; 2: 235.*
2. *Maue-Dickson W, Dickson DR. Anatomy and physiology related to cleft palate: current research and clinical implications. Plast Reconstr Surg 1980; 65: 83.*
3. *Boorman JG, Freedlander E. Surgical anatomy of the velum and pharynx. In Jackson IT, Sommerlad BC, eds: Recent advances in Plastic Surgery, No. 4. Edinburgh, Churchill Livingstone, 1992: 17.*

33. The correct response is C.

The musculus uvulae is the only intrinsic muscle of the palate. It is a paired muscle that is the most superiorly located of the muscles of the velum. It is orientated longitudinally on the nasal side of the levator veli palatini.The muscle takes origin from the palatine aponeurosis and ends in the uvula. It helps in speech and regulates the length of the posterior portion of the soft palate and uvula, probably like the lumbrical muscles of the hand. It can bend the uvula forwards.

Reference:

1. *Dickson DR. Anatomy of the normal velopharyngeal mechanism. Clin Plast Surg 1975; 2:235.*
2. *Maue-Dickson W, Dickson DR. Anatomy and physiology related to cleft palate: current research and clinical implications. Plast Reconstr Surg 1980; 65: 83.*

34. The correct response is A.

The palatoglossus muscle forms the anterior pillar of the tonsil. It forms the anterior arch. It arises from the palatine aponeurosis and is inserted into the side of the tongue. It helps to pull the tongue up to narrow the oral cavity and separates the oral cavity from the oropharynx.

Reference:

1. *Dickson DR. Anatomy of the normal velopharyngeal mechanism. Clin Plast Surg 1975; 2: 235.*
2. *Maue-Dickson W, Dickson DR. Anatomy and physiology related to cleft palate: current research and clinical implications. Plast Reconstr Surg 1980; 65: 83.*

35. The correct response is B.

The palatopharyngeus forms the posterior arch. It arises from the posterior border of hard palate and palatine aponeurosis and is inserted into the posterior border of thyroid cartilage. It forms the longitudinal muscle coat of the pharynx. It pulls the pharynx upwards and helps in swallowing. It forms the palatopharyngeal arch which lies behind the tonsils.

Reference:

1. *Dickson DR. Anatomy of the normal velopharyngeal mechanism. Clin Plast Surg 1975; 2: 235.*
2. *Maue-Dickson W, Dickson DR. Anatomy and physiology related to cleft palate: current research and clinical implications. Plast Reconstr Surg 1980; 65: 83.*

36. The correct response is B.

The highest incidence of familial occurrence of 2% is with sagittal craniosynostosis.

Reference:

1. *Posnick JC. Craniofacial and maxillofacial surgery. Philadelphia, WB Saunders, 2000: 127.*
2. *Cohen MM Jr, Kreiborg S. Birth prevalence studies of the Crouzon syndrome: comparison of direct and indirect methods. Clin Genet 1992; 41:12-15.*

37. The correct response is E.

All of the above are features of Apert's syndrome that is characterised by craniosynostosis and anomalies of hands and feet.

Reference:

Kreiborg S, Aduss H. Pre- and postsurgical facial growth in patients with Crouzon's and Apert's syndromes. Cleft Palate J 1986; 23 (suppl 1): 78-90.

38. The correct response is A.

Tessier ranked the severity of deformity in adults by measuring the interorbital distance and placed it in three categories - first, second and third degrees. The intercanthal distance of 30-34 mm will be classified as first degree. The second degree will have 34-40 mm and third degree will have over 40 mm of intercanthal distance.

Hypertelorism has also been classified into four types based on C.T. scan findings as below :

A. Type I = Parallel orbital walls
B. Type II = Wedge shaped posteriorly
C. Type III = Oval
D. Type IV = Wedge shaped anteriorly

Reference:

1. *Tessier P. Orbital hypertelorism.I. Successive surgical attempts. Material and Methods. Causes and mechanisms. Scand J Plast Reconstr Surg 1972; 6: 135-155.*
2. *Farkas LG. Anthropometry of the Head and Face, 2nd ed. New York, Raven Press, 1994.*

39. The correct response is D.

An encephalocoele is a herniation of dura, cerebrospinal fluid and brain tissue through a defect in the cranium.

Reference:

1. *Charoonsmith T, Suwanwela C. Frontoethmoidal encephalomeningocoele with special reference to plastic reconstruction. Clin Plast Surg 1974; 1: 27-47.*
2. *Bauer BS. Benign tumours and conditions of the head and neck. In Coleman JJ, Wilkins EG, VanderKam VM. Head and Neck Surgery. St. Louis, Mosby, 2000: 1135.*

40. The correct response is C.

The common pathway for frontonasal malformations including dermal glioma and encephalocoele is an evagination of dura through the foramen cecum. This occurs in the prenasal space between the skin and the nasal cartilages.

Reference:

1. *Bauer BS. Benign tumours and conditions of the head and neck. In Coleman JJ, Wilkins EG, VanderKam VM. Head and Neck Surgery. St. Louis, Mosby, 2000: 1135.*
2. *Charoonsmith T, Suwanwela C. Frontoethmoidal encephalomeningocoele with special reference to plastic reconstruction. Clin Plast Surg 1974; 1: 27-47.*

41. The correct response is C.

Van der Woude syndrome is the commonest syndrome associated with cleft lip and palate. The incidence is between 1 in 35,000 and 1 in 100,000 white in individuals and it occurs in 1% to 2% of patients with facial clefts. The diagnostic finding in this syndrome is bilateral paramedian lower lip pits.

Reference:

Burdick AB. Genetic epidemiology and control of genetic expression in van der Woude syndrome. J Craniofac Genet Dev Biol Suppl 1986; 2: 99-105.

42. The correct response is C.

Van der Woude syndrome is the commonest syndrome associated with cleft lip and palate. The incidence is between 1 in 35,000 and 1 in 100,000 white in individuals and it occurs in 1% to 2% of patients with facial clefts. The diagnostic finding in this syndrome is bilateral paramedian lower lip pits. These pits are oval or transverse sinuses that are present at the dry and wet vermilion junctions. They typically traverse the underlying orbicularis muscle and end in a blind pouch that communicates with the underlying minor salivary glands.

Reference:

Burdick AB. Genetic epidemiology and control of genetic expression in van der Woude syndrome. J Craniofac Genet Dev Biol Suppl 1986; 2: 99-105.

43. The correct response is D.

The velocardiofacial syndrome is associated with palate abnormality, mandibular retrusion, narrow palpebral fissures, ventricular septal defect and other abnormalities. The most important finding for surgeons is a medial displacement of the carotid artery into the pharynx which must be considered in planning for pharyngeal flap surgery.

Reference:

1. *D'Antonio LL, Marsh JL. Abnormal carotid arteries in the velocardiofacial syndrome. Plast Reconstr Surg 1987; 80: 471-472.*
2. *Shprintzen RA. New syndrome involving cleft palate, cardiac anomalies, typical facies, and learning disabilities: velocardiofacial syndrome. Cleft Palate Craniofac J 1978; 15: 56-62.*

44. The correct response is C.

Epibulbar dermoid is a characteristic feature of Goldenhar syndrome by which it can be differentiated from hemifacial microsomia. The rest of the features are found in hemifacial microsomia.

Reference:

1. *Feingold M, Baum J. Goldenhar's syndrome. Am J Dis Child 1978; 132: 136-138.*
2. *Gorlin RJ, Pindborg JJ, Cohen MM. Syndromes of the Head and Neck, 2nd ed. New York, McGraw-Hill, 1976.*

45. The correct response is E.

The deformities in craniofacial microsomia involve ear, mandible, maxilla, pterygoid process of sphenoid bone, temporal bone, frontal bone and facial nerve besides other structures.

Reference:

1. *Feingold M, Baum J. Goldenhar's syndrome. Am J Dis Child 1978; 132: 136-138.*
2. *Cousley RR, Calvert ML. Current concepts in the understanding and management of hemifacial microsomia. Br J Plast Surg 1997; 50: 536-551.*

46. The correct response is B.

In craniofacial microsomia, the jaw deviates towards the affected side because of the weakness of the jaw muscles (masseter and medial pterygoid) and hypoplasia of the mandible.

Reference:

1. *Feingold M, Baum J. Goldenhar's syndrome. Am J Dis Child 1978; 132: 136-138.*
2. *Cousley RR, Calvert ML. Current concepts in the understanding and management of hemifacial microsomia. Br J Plast Surg 1997; 50: 536-551.*

47. The correct response is E.

All of the above may be observed in cases with craniofacial microsomia, besides the three major features of auricular, mandibular and maxillary hypoplasia. The mandible, maxilla, zygomatic bone and orbit show hypoplasia. Soft tissue hypoplasia includes masseter, medial pterygoid and lateral pterygoid muscles. The ear deformities include preauricular sinus, skin tags, microtia, hearing loss and abnormally placed and deformed ears.

Reference:

1. *Grayson BH, McCarthy JG, Bookstein F. Analysis of craniofacial asymmetry by multiplane cephalometry. Am J Orthod 1983; 84: 217-224.*
2. *Cousley RR, Calvert ML. Current concepts in the understanding and management of hemifacial microsomia. Br J Plast Surg 1997; 50: 536-551.*

48. The correct response is D.

Boat head shape of the skull is seen in scaphocephaly. The sagittal suture is involved which leads to characteristic development of the head in the form of a boat.

Reference:

1. *Cohen MM. Syndromes with craniosynostosis. In Cohen MM, MacLean RE, eds: Craniosynostosis: Diagnosis, Evaluation and Management. New York, Oxford University Press, 2000: 309-440.*
2. *Cohen MM. Sutural biology. In Cohen MM, MacLean RE, eds: Craniosynostosis: Diagnosis, Evaluation and Management. New York, Oxford University Press, 2000: 11-23.*

49. The correct response is E.

Tower head shape of the head is seen in turricephaly. Multiple sutures are involved which leads to characteristic development of the tower head shape of the skull.

Reference:

1. *Cohen MM. Syndromes with craniosynostosis. In Cohen MM, MacLean RE, eds: Craniosynostosis: Diagnosis, Evaluation and Management. New York, Oxford University Press, 2000: 309-440.*
2. *Cohen MM. Sutural biology. In Cohen MM, MacLean RE, eds: Craniosynostosis: Diagnosis, Evaluation and Management. New York, Oxford University Press, 2000: 11-23.*

50. The correct response is A.

Sagittal craniosynostosis is the commonest nonsyndromic synostoses characterised by boat shaped skull, frontal bossing, long anterior and posterior cranial fossa and occipital protuberance.

Reference:

1. *Cohen MM. Syndromes with craniosynostosis. In Cohen MM, MacLean RE, eds: Craniosynostosis: Diagnosis, Evaluation and Management. New York, Oxford University Press, 2000: 309-440.*
2. *Cohen MM. Sutural biology. In Cohen MM, MacLean RE, eds: Craniosynostosis: Diagnosis, Evaluation and Management. New York, Oxford University Press, 2000: 11-23.*

51. The correct response is B.

Brow recession is common in unilateral coronal synostosis. The individuals with coronal synostosis have progressively stigmatising facial deformity. They can have raised eyebrow on the same side due to ipsilateral frontal recession, wide eye on the same side and smaller on the normal side due to frontal bossing and affected side face may be expanded with the normal side of face being compressed.

Reference:

1. *Cohen MM. Syndromes with craniosynostosis. In Cohen MM, MacLean RE, eds: Craniosynostosis: Diagnosis, Evaluation and Management. New York, Oxford University Press, 2000: 309-440.*
2. *Cohen MM. Sutural biology. In Cohen MM, MacLean RE, eds: Craniosynostosis: Diagnosis, Evaluation and Management. New York, Oxford University Press, 2000: 11-23.*

52. The correct response is A.

Coronal craniosynostosis results in a skull which does not grow anteroposteriorly leading to recessed frontal bones and flattened occiput. This condition is known as brachycephaly. Brachycephaly hence occurs following decreased anteroposterior diameter and an increased temporoparietal width as demonstrated on CT. The fused coronal suture is also clearly visible on both the sides. Turricephaly and acrocephaly occur because of increased vertical height of the skull although these occur in syndromic individuals with multiple suture involvement.

Plagiocephaly or "twisted head" is used to describe anterior or posterior deformities. Plagiocephaly is classified as anterior or posterior as well as synostotic and nonsynostotic or deformational. Anterior synostotic plagiocephaly refers to coronal craniosynostosis and posterior synostotic plagiocephaly refers to lambdoid craniosynostosis.

Reference:

1. *Marsh JL, Kaufman B. Bilateral coronal craniosynostosis. In Lin KY, Ogle RC, Jane JA, eds: Craniofacial Surgery: Science and Surgical Technique. Philadelphia, WB Saunders, 2001: 218-224.*
2. *Cohen MM. Syndromes with craniosynostosis. In Cohen MM, MacLean RE, eds: Craniosynostosis: Diagnosis, Evaluation and Management. New York, Oxford University Press, 2000: 309-440.*

53. The correct response is D.

Metopic synostosis is most common in newborns and is often associated with behavioural impairment because of a greater frequency of central nervous system anomalies and chromosome defects detectable on routine karyotyping. It is characterised by triangular head with bifrontal narrowing and parieto-occipital protrusion. The cranium has a midfrontal keel like projection.

Reference:

1. *Shuper A, Merlob P, Grunebaum M et al. The incidence of isolated craniosynostosis in the newborn infant. Am J Dis Child 1985; 139: 85-86.*
2. *Lajeunie F, Le Merrer M, Marchac D, Renier D. Syndromal and monosyndromal primary trigonocephaly: analysis of a series of 237 patients. Am J Med Genet 1998; 75: 211-215.*

54. The correct response is C.

Excessive caudal protrusion of one mastoid with minimalization of the other is a pathognomonic clinico-radiologic sign of unilateral lambdoid synostosis. The combination of frontal dominance and pathognomonic facial dysmorphism can clinically separate unilateral coronal synostosis from other causes of plagiocephaly.

Reference:

1. *Ellenbogen RG, Gruss JS, Cunningham ML. Update on craniofacial surgery: the differential diagnosis of lambdoid synostosis/posterior plagiocephaly. Clin Neurosurg, 2000; 47: 303-318.*
2. *Mulliken JB, Vander Woude DL, Hansen M, et al. Analysis of posterior plagiocephaly: deformational versus synostotic. Plast Reconstr Surg 1999;103: 371-380.*

55. The correct response is D.

Lip adhesion surgery advocated by Johnson (1960) was for wide unilateral clefts with a view to mould the arches and to reduce the gap for final correction at a later stage. It is however associated with complications like dehiscence and its acceptability varies from centre to centre and patient to patient.

Reference:

1. *Takahashi S. Lip adhesion operation. Jpn J Oral Surg 1970; 16: 68.*
2. *Randall P. A lip adhesion operation in cleft lip surgery. Plast Reconstr Surg 1965; 35: 371.*

56. The correct response is D.

The Mohler repair is a versatile technique of unilateral cheiloplasty that is useful for most type of clefts. It is especially useful for staged reconstruction of the bilateral asymmetric cleft lip owing to the design of the incisions. It also places the cleft side philtral column in a more ideal anatomic position as compared to the other techniques.

Reference:

1. *Mohler L. Unilateral cleft lip repair. Operative Techniques Plast Reconstr Surg 1995; 2: 193-199.*
2. *Mohler L. Unilateral cleft lip repair. Plast Reconstr Surg 1987; 80: 511-517.*

57. The correct response is A.

The levator labii superioris is responsible for initiating the smile by raising the upper lip. A full smile however requires actions of zygomaticus major and the superior fibres of the buccinator.

Reference:

1. *Zachrisson B. Esthetic factors involved in anterior tooth display and the smile vertical dimension. J Clin Orthod 1998; 32: 432-445.*
2. *Peck S, Peck L, Kataina M. The gingival smile line. Angle Orthod 1992; 62: 91-100, discussion 101-102.*

58. The correct response is D.

All the factors as mentioned in A,B,C are responsible to a variable extent for the peaking. Correction is done by incorporating a triangular flap from just above the white roll from the lateral lip element. Peaking as a complication is not seen in cases managed by triangular flap methods of repair.

Reference:

1. *Noordhoff MS, Chen YR, Chen KT et al. The surgical technique for the complete unilateral cleft lip-nasal deformity. Operative Techniques Plast Reconstr Surg 1995; 2: 167-174.*
2. *Mulliken JB, Martinez-Perez D. The principle of rotation advancement for repair of unilateral complete cleft lip and nasal deformity: technical variations and analysis of results. Plast Reconstr Surg 1999; 104: 1247-1260.*

59. The correct response is E.

All of the above deformities can be corrected by V-Y plasty.

Reference:

1. *Noordhoff MS, Chen YR, Chen KT et al. The surgical technique for the complete unilateral cleft lip-nasal deformity. Operative Techniques Plast Reconstr Surg 1995; 2: 167-174.*
2. *Salyer KE. Early and late treatment of the unilateral cleft nasal deformity. Cleft Palate Craniofac J 1992; 29: 556-569.*

60. The correct response is D.

All of the above factors mentioned at A,B,C contribute to a variable extent in the development of vermilion notching in the postoperative result following cleft lip repair.

Reference:

1. *Noordhoff MS, Chen YR, Chen KT et al. The surgical technique for the complete unilateral cleft lip-nasal deformity. Operative Techniques Plast Reconstr Surg 1995; 2: 167-174.*
2. *Salyer KE. Early and late treatment of the unilateral cleft nasal deformity. Cleft Palate Craniofac J 1992; 29: 556-569.*

61. The correct response is C.

The alar web in cleft lip nose deformity consists of a fold of vestibular skin along with prolapsed lower alar cartilage. Successful treatment of alar webbing needs to address both these issues relating to excision of skin and repositioning the alar cartilage after ellliptical trimming.

Reference:

1. *Agarwal R, Chandra R. The alar web in cleft lip nose deformity: Study in adult unilateral clefts. J Craniofac Surg. 2012 [In Press].*
2. *Agarwal R, Chandra R. The Septospinal Ligament in Cleft lip Nose Deformity: Study in Adult Unilateral Clefts. Plast Reconstr Surg 2007; 120(6): 1633-1640.*

62. The correct response is E.

All of the above factors have a role in protrusion of the premaxilla.

Reference:

1. *Salyer KE. Primary unilateral cleft-lip/nose repair. In Bardach J, Salyer KE. eds: Atlas of Craniofacial and Cleft Surgery, vol2. Philadelphia. Lippincott-Raven. 1999; 423-433.*
2. *Latham RA. Development and structure of the premaxillary deformity in bilateral cleft lip palate. Br J Plast Surg 1973; 26: 1.*

63. The correct response is B.

Resection of the projecting premaxilla should be condemned. The reason is that the long term effects on dentofacial development are detrimental and devastating following the resection. The rest of the methods can be used for the management of projecting premaxilla.

Reference:

1. *Motohashi N, Pruzansky S. Long term effects of premaxillary excision in patients with complete bilateral cleft lips and palates. Cleft Palate J 1981; 18: 177.*
2. *Cronin TD. Surgery of the double cleft lip and protruding premaxilla. Plast Reconstr Surg 1957; 19: 389.*

64. The correct response is C.

The forked flap recruits skin from the prolabial skin for columella reconstruction. The prolabial skin is divided into three parts. The central part is used for constructing the midline skin of the lip while the two lateral forks are banked under the alar base for later use.

Reference:

1. *Millard DR Jr. Closure of bilateral cleft lip and elongation of columella by two operations in infancy. Plast Reconstr Surg 1971; 47: 324.*
2. *Schultz LW. Bilateral cleft lips. Plast Reconstr Surg 1946; 1: 338.*

65. The correct response is C.

Airway obstruction is the most serious complication following bilateral cleft lip and nose repair in the immediate postoperative period. Haematoma and oedema of a bilaterally dissected nose can produce a transient but complete nasal obstruction. Haemorrhage can also be a significant problem. The other options dehiscence, infection and scarring can also occur following bilateral cleft lip nose repair.

Reference:

1. *Millard DR Jr. Closure of bilateral cleft lip and elongation of columella by two operations in infancy. Plast Reconstr Surg 1971; 47: 324.*
2. *Schultz LW. Bilateral cleft lips. Plast Reconstr Surg 1946; 1: 338.*

66. The correct response is B.

Cronin et al in 1990 described a conchal cartilage graft to lengthen the medial crus.

Reference:

Cronin T, Cronin E, Roper P, et al. Bilateral cleft. In McCarthy JG, ed: Reconstructive Plastic Surgery, vol 4. Philadelphia, WB Saunders, 1990: 2653.

67. The correct response is E.

The anterior nasal spine is poorly formed or absent in the bilateral cleft lip deformity, resulting in a retruded area under the base of the septal cartilage and recession of the footplates of the medial crura. It is present in the rest of the conditions.

Reference:

1. *Millard DR Jr. Closure of bilateral cleft lip and elongation of columella by two operations in infancy. Plast Reconstr Surg 1971; 47: 324.*
2. *Cronin T, Cronin E, Roper P, et al. Bilateral cleft. In McCarthy JG, ed: Reconstructive Plastic Surgery, vol 4. Philadelphia, WB Saunders, 1990: 2653.*

68. The correct response is D.

The submucous cleft palate is traditionally defined by a triad of deformities: a bifid uvula, a notched posterior hard palate, and muscular diastasis of the velum. Submucous clefts vary considerably, however, and muscular diastasis can occur in the absence of a bifid uvula. The other conditions listed do not have a notch in the posterior palate.

Reference:

1. *Millard DR Jr. Closure of bilateral cleft lip and elongation of columella by two operations in infancy. Plast Reconstr Surg 1971; 47: 324.*
2. *Cronin T, Cronin E, Roper P, et al. Bilateral cleft. In McCarthy JG, ed: Reconstructive Plastic Surgery, vol 4. Philadelphia, WB Saunders, 1990: 2653.*

69. The correct response is B.

von Langenbeck is credited with the description of the mucoperiosteal plane of dissection for closure of the cleft palate. He described the use of this plane of dissection for ease in mobilising the flaps.

Reference:

Goldwyn RM. Bernhard von Langenbeck. His life and legacy. Plast Reconstr Surg 1969;44: 248-254.

70. The correct response is C.

The time for repair of cleft palate depends on the optimal speech outcome. A growing body of opinion now supports and advocates repair of the cleft palate around 9-10 months of age for children with apparently normal development. However the optimal time for palatoplasty still remains scientifically unproven.

Reference:

1. *Peterson-Falzone SJ. The relationship between timing of cleft palate surgery and speech outcome: what have we learned, and where do we stand in the 1990s? Semin Orthod 1996; 2: 185-191.*
2. *Evans D, Renfrew C. The timing of primary cleft palate repair. Scand J Plast Reconstr Surg 1974; 8: 153-155.*

71. The correct response is C.

The Veau-Wardill-Kilner technique helps to push the palate back and achieve greater length for the palate and also places the levator in a more favourable position. However this repair leaves large open areas anteriorly which may lead to scarring and loss of maxillary width anteriorly.

Reference:

1. *Wallace AF. A history of the repair of cleft lip and palate in Britain before World War II. Ann Plast Surg 1987; 19: 266-273.*
2. *Cronin TD. Method of preventing raw areas on the nasal surface of soft palate in push-back surgery. Plast Reconstr Surg 1957; 20: 474.*

72. The correct response is C.

Furlow adapted the principle of Z-plasty for closure of cleft palate. Z-plasty is performed on both the nasal and oral surfaces of the soft palate in opposite directions. The cleft margin is used for placing the central limb of the Z and the levator muscle is included in the posteriorly based flap.

Reference:

1. *Furlow LT Jr. Cleft palate repair by double opposing Z-plasty. Plast Reconstr Surg 1986; 78: 724.*
2. *Randall P, LaRossa D, Solomon M. Experience with the Furlow double-reversing Z-plasty for cleft palate repair. Plast Reconstr Surg 1986; 77: 569-576.*

73. The correct response is D.

The nasal septum needs to be incised so as to be able to raise the vomer flap. This flap is commonly used to close the nasal lining in repair of the cleft palate. In unilateral clefts, the flap is reflected down after incising the nasal septum, whereas in bilateral clefts, two vomer flaps are needed to close the nasal lining.

Reference:

1. *Friede H, Johanson B. A follow up study of cleft children treated with vomer flap as part of a three stage soft tissue surgical procedure. Facial morphology and dental occlusion. Scand J Plast Reconstr Surg 1977; 11: 45-47.*
2. *Delaire J, Precious D. Avoidance of the use of vomerine mucosa in primary surgical management of velopalatine clefts. Oral Surg Oral Med Oral Pathol 1985; 60: 589-597.*

74. The correct response is E.

All of the above are valid reasons for performing alveolar bone graft in clefts.

Reference:

1. *Dado DV, Rosenstein SW, Alder ME et al. Long term assessment of early alveolar bone grafts using three dimensional computer assisted tomography: a pilot study. Plast Reconstr Surg 1997; 99: 1840-1845.*
2. *Eppley BL. Alveolar cleft bone grafting. Part I. Primary bone grafting. J Oral Maxillofac Surg 1996; 54: 74-82.*

75. The correct response is B.

Primary alveolar bone grafting refers to the placement of bone in the alveolar and hard palate cleft usually at the time of cleft palate repair. This has been proposed to avoid a later operation. However most investigators have found that there is a negative effect on maxillary growth from primary bone grafting.

Reference:

1. *Dado DV, Rosenstein SW, Alder ME et al. Long term assessment of early alveolar bone grafts using three dimensional computer assisted tomography: a pilot study. Plast Reconstr Surg 1997; 99: 1840-1845.*
2. *Eppley BL. Alveolar cleft bone grafting. Part I. Primary bone grafting. J Oral Maxillofac Surg 1996; 54: 74-82.*

76. The correct response is E.

Secondary alveolar bone grafting refers to the placement of bone in the alveolar and hard palate cleft before eruption of the cuspid into the cleft. If the grafting is done after eruption of the cuspid, there is a greater possibility of late root resorption.

Reference:

1. *Bergland O, Semb G, Abyholm FE. Elimination of the residual alveolar cleft by secondary bone grafting and subsequent orthodontic treatment. Cleft Palate J 1986; 23: 175-205.*
2. *Enemark H, Sindet-Pedersen S, Bundgaard M. Long term results after secondary bone grafting of alveolar clefts. J Oral Maxillofac Surg 1987; 45: 913-919.*

77. The correct response is E.

Bilateral complete cleft lip and palate is one of the most challenging condition for the orthodontist as it may pose the greatest degree of orthodontic problems including malalignment of the arches and protrusion of the premaxilla. In contrast the incomplete cleft lip usually poses the least challenge for the orthodontist.

Reference:

1. *Figueroa AA, Reisberg DJ, Polley JW, Cohen M. Intraoral appliance modification to retract the premaxilla in patients with bilateral cleft lip. Cleft Palate Craniofac J 1996; 33: 497-500.*
2. *Aduss H, Figueroa AA. Stages of orthodontic treatment in complete unilateral cleft lip and palate. In Bardach J, Morris HL. eds: Multidisciplinary management of cleft lip and palate. Philadelphia, WB Saunders, 1990: 607-615.*

78. The correct response is A.

In the cleft patient with posterior cross-bite, the arch form changes before the eruption of the primary canines, therefore at the time of eruption of these teeth the maxillary cleft-side primary canine erupts medially to the lower one. In addition, there is minor palatal displacement of the maxillary primary canine and labial displacement of the mandibular one.

Reference:

1. *Figueroa AA, Polley JW, Cohen M. Orthodontic management of the cleft lip and palate patient. Clin Plast Surg 1993; 20: 733-753.*
2. *Aduss H, Figueroa AA. Stages of orthodontic treatment in complete unilateral cleft lip and palate. In Bardach J, Morris HL. eds: Multidisciplinary management of cleft lip and palate. Philadelphia, WB Saunders, 1990: 607-615.*

79. The correct response is E.

The technique of maxillary distraction using rigid external device requires all of the above steps for a successful result. The distracted maxilla has to be retained and hence a rigid appliance should be used for 'retention' for 4-8 weeks or more as required.

Reference:

1. *Figueroa AA, Polley JW. Management of severe cleft maxillary deficiency with distraction osteogenesis: procedure and results. Am J Orthod Dentofacial Orthop 1999; 115: 1-12.*
2. *Figueroa AA, Polley JW, Ko EW. Maxillary distraction for the management of cleft maxillary hypoplasia with a rigid external distraction system. Semin Orthod 1999; 5: 46-51.*

80. The correct response is B.

The perception of inordinate nasal resonance during the production of vowels is termed as hypernasality. Nasal emission is the escape of nasal air associated with the production of consonants. Hyponasality is a decrease in normal nasal resonance and mixed hypernasality and hyponasality is presence of hypernasality and hyponasality in the same individual.

Reference:

Loney RW, Bloem TJ. Velopharyngeal dysfunction: recommendations for use of nomenclature. Cleft Palate J 1987; 24: 334-335.

81. The correct response is E.

The hard palate is not involved in velopharyngeal closure.

Reference:

Loney RW, Bloem TJ. Velopharyngeal dysfunction: recommendations for use of nomenclature. Cleft Palate J 1987; 24: 334-335.

82. The correct response is C.

The submucous cleft palate is characterised by a triad described by Calnan and consisting of bifid uvula, separation of the soft palate musculature in the midline and a notch in the bony posterior hard palate.

Reference:

Calnan JS. Submucous cleft palate. Br J Plast Surg 1954; 6: 264-282.

83. The correct response is E.

All of the above complications may be seen after posterior pharyngeal flap surgery.

Reference:

1. *Lesavoy MA, Borud LJ, Thorson T et al. Upper airway obstruction after pharyngeal flap surgery. Ann Plast Surg 1996; 36: 26-32.*
2. *Hynes W. The results of pharyngoplasty by muscle transplantation in "failed cleft palate" cases, with special reference to the influence of the pharynx on voice production. Ann R Coll Surg Engl 1953; 13: 17-35.*

84. The correct response is D.

The low level of inset of the pharyngoplasty flaps was the greatest criticism of Orticochea's sphincter pharyngoplasty. The flaps were inset much below the level of usual velopharyngeal closure.

Reference:

1. *Riski JE, Serafin D, Riefkohl R et al. A rationale for modifying the site of insertion of the Orticochea pharyngoplasty. Plast Reconstr Surg 1984; 73: 882-890.*
2. *Orticochea M. The timing and management of dynamic muscular pharyngeal sphincter construction in velopharyngeal insufficiency. Br J Plast Surg 1999; 52: 85-87.*

85. The correct response is B.

The nose almost stops growing around the age of 11-12 years in girls as per cephalometric evidence. The nose in boys stops growing around the age of 13-14 years. Henceforth full osseocartilaginous vault surgery and septal modifications should be performed after these ages.

Reference:

1. *Akguner M, Barutcu A, Karaca C. Adolescent growth patterns of the bony and cartilaginous framework of the nose: a cephalometric study. Ann Plast Surg 1998; 41: 66-69.*
2. *Bardach J, Salyer KE. Correction of secondary unilateral cleft lip deformities. In Bardach J, Salyer KE, eds: Surgical Techniques in Cleft Lip and Palate. Chicago, Year Book, 1987: 225 246.*

86. The correct response is C.

The width of philtrum in a normal adult male at the level of Cupid's bow is 8-12 mm. The philtral ridges are not parallel, they gradually narrow as they approach the columella from the Cupid's bow.

Reference:

1. *McCarthy JG, Cutting C. Secondary deformities of cleft lip and palate. In Georgiade NG, Riefkohl R, Barwick W, eds: Textbook of Plastic, Maxillofacial and Reconstructive Surgery. Baltimore, Williams and Wilkins, 1992: 307-319.*
2. Bardach J, Salyer KE. Correction of secondary unilateral cleft lip deformities. In Bardach J, Salyer KE, eds: Surgical Techniques in Cleft Lip and Palate. Chicago, Year Book, 1987: 225-246.

87. The correct response is B.

The width of philtrum in a child at the level of Cupid's bow is 6 mm. The philtral ridges are not parallel, they gradually narrow as they approach the columella from the Cupid's bow.

Reference:

1. *McCarthy JG, Cutting C. Secondary deformities of cleft lip and palate. In Georgiade NG, Riefkohl R, Barwick W, eds: Textbook of Plastic, Maxillofacial and Reconstructive Surgery. Baltimore, Williams and Wilkins, 1992: 307-319.*
2. *Bardach J, Salyer KE. Correction of secondary unilateral cleft lip deformities. In Bardach J, Salyer KE, eds: Surgical Techniques in Cleft Lip and Palate. Chicago, Year Book, 1987: 225-246.*

88. The correct response is B.

The philtral ridges are not parallel, they gradually narrow as they approach the columella from the Cupid's bow.

Reference:

1. *McCarthy JG, Cutting C. Secondary deformities of cleft lip and palate. In Georgiade NG, Riefkohl R, Barwick W, eds: Textbook of Plastic, Maxillofacial and Reconstructive Surgery. Baltimore, Williams and Wilkins, 1992: 307-319.*
2. *Bardach J, Salyer KE. Correction of secondary unilateral cleft lip deformities. In Bardach J, Salyer KE, eds: Surgical Techniques in Cleft Lip and Palate. Chicago, Year Book, 1987: 225-246.*

89. The correct response is C.

The 'whistle' deformity refers to notching of the vermilion. This occurs when there is less vermilion on the medial portion of the lip than on the lateral lip segment.

Reference:

1. *McCarthy J, Cutting C. Secondary deformities of cleft lip and palate. In Georgiade NG, Riefkohl R, Barwick W. eds: Textbook of Plastic, Maxillofacial and Reconstructive Surgery. Baltimore, Williams and Wilkins, 1992: 307-319.*
2. *Kapetansky DI. Double pendulum flaps for whistling deformities in bilateral cleft lips. Plast Reconstr Surg 1971; 47: 321-323.*

90. The correct response is D.

Secondary deformities of the cleft lip and palate are common. Deficiencies of the labial sulcus are most common after bilateral cleft lip repair. This is due to the underlying anatomy of the deformity rather than on the particular technique.

Reference:

1. *McCarthy J, Cutting C. Secondary deformities of cleft lip and palate. In Georgiade NG, Riefkohl R, Barwick W. eds: Textbook of Plastic, Maxillofacial and Reconstructive Surgery. Baltimore, Williams and Wilkins, 1992:307-319.*
2. *Kapetansky DI. Double pendulum flaps for whistling deformities in bilateral cleft lips. Plast Reconstr Surg 1971; 47: 321-323.*

91. The correct response is A.

The tight upper lip deformity is best corrected by an Abbe flap. Other flaps listed are for correction of bigger lip defects.

Reference:

1. *McCarthy J, Cutting C. Secondary deformities of cleft lip and palate. In Georgiade NG, Riefkohl R, Barwick W. eds: Textbook of Plastic, Maxillofacial and Reconstructive Surgery. Baltimore, Williams and Wilkins, 1992:307-319.*
2. *Bardach J, Salyer KE. Correction of secondary unilateral cleft lip deformities. In Bardach J, Salyer KE, eds: Surgical Techniques in Cleft Lip and Palate. Chicago, Year Book, 1987: 225-246.*

92. The correct response is C.

Tight lip is the commonest secondary deformity seen in patients with bilateral cleft lip. This is due to the inherent severity of the deformity rather than because of the type of repair. This problem is further compounded in presence of protruding premaxilla or a wide cleft. It can be treated well using the Abbe flap.

Reference:

1. *McCarthy J, Cutting C. Secondary deformities of cleft lip and palate. In Georgiade NG, Riefkohl R, Barwick W. eds: Textbook of Plastic, Maxillofacial and Reconstructive Surgery. Baltimore, Williams and Wilkins, 1992: 307-319.*
2. *Bardach J, Salyer KE. Correction of secondary unilateral cleft lip deformities. In Bardach J, Salyer KE, eds: Surgical Techniques in Cleft Lip and Palate. Chicago, Year Book, 1987: 225-246.*

93. The correct response is D.

The anatomy of the septum is important in the correction of cleft lip nose deformity. The caudal septum in unilateral cleft lip nose deformity is deviated towards the non-cleft side while the body of the septum often blocks the cleft side vestibule.

Reference:

1. *Agarwal R, Chandra R. The Septospinal Ligament in Cleft lip Nose Deformity: Study in Adult Unilateral Clefts. Plast Reconstr Surg 2007; 120(6): 1633-1640.*
2. *Millard D,* Morovic C. Primary unilateral cleft nose correction: a ten year follow-up. Plast Reconstr Surg 1998; 102: 1331-1338.*

94. The correct response is C.

The septospinal ligament is a structure which develops in the milieu of unilateral cleft lip nose deformity extending between the caudal border of the nasal septum and the anterior nasal spine. It is responsible for the deformity of the tip of the nose. This ligament needs to be excised in order to be able to straighten the septum for correcting the tip in unilateral cleft lip nose deformity.

Reference:

1. *Agarwal R, Chandra R. The Septospinal Ligament in Cleft lip Nose Deformity: Study in Adult Unilateral Clefts. Plast Reconstr Surg 2007; 120(6): 1633-1640.*
2. *Agarwal R, Bhatnagar S.K, Pandey S.D, Singh A.K, Chandra R. Nasal Sill Augmentation in Adult Incomplete Cleft Lip Nose Deformity using Superiorly Based Turn Over Orbicularis Oris Muscle Flap. An Anatomic Approach. Plast. Reconstr. Surg 1998; 102(5): 1350-1357.*

95. The correct response is D.

The nasal sill in unilateral cleft lip nose deformity is affected due to both skeletal and soft tissue hypoplasia. The abnormal insertion of muscles further contribute to the deformity of nose sill in addition to the other features of cleft lip nose deformity. The nasal sill in such cases is widened and depressed due to the above abnormalities.

Reference:

1. *Agarwal R, Chandra R. The Septospinal Ligament in Cleft lip Nose Deformity: Study in Adult Unilateral Clefts. Plast Reconstr Surg 2007; 120(6): 1633-1640.*
2. *Agarwal R, Bhatnagar S.K, Pandey S.D, Singh A.K, Chandra R. Nasal Sill Augmentation in Adult Incomplete Cleft Lip Nose Deformity using Superiorly Based Turn Over Orbicularis Oris Muscle Flap. An Anatomic Approach. Plast. Reconstr. Surg 1998; 102(5): 1350-1357.*

96. The correct response is E.

All of the above findings may be observed in varying grades of severity in patients with unilateral cleft lip nose deformity.

Reference:

1. *Agarwal R, Mandhani PA, Parihar A , Chandra R. Three dimensional computed tomographic analysis of the maxilla in unilateral cleft lip and palate: Implications for rhinoplasty. J Craniofac Surg. 2012 [In Press].*
2. *Agarwal, R, Chandra, R. The Unrecognized Skeletal Components of the Cleft Lip Nose Deformity. Plast Reconstr Surg 2008; 122(1): 313-315.*

97. The correct response is B.

Tessier classified interorbital distances as follows.

Grade I – 30-34 mm

Grade II – 34-40 mm

Grade III – 40 mm and above

The average inter orbital distance in males is 28 mm and 25 mm in women.

Reference:

1. *Converse JM, Ransohoff J, Mathews ES, et al. Ocular hypertelorism and pseudohypertelorism. Advances in surgical treatment. Plast Reconstr Surg 1970; 45:1.*
2. *Tessier P, Guiot G, Derome P. Orbital hypertelorism. II. Definite treatment of orbitalhypertelorism (OR.H.) by craniofacial or by extracranial osteotomies. Scan J Plast Reconstr Surg 1973; 7: 39.*

98. The correct response is D.

The posterior ethmoidal cells are not enlarged in orbital hypertelorism. The rest are features found in orbital hypertelorism.

Reference:

1. *Converse JM, Ransohoff J, Mathews ES, et al. Ocular hypertelorism and pseudohypertelorism. Advances in surgical treatment. Plast Reconstr Surg 1970; 45: 1.*
2. *Tessier P, Guiot G, Derome P. Orbital hypertelorism. II. Definite treatment of orbitalhypertelorism (OR.H.) by craniofacial or by extracranial osteotomies. Scan J Plast Reconstr Surg 1973; 7: 39.*

99. The correct response is E.

The bipartition procedure is used to treat all the above deformities. This procedure is also done through a combined craniofacial route to mobilise the circumferential orbit and avoid injury to the frontal lobe of the brain.

Reference:

van der Meulen JC. Medial faciotomy. Br J Plast Surg 1979; 32: 339.

100. The correct response is D.

Subcranial osteotomy entails a U-shaped osteotomy with paramedian bone resection. The orbits are mobilised and bone grafts are placed in the lateral defects. The other osteotomies do not fall in the description of U-shaped osteotomy.

Reference:

McCarthy JG, Thorne CHM, Woodsmith D. Principles of craniofacial surgery: orbital hypertelorism. In McCarthy JG, ed: Plastic Surgery. Philadelphia, WB Saunders, 1990: 2974.

101. The correct response is C.

The number 0 cleft involves the midline structures and the soft tissue and skeletal characteristics also involve these structures. The nasal process of maxilla are broad, flattened and displaced laterally from the midline. The nasal septum is thickened. Cleft of the lip and downslanting of the eyes are not observed in number 0 cleft.

Reference:

1. *Tessier P. Anatomical classification of facial, craniofacial and laterofacial clefts. J Maxillofac Surg 1976; 4: 69.*
2. *Tessier P. Anatomical classification of facial, craniofacial and laterofacial clefts. In Tessier P, ed: Symposium on Plastic Surgery in the Orbital Region. St. Louis, CV Mosby, 1976: 189-198.*

102. The correct response is C.

The number 1 cleft, similar to the common cleft lip, passes through the Cupid's bow and then through the alar cartilage dome. Notching in the area of the soft triangle of the nose is a distinct feature. The columella may be short and broad. The nasal tip and nasal septum deviate away from the cleft.

Reference:

1. *Tessier P. Anatomical classification of facial, craniofacial and laterofacial clefts. J Maxillofac Surg 1976; 4: 69.*
2. *David DJ, Moore MH, Cooter RD. Tessier clefts revisited with a third dimension. Cleft Palate J. 1989; 26: 163.*

103. The correct response is A.

The nasal deformity is in the middle third of the alar rim and distinguishes the number 2 cleft from other clefts. The rest of the options coincide with the number 3 cleft.

Reference:

1. *Tessier P. Anatomical classification of facial, craniofacial and laterofacial clefts. J Maxillofac Surg 1976; 4: 69.*
2. *David DJ, Moore MH, Cooter RD. Tessier clefts revisited with a third dimension. Cleft Palate J. 1989; 26: 163.*

104. The correct response is E.

Osseous characteristics of this facial cleft include involvement of the orbit and direct communication of the oral, nasal, and orbital cavities. The cleft begins between the lateral incisor and the canine. In contrast to the number 1 and number 2 facial clefts, the anterior maxillary arch is flat in the number 3 cleft. The number 3 cleft disrupts the frontal process of the maxilla and then terminates in the lacrimal groove.

Reference:

1. *Tessier P. Anatomical classification of facial, craniofacial and laterofacial clefts. J Maxillofac Surg 1976; 4: 69.*
2. *David DJ, Moore MH, Cooter RD. Tessier clefts revisited with a third dimension. Cleft Palate J. 1989; 26: 163.*

105. The correct response is D.

The number 4 cleft begins between the lateral incisor and the canine. The cleft extends lateral to the pyriform aperture to involve the maxillary sinus. The medial wall of the maxillary sinus, is intact. A confluence exists between the oral cavity, maxillary sinus, and orbital cavity but not the nasal cavity as is seen in number 3 cleft. The cleft then passes medial to the infraorbital foramen. This landmark defines the boundary between the medial number 4 facial cleft and lateral number 5 facial cleft. The number 4 cleft terminates at the medial aspect of the inferior orbital rim. With an absent medial orbital floor and rim, the globe may prolapse inferiorly.

Reference:

1. *Tessier P. Anatomical classification of facial, craniofacial and laterofacial clefts. J Maxillofac Surg 1976; 4: 69.*
2. *Longaker MT, Lipshutz GS, Kawamoto HK Jr. Reconstruction of Tessier no. 4 clefts revisited. Plast Reconstr Surg. 1997; 99: 1501.*

106. The correct response is E.

All of the above features may be seen in number 6 cleft. The number 6 facial cleft is along the zygomatico–maxillary suture separating the maxilla and zygoma. There is no alveolar cleft, but a short posterior maxilla may result in an occlusal tilt. Choanal atresia is common. The cleft enters the orbit at the lateral third of the orbital rim and floor. It connects to the inferior orbital fissure. The zygoma is hypoplastic with an intact zygomatic arch. There is narrowing of the anterior cranial fossa. The sphenoid is normal.

Reference:

1. *Tessier P. Anatomical classification of facial, craniofacial and laterofacial clefts. J Maxillofac Surg 1976; 4: 69.*
2. *Kawamoto HK Jr. The kaleidoscopic world of rare craniofacial clefts: order out of chaos (Tessier classification). Clin Plast Surg. 1976; 3: 529.*

107. The correct response is D.

There is a wide range of osseous anomalies in number 7 cleft. The skeletal cleft passes through the pterygomaxillary junction. Tessier believed that the cleft is centered in the region of the zygomaticotemporal suture. The posterior maxilla and mandibular ramus are hypoplastic in the vertical dimension, creating an occlusal plane that is canted cephalad on the affected side. The coronoid process and condyle are also often hypoplastic and asymmetric, which contributes to a posterior open bite on the affected side.

Reference:

1. *Tessier P. Anatomical classification of facial, craniofacial and laterofacial clefts. J Maxillofac Surg 1976; 4: 69.*
2. *Kawamoto HK Jr. The kaleidoscopic world of rare craniofacial clefts: order out of chaos (Tessier classification). Clin Plast Surg. 1976; 3: 529.*

108. The correct response is D.

The bony component of the 8 cleft occurs at the frontozygomatic suture. Tessier noted a notch in this region in patients with Goldenhar syndrome. In the complete form of Treacher Collins syndrome' the zygoma may be hypoplastic or absent.

Reference:

1. *Tessier P. Anatomical classification of facial, craniofacial and laterofacial clefts. J Maxillofac Surg 1976;4:69.*
2. *David DJ, Moore MH, Cooter RD. Tessier clefts revisited with a third dimension. Cleft Palate J. 1989; 26: 163.*

109. The correct response is D.

The number 8 cleft extends from the lateral canthus to the temporal region. A dermatocele may occupy the coloboma of the lateral commissure. Occasionally, abnormal hair manifestations can be seen along a line between the temporal area and the lateral canthus. The soft-tissue malformation presents as a true lateral commissure coloboma (dermatocele) with absence of the lateral canthus. Abnormalities of the globe, in the form of epibulbar dermoids may also be present.

Reference:

1. *Tessier P. Anatomical classification of facial, craniofacial and laterofacial clefts. J Maxillofac Surg 1976; 4: 69.*
2. *David DJ, Moore MH, Cooter RD. Tessier clefts revisited with a third dimension. Cleft Palate J. 1989; 26: 163.*

110. The correct response is D.

Changes in the cribriform plate are the hallmark of number 13 cleft. The paramedian bony cleft traverses the frontal bone before coursing along the olfactory groove. There is widening of the olfactory groove, the cribriform plate, and the ethmoid sinus, which results in hypertelorism. A paramedian frontal encephalocele can cause the cribriform plate to be displaced inferiorly, leading to orbital dystopia.

Reference:

1. *Tessier P. Anatomical classification of facial, craniofacial and laterofacial clefts. J Maxillofac Surg 1976; 4: 69.*
2. *David DJ, Moore MH, Cooter RD. Tessier clefts revisited with a third dimension. Cleft Palate J. 1989; 26: 163.*

111. The correct response is E.

The frontonasal angle is obtuse due to the cleft which is medial to the medial canthus. The rest of the features are present in the number 12 cleft.

Reference:

1. *Tessier P. Anatomical classification of facial, craniofacial and laterofacial clefts. J Maxillofac Surg 1976; 4: 69.*
2. *David DJ, Moore MH, Cooter RD. Tessier clefts revisited with a third dimension. Cleft Palate J. 1989; 26: 163.*

112. The correct response is D.

There is typically a paramedian frontal encephalocele, in number 13 cleft which is located between the nasal bone and the frontal process of the maxilla. The soft-tissue cleft is medial to intact eyelids and eyebrows. The medial end of the eyebrow, however, can be displaced inferiorly. A V-shaped frontal hair projection can also be seen.

Reference:

1. *Tessier P. Anatomical classification of facial, craniofacial and laterofacial clefts. J Maxillofac Surg 1976; 4: 69.*
2. *David DJ, Moore MH, Cooter RD. Tessier clefts revisited with a third dimension. Cleft Palate J. 1989; 26: 163.*

113. The correct response is E.

All of the above features are seen in number 14 cleft. The number 14 cleft may produce an agenesis or an overabundance of tissue. When agenesis occurs, orbital hypotelorism is generally seen. Included in this group of craniofacial malformations are the holoprosencephalic disorders, which include cyclopia, ethmocephaly, and cebocephaly. The cranium is typically microcephalic and there is hypotelorism. Malformations of the forebrain are usually proportional to the degree of facial abnormality. At the other end of the spectrum, hypertelorism is associated with the number 14 cleft. Lateral displacement of the orbits can be produced by midline masses such as a frontonasal encephalocele or a midline frontal encephalocele.

Reference:

1. *Tessier P. Anatomical classification of facial, craniofacial and laterofacial clefts. J Maxillofac Surg 1976; 4: 69.*
2. *David DJ, Moore MH, Cooter RD. Tessier clefts revisited with a third dimension. Cleft Palate J. 1989; 26: 163.*

114. The correct response is D.

The median cleft of the lower jaw was first described by Couronne. These median clefts of the lower lip and mandible are caudal extensions of the number 14 cranial cleft and number 0 facial cleft.

Reference:

1. *Tessier P. Anatomical classification of facial, craniofacial and laterofacial clefts. J Maxillofac Surg 1976; 4: 69.*
2. *David DJ, Moore MH, Cooter RD. Tessier clefts revisited with a third dimension. Cleft Palate J. 1989; 26: 163.*

115. The correct response is E.

Ankyloglossia and total absence of the tongue have been reported with midline mandibular clefts- number 30 cleft.

Reference:

1. *Tessier P. Anatomical classification of facial, craniofacial and laterofacial clefts. J Maxillofac Surg 1976; 4: 69.*
2. *David DJ, Moore MH, Cooter RD. Tessier clefts revisited with a third dimension. Cleft Palate J. 1989; 26: 163.*

116. The correct response is E.

Ankyloglossia and total absence of the tongue have been reported with midline mandibular clefts- number 30 cleft.

Reference:

1. *Tessier P. Anatomical classification of facial, craniofacial and laterofacial clefts. J Maxillofac Surg 1976; 4: 69.*
2. *David DJ, Moore MH, Cooter RD. Tessier clefts revisited with a third dimension. Cleft Palate J. 1989; 26: 163.*

117. The correct response is A.

Abnormalities of the lateral third of the upper eyelid and eyebrow are the hallmarks of the number 9 cleft. This upper lateral orbit cleft is the rarest of the craniofacial clefts. The number 9 cleft begins the march from lateral to medial of the cranial clefts. The lateral canthus is also distorted. In the severe form, microphthalmia is present. The superolateral bony deficiency of the orbits allows for a lateral displacement of the globes. The cleft then extends cephalad into the temporoparietal hair-bearing scalp. The temporal hairline is anteriorly displaced and a temporal hair projection is often seen in the number 9 cleft. Furthermore, a cranial nerve VII palsy in the forehead and upper eyelid is common.

Reference:

1. *Tessier P. Anatomical classification of facial, craniofacial and laterofacial clefts. J Maxillofac Surg 1976; 4: 69.*
2. *Kawamoto HK Jr. Rare craniofacial clefts. In: McCarthy JG, ed. Plastic Surgery. Philadelphia: WB Saunders; 1990: 2922–2973.*

118. The correct response is C.

Tessier cleft no. 3 is medial to the lower lacrimal punctum.

Reference:

1. *Tessier P. Anatomical classification of facial, craniofacial and laterofacial clefts. J Maxillofac Surg 1976; 4: 69.*
2. *Kawamoto HK Jr. Rare craniofacial clefts. In: McCarthy JG, ed. Plastic Surgery. Philadelphia: WB Saunders; 1990: 2922–2973.*

119. The correct response is E.

Tessier cleft no. 12 lies medial to the medial canthus and the colobomas extend to the root of the eyebrow. There is a lateral displacement of the medial canthus with an aplasia of the medial end of the eyebrow. There are no eyelid clefts. The forehead skin is normal with a short, downward projection of the paramedian frontal hairline.

Reference:

1. *Tessier P. Anatomical classification of facial, craniofacial and laterofacial clefts. J Maxillofac Surg 1976; 4: 69.*
2. *Kawamoto HK Jr. Rare craniofacial clefts. In: McCarthy JG, ed. Plastic Surgery. Philadelphia: WB Saunders; 1990: 2922–2973.*

120. The correct response is C.

Tessier cleft no. 9 may be commonly associated with a palsy of the seventh nerve. This is due to soft tissue furrow from the lateral canthus of the eye to the temporal region.

Reference:

1. *Tessier P. Anatomical classification of facial, craniofacial and laterofacial clefts. J Maxillofac Surg 1976; 4: 69.*
2. *Kawamoto HK Jr. Rare craniofacial clefts. In: McCarthy JG, ed. Plastic Surgery. Philadelphia: WB Saunders; 1990: 2922–2973.*

121. The correct response is D.

Tessier cleft no. 13 may be associated with midline clefting of the frontal bone. There is widening of the olfactory groove, the cribriform plate, and the ethmoid sinus, which results in hypertelorism. A paramedian frontal encephalocele can cause the cribriform plate to be displaced inferiorly leading to orbital dystopia.

Reference:

1. *Tessier P. Anatomical classification of facial, craniofacial and laterofacial clefts. J Maxillofac Surg 1976; 4: 69.*
2. *Kawamoto HK Jr. Rare craniofacial clefts. In: McCarthy JG, ed. Plastic Surgery. Philadelphia: WB Saunders; 1990: 2922–2973.*

122. The correct response is E.

Orbital dystopia may be either vertical or horizontal. The midline number 14 cleft may have horizontal or transverse dystopia with the bony orbits displaced laterally (orbital hypertelorism) or medially (hypotelorism), whereas, the lateral number 10 through 13 clefts may have a component of vertical dystopia or asymmetric orbital hypertelorism with the orbits on different horizontal planes.

Reference:

1. *Tessier P. Anatomical classification of facial, craniofacial and laterofacial clefts. J Maxillofac Surg 1976; 4: 69.*
2. *Kawamoto HK Jr. Rare craniofacial clefts. In: McCarthy JG, ed. Plastic Surgery. Philadelphia: WB Saunders; 1990: 2922–2973.*

123. The correct response is C.

Diprosopus refers to facial duplication which is rare and consists of two complete faces on a single head. The other options are incorrect.

Reference:

1. *Verdi GD, Hersh JH, Russell LJ. Partial duplication of the face: case report and review. Plast Reconstr Surg 1991; 87: 759-762.*
2. *Fearon JA, Mulliken JB. Midfacial duplication: a rare malformation sequence. PlastReconstr Surg 1987; 79: 260-264.*

124. The correct response is B.

The genetic nature of Treacher Collins syndrome is well established as a dominant disorder of craniofacial development that results from mutation of TCOF1 gene on chromosome 5. A mouse model of this syndrome has been generated by ablation of the murine equivalent of the human TCOF1 gene.

Reference:

1. *The Treacher Collins Syndrome Collaborative Group: Positional cloning of a gene involved in the pathogenesis of Treacher Collins syndrome. Nat Genet 1996; 12: 124-129.*
2. *Edwards SJ, Gladwin AJ, Dixon MJ. The mutational spectrum in Treacher Collins syndrome reveals a predominance of mutations that create a premature-termination codon. Am J Hum Genet 1997; 60: 515-524.*

125. The correct response is A.

The Pi procedure is used to correct scaphocephaly, whereby the anteroposterior length of the skull is reduced by an osteotomy in the shape of a Pi. This leaves a stable central strut that is secured to the frontal segment with resorbable plates and screws after slowly advancing it anteriorly, thus diminishing the anteroposterior length.

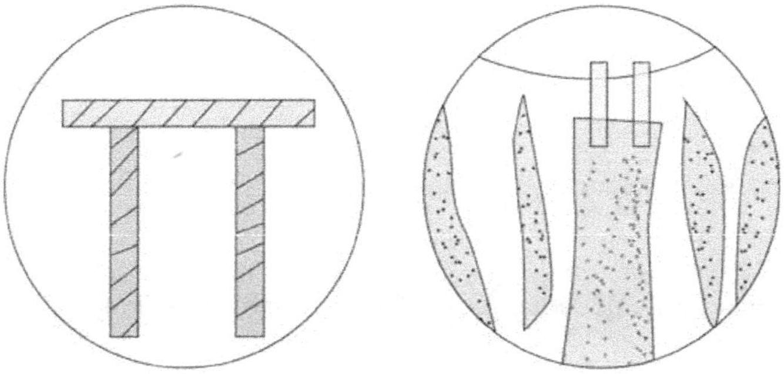

Pi procedure

Reference:

Jane JA, Edgerton M, Futrell J et al. Immediate correction of sagittal synostosis. J Neurosurg 1978; 49: 7-5-710.

126. The correct response is A.

The Hung span technique is used to treat patients with scaphocephaly with increased intracranial volume. It works by widening the biparietal dimension while reducing the anteroposterior dimension. In this, barrel shaped osteotomies are made in the temporoparietal area. These are fractured and then fixed along with the central strut of bone.

Reference:

McCarthy JG, Bradley JP, Stelnicki E et al. Hung span method of scaphocephaly reconstruction in patients with elevated intracranial pressure. Plast Reconstr Surg 2002; 109: 2009-2018.

127. The correct response is B.

Brachycephaly is seen in bilateral coronal craniosynostosis where the bitemporal diameter of the skull is more. The anterioposterior diameter is less due to lack of growth and foreshortening.

Reference:

Munro I. Craniofacial syndromes. In McCarthy JG, ed: Plastic Surgery vol 4. Philadelphia, WB Saunders, 1990: 3101.

128. The correct response is C.

Unilateral coronal stenosis produces a malformed skull (plagiocephaly) which looks like a twisted skull. In this, when a posteroanterior skull radiograph is taken, the classic 'Harlequin sign' is seen as an oblique line through the orbit. This is produced by the greater wing of the sphenoid, which gets elevated due to the deformity.

Reference:

Munro I. Craniofacial syndromes. In McCarthy JG, ed: Plastic Surgery vol 4. Philadelphia, WB Saunders, 1990: 3101.

129. The correct response is B.

The classic 'Harlequin' sign is seen on a posteroanterior skull radiograph. It is seen in plagiocephaly and is produced by the greater wing of the sphenoid which is seen as an oblique line through the orbit due to sutural fusion.

Reference:

Munro I. Craniofacial syndromes. In McCarthy JG, ed: Plastic Surgery vol 4. Philadelphia, WB Saunders, 1990: 3101.

130. The correct response is B.

The classic 'Harlequin' sign is seen on a posteroanterior skull radiograph. It is seen in plagiocephaly and is produced by the greater wing of the sphenoid which is seen as an oblique line through the orbit due to sutural fusion.

Reference:

Munro I. Craniofacial syndromes. In McCarthy JG, ed: Plastic Surgery vol 4. Philadelphia, WB Saunders, 1990: 3101.

131. The correct response is A.

Crouzon syndrome is not associated with limb abnormalities. The other syndromes listed in the options are all associated with limb abnormalities.

Reference:

Munro I. Craniofacial syndromes. In McCarthy JG, ed: Plastic Surgery vol 4. Philadelphia, WB Saunders, 1990: 3101.

4

132. The correct response is C.

The classic "copper beaten" skull is frequently though nonspecifically associated with elevated intracranial pressure. The other options are incorrect.

Reference:

Munro I. Craniofacial syndromes. In McCarthy JG, ed: Plastic Surgery vol 4. Philadelphia, WB Saunders, 1990: 3101.

133. The correct response is E.

The "Cloverleaf skull" deformity is seen in all of the syndromic or multiple sutural synostoses. These patients have a trilobar cranial vault deformity due to stenosed sutures and they frequently have intracranial hypertension. The other options are incorrect.

Reference:

1. *Munro I. Craniofacial syndromes. In McCarthy JG, ed: Plastic Surgery vol 4. Philadelphia, WB Saunders, 1990: 3101.*
2. *O'Keefe M, Algawi K, Fitzsimmon S et al. Ocular complications of cloverleaf skull syndrome. J Pediatr Ophthalmol Strabismus 1998; 35: 292-293.*

134. The correct response is E.

The "Cloverleaf skull" deformity is seen in all of the syndromic or multiple sutural synostoses. These patients have a trilobar cranial vault deformity due to stenosed sutures and they frequently have intracranial hypertension. It is best treated with radical craniectomy. The other options are incorrect.

Reference:

1. *Turner P, Reynolds A. Generous craniectomy for Kleeblattschadel anomaly. Neurosurgery 1980; 6: 555-558.*
2. *O'Keefe M, Algawi K, Fitzsimmon S et al. Ocular complications of cloverleaf skull syndrome. J Pediatr Ophthalmol Strabismus 1998; 35: 292-293.*

135. The correct response is D.

The zygomatic bone is hypoplastic or absent in cases of Treacher Collins syndrome. The zygoma forms the inferior and lateral wall of the orbit. The lateral canthus attachment is floating or uncertain. The greater wing of the sphenoid compensates for the deformity of the lateral orbital wall.

Reference:

1. *Posnick J. Treacher Collins syndrome. In Aston S, ed: Grabb and Smith's Plastic Surgery, 5th ed. Philadelphia, Lippincott-Raven, 1977.*
2. *Hertle RW, Ziyland S, Katowitz JA. Ophthalmic features and visual prognosis in theTreacher-Collins syndrome. Br J Ophthalmol 1993; 77: 642.*

136. The correct response is E.

Egg shaped orbit is seen in Treacher Collins syndrome. Its base is located superomedially and its axis is oriented inferolaterally. This is also contributed by hypoplasia/ absence of zygoma in this syndrome.

Reference:

1. *Posnick J. Treacher Collins syndrome. In Aston S, ed: Grabb and Smith's Plastic Surgery, 5th ed. Philadelphia, Lippincott-Raven, 1977.*
2. *Hertle RW, Ziyland S, Katowitz JA. Ophthalmic features and visual prognosis in the Treacher-Collins syndrome. Br J Ophthalmol 1993; 77: 642.*

137. The correct response is E.

A concave antegonial notch with markedly obtuse gonial angle of the mandible is a distinguishing feature of Treacher Collins syndrome. The chin is retrusive and vertically long and points backward.

Reference:

1. *Raulo Y, Tessier P. Mandibulo-facial dysostosis, analysis: principles of surgery. Scand J Plast Reconstr Surg 1981; 15: 251.*
2. *Roberts F, Pruzansky S, Aduss H. An X-radiocephalometric study of mandibulofacial dysostosis in man. Arch Oral Biol 1975; 20: 265.*

138. The correct response is E.

Colobomas or pseudocolobomas of the lower eyelid are pathognomonic of Treacher Collins syndrome. The medial two thirds of the lower lid is without cilia. The inferolateral orbital dystopia results in a classic obliquity and antimongoloid slant to the palpebral fissure.

Reference:

1. *Raulo Y, Tessier P. Mandibulo-facial dysostosis, analysis: principles of surgery. Scand J Plast Reconstr Surg 1981; 15: 251.*
2. *Roberts F, Pruzansky S, Aduss H. An X-radiocephalometric study of mandibulofacial dysostosis in man. Arch Oral Biol 1975; 20: 265.*

139. The correct response is D.

The triad of glossoptosis, micrognathia and airway obstruction is characteristic of Pierre Robin sequence. Although cleft palate is not included, it is commonly associated with this disorder and may also increase the intensity of obstruction.

Reference:

1. *Munro I. Craniofacial syndromes. In McCarthy JG, ed: Plastic Surgery vol 4. Philadelphia, WB Saunders, 1990:3101.*
2. *Sadewitz VL. Robin sequence: changes in thinking leading to changes in patients care. Cleft Palate Craniofac J 1992; 29: 246.*

140. The correct response is E.

The triad of glossoptosis, micrognathia and airway obstruction is characteristic of Pierre Robin sequence but is also found in other syndromes. Stickler, 22q11 deletion and foetal alcohol syndrome can all have the features of the Robin sequence.

Reference:

1. *Shprintzen RJ. The implications of the diagnosis of Robin sequence. Cleft Palate Craniofac J 1992; 29: 205.*
2. *Munro I. Craniofacial syndromes. In McCarthy JG, ed: Plastic Surgery vol 4. Philadelphia, WB Saunders, 1990: 3101.*

141. The correct response is E.

All of the above contribute to the airway obstruction in Pierre Robin sequence.

Reference:

1. *Shprintzen RJ. The implications of the diagnosis of Robin sequence. Cleft Palate Craniofac J 1992; 29: 205.*
2. *Munro I. Craniofacial syndromes. In McCarthy JG, ed: Plastic Surgery vol 4. Philadelphia, WB Saunders, 1990: 3101.*

142. The correct response is E.

All of the above features may be seen in the nose in cases of Treacher Collins syndrome. The nose though is one of the facial feature in this syndrome which is rather normal when compared to abnormalities of the other parts of the face.

Reference:

1. *Farkas LG, Posnick JC. Detailed morphometry of the nose in patients with Treacher Collins syndrome. Ann Plast Surg 1989; 22: 211.*
2. *Roddi R, Vaandrager M, van der Meulen JC. Treacher Collins syndrome: early surgical treatment of orbitomalar malformations. J Craniofac Surg 1995; 6: 211.*

143. The correct response is D.

The children with Pierre Robin syndrome should be nursed preferably in 'prone position' after a feed. Prone positioning allows gravity to keep the tongue forward and decrease the chance of its falling into the hypopharynx.

Reference:

1. *Shprintzen RJ. The implications of the diagnosis of Robin sequence. Cleft Palate Craniofac J 1992; 29: 205.*
2. *Munro I. Craniofacial syndromes. In McCarthy JG, ed: Plastic Surgery vol 4. Philadelphia, WB Saunders, 1990: 3101.*

144. The correct response is E.

All of the above are valid physiologic criteria for surgical intervention in Pierre Robin sequence. Conservative treatment is recommended for infants demonstrating improvements in weight gain, strength, and tongue coordination.

Reference:

1. *Shprintzen RJ. The implications of the diagnosis of Robin sequence. Cleft Palate Craniofac J 1992; 29: 205.*
2. *Munro I. Craniofacial syndromes. In McCarthy JG, ed: Plastic Surgery vol 4. Philadelphia, WB Saunders, 1990: 3101.*

145. The correct response is E.

The tongue-lip adhesion procedure is done in patients with Robin sequence. The goal of this procedure is to relieve the airway obstruction by pulling a low and posteriorly positioned tongue forward and suturing it to the lower lip. The other options are incorrect.

Reference:

1. *Parsons RW, Smith DJ. A modified tongue-lip adhesion for Pierre Robin anomalad. Cleft Palate J 1980; 17: 144.*
2. *Argamaso RV. Glossopexy for upper airway obstruction in Robin sequence. Cleft Palate Craniofac J 1992; 29: 232.*

146. The correct response is D.

Reconstruction of the mandibular ramus, condyle and the glenoid fossa is required in Pruzansky type III mandibular deformity where there is absence of the ramus and temporomandibular joint. The traditional technique has been to use the rib graft for glenoid fossa and a costochondral rib graft for the condyle.

Reference:

1. *Pruzansky S. Not all dwarfed mandibles are alike. Birth Defects 1969; 1: 120.*
2. *Kaban LB, Moses MH, Mulliken JB. Surgical correction of hemifacial microsomia in the growing child. Plast Reconstr Surgery 1998; 82: 9.*

147. The correct response is E.

The exact aetiology of Romberg's disease is unknown but all the above have been proposed as theories for its pathogenesis.

Reference:

1. *Pensler JM, Murphy JB. Clinical and ultrastructural studies of Romberg's hemifacial atrophy. Plast Reconstr Surg 1990; 85: 669-674, discussion 675-676.*
2. *Wells JH, Edgerton MT. Correction of severe hemifacial atrophy with a free dermis-fat from the lower abdomen. Plast Reconstr Surg 1977; 59: 223-230.*

148. The correct response is E.

Romberg's disease is distinct from scleroderma but may represent a localised form of this disease. All the tissues are involved from skin to bone and there is diffuse fibrosis of the skin, blood vessels, synovia and the vital organs such as the kidneys. A combination of vascular abnormalities, excess collagen and deposition of matrix substance are the possible causes of this disorder.

Reference:

1. *Pensler JM, Murphy JB. Clinical and ultrastructural studies of Romberg's hemifacial atrophy. Plast Reconstr Surg 1990; 85: 669-674, discussion 675-676.*
2. *Wells JH, Edgerton MT. Correction of severe hemifacial atrophy with a free dermis-fat from the lower abdomen. Plast Reconstr Surg 1977; 59: 223-230.*

149. The correct response is D.

The circumflex scapular flap has been found to be most versatile for restoration of facial contour. The omentum has disadvantage of having no dermal or facial attachments to fix the tissue to the desired location. The groin and superficial inferior epigastric flaps are useful when large amounts of skin coverage is also required, which limits the possibility of using pliable fascia beyond the width of the skin paddle design.

Reference:

1. *Wells JH, Edgerton MT. Correction of severe hemifacial atrophy with a free dermis-fat from the lower abdomen. Plast Reconstr Surg 1977; 59: 223-230.*
2. *Sibert JW, Longaker MT, Angrigiani C. The inframammary extended circumflex scapular flap: an aesthetic improvement of the parascapular flap. Plast Reconstr Surg 1997; 99: 70-77.*

150. The correct response is A.

The results of facial contouring with silicone have been unsatisfactory with the possibility of delayed scar and contracture formation. Removal of free silicone is also a difficult task. The rest of the options are suitable alternatives for facial contouring.

Reference:

1. *Rees TD, Ashley FL. Treatment of facial atrophy with liquid silicone. Am J Surg 1966; 111: 531-535.*
2. *Rees TD, Ashley FL, Delgado JP. Silicone fluid injections for facial atrophy. A ten-year study. Plast Reconstr Surg 1973; 52: 118-127.*

151. The correct response is D.

The diagnosis in this lady is a pyogenic granuloma. These lesions are common in young adults. These are rapidly developing and are prone to bleeding and local irritation. Treatment consists of excision and cauterization of the base. This site is uncommon for implantation dermoid which usually occur on the fingers with a history of skin puncture. Nevus sebaceus of Jadassohn is present at birth and presents as salmon-coloured and waxy in nature. A vascular malformation is also a possibility but the clinical features consist of a long standing lesion with slow growth.

Reference:

1. *Fitzpatrick TB, Johnson RA, Wolff K et al. Color Atlas and Synopsis of Clinical Dermatology. 4th ed. New York: McGraw-Hill; 2001: 172-173.*
2. *Popkin GL. Tumors of the skin. In: McCarthy JG, ed. Plastic Surgery. Philadelphia: WB Saunders; 1990: 3560-3613.*

152. The correct response is C.

The lesion in the picture is most likely an earlobe keloid which is clinically characterized by exuberant growth of proliferative scar outside the boundaries of the initial scar bed. It is common in the ear especially after ear piercing in susceptible individuals having predilection for this type of tendency. The lesions keep on growing and do not regress and are of recurrent nature.

Reference:

1. *Niessen FB, Spauwen PH, Schalkwijk J et al. On the nature of hypertrophic scars and keloids: a review. Plast Reconstr Surg. 1999; 104: 1435-1458.*
2. *Marneros AG, Norris JEC, Olsen BR et al. Clinical genetics of familial keloids. Arch Dermatol. 2001; 137: 1429-1434.*

153. The correct response is D.

The presenting clinical features combined with the CT finding of zygomatic deformity is characteristic of Treacher Collins syndrome which is a combination of Tessier no. 6,7,8 cleft. Pierre Robin syndrome is characterised by high arched palate, microgenia and airway obstruction. There is no zygomatic abnormality in this syndrome.

Reference:

1. *Farkas LG, Posnick JC. Detailed morphometry of the nose in patients with Treacher Collins syndrome. Ann Plast Surg 1989; 22: 211.*
2. *Roddi R, Vaandrager M, van der Meulen JC. Treacher Collins syndrome: early surgical treatment of orbitomalar malformations. J Craniofac Surg 1995; 6: 211.*
3. *Shprintzen RJ. The implications of the diagnosis of Robin sequence. Cleft Palate Craniofac J 1992; 29: 205.*

154. The correct response is C.

The presenting clinical features and facial appearance is consistent with the diagnosis of Pierre Robin sequence. Tongue-lip adhesion is performed in patients with retrognathia and glossoptosis to improve the airway. Pierre Robin sequence describes the clinical triad of microretrognathia, glossoptosis, and upper airway obstruction. Patients may present with airway obstruction, feeding difficulties, or both immediately after birth or during the following weeks of life. If left untreated, many of these infants experience failure to thrive, chronic hypoxemia, and cor pulmonale. Pierre Robin sequence may be nonsyndromic or associated with syndromes such as bifacial or hemifacial microsomia. Tongue-lip adhesion was first described as a treatment of upper airway obstruction in Pierre Robin sequence by Douglas in 1946. There has been a recent trend toward distraction osteogenesis of the infant mandible in patients who present with microretrognathia and airway obstruction with good initial results.

Reference:

1. *Farkas LG, Posnick JC. Detailed morphometry of the nose in patients with Treacher Collins syndrome. Ann Plast Surg 1989; 22: 211.*
2. *Roddi R, Vaandrager M, van der Meulen JC. Treacher Collins syndrome: early surgical treatment of orbitomalar malformations. J Craniofac Surg 1995; 6: 211.*
3. *Shprintzen RJ. The implications of the diagnosis of Robin sequence. Cleft Palate Craniofac J 1992; 29: 205.*

155. The correct response is A.

This patient has severe maxillary retrusion associated with bilateral cleft lip and palate. Such patients need constant orthodontic care for growth monitoring of the face and to institute corrective measures exigently. At this stage he is a good candidate for a LeFort osteotomy combined with distraction. This would allow gradual skeletal and soft tissue correction of his deformity.

Reference:

1. *Yu JC, Fearon J, Havlik RJ, et al. Distraction osteogenesis of the craniofacial skeleton. Plast Reconstr Surg. 2004; 114: 1e-20e.*
2. *Figueroa AA, Polley JW, Friede H, et al. Long-term skeletal stability after maxillary advancement with distraction osteogenesis using a rigid external distraction device in cleft maxillary deformities. Plast Reconstr Surg. 2004; 114: 1382-1392.*

5

ONCOPLASTIC SURGERY

QUESTIONS

1. Scrofula is a type of?

A. Neoplasm
B. Tubercular adenitis
C. Vascular malformation in the neck
D. Retropharyngeal abscess
E. Congenital cyst

2. Pyogenic granulomas are characterized by which one of the following features?

A. Pin head to 2-3 cm size lesions
B. Rapidly growing
C. History of bouts of bleeding
D. Pulpy lesions
E. All of the above

3. Proliferating capillaries in a fibromyxomatous stroma is characteristic of which one of the following?

A. Dermoid cyst
B. Branchial cyst
C. Pyogenic granuloma
D. Teratoma
E. Scrofula

4. The lateral brow is a common place for dermoid due to which one of the following?

A. Site of embryological rests of tissue
B. Genetic predeliction
C. Zygomaticofrontal suture
D. Branchial arch fusion plane
E. Incidental

5. Which one of the following is true about haemangiomas?

A. Endothelial tumours
B. Rapid growth
C. Slow regression
D. No recurrence
E. All of the above

6. Giant haemangiomas of childhood associated with thrombocytopenia, petechial haemorrhages and bleeding are found in which one of the following?

A. Sturge Weber syndrome
B. Kasabach Merritt phenomenon
C. Turner syndrome
D. Mafucci syndrome
E. Proteus syndrome

7. Which one of the following syndrome is commonly associated with ocular and leptomeningeal vascular anomalies?

A. Sturge Weber syndrome
B. Kasabach Merritt phenomenon
C. Turner syndrome
D. Mafucci syndrome
E. Proteus syndrome

8. Haemangiomas occur most commonly in which one of the following region?

A. Trunk
B. Upper limb
C. Craniofacial
D. Lower limb
E. Abdomen

9. Which one of the following is a local complication of sclerotherapy for vascular malformations?

A. Blistering
B. Necrosis
C. Ulceration
D. Nerve damage
E. All of the above

10. Which one of the following modality is the mainstay of treatment for lymphatic malformation?

A. Antibiotic therapy
B. Sodium morrhuate sclerotherapy
C. Intralesional bleomycin
D. Argon laser
E. Resection

11. Which one of the following investigative modality is most sensitive for delineating aneurysmal dysplastic changes in the involved vessels in patients with arteriovenous malformations?

A. Ultrasonography
B. Colour Doppler study
C. Computed Tomography
D. Magnetic Resonance Imaging
E. Digital Subtraction Angiography

12. Which one of the following syndrome is commonly associated with bone exostoses and enchondromas in combination with exophytic cutaneous venous malformations?

A. Sturge Weber syndrome
B. Kasabach Merritt phenomenon
C. Turner syndrome
D. Mafucci syndrome
E. Proteus syndrome

13. Which one of the following syndrome is commonly associated with skeletal hypertrophy of an extremity in combination with a slow flow capillary-lymphatic-venous malformation?

A. Sturge Weber syndrome
B. Kasabach Merritt phenomenon
C. Klippel-Trenaunay syndrome
D. Mafucci syndrome
E. Proteus syndrome

14. Which one of the following syndrome is a fast flow capillary-arteriovenous malformation ?

A. Sturge Weber syndrome
B. Kasabach Merritt phenomenon
C. Klippel-Trenaunay syndrome
D. Parkes-Weber syndrome
E. Proteus syndrome

15. The Wharton's duct is related to which one of the following gland?

A. Parotid
B. Submandibular
C. Sublingual
D. Meibomian gland
E. Lacrimal gland

16. Technetium scan is based on the ability of the salivary glands to concentrate this element. Which one of the following tumour of salivary gland is best diagnosed with this method?

A. Mucoepidermoid carcinoma
B. Monomorphic adenoma
C. Papillary cystadenoma lymphomatosum
D. Adenoid cystic carcinoma
E. Acinic cell carcinoma

17. The characteristic "Swiss cheese" appearance on histological examination is seen in which one of the following salivary gland neoplasm?

A. Mucoepidermoid carcinoma
B. Monomorphic adenoma
C. Papillary cystadenoma lymphomatosum
D. Adenoid cystic carcinoma
E. Acinic cell carcinoma

18. A cystic swelling at the site of an unerupted tooth is which one of the following?

A. Gingival cyst
B. Dental cyst
C. Periodontal cyst
D. Dentigerous cyst
E. Gorlin cyst (Calcifying odontogenic cyst)

19. Which one of the following type of ameloblastoma is treated by enucleation and curettage?

A. Unicystic
B. Extraosseous
C. Intraosseous
D. Maxillary
E. All of the above

20. The presenting features of a case of tumour of the jaw, histologically characterised by proliferation of fibroblasts producing a dense collagen matrix containing trabeculae of osteoid and bone are characteristic of which one of the following?

A. Osteoid osteoma
B. Osteoblastoma
C. Fibrous dysplasia
D. Cementoblastoma
E. Odontogenic carcinoma

21. Which one of the following tumour of the oral cavity is best resected using a mandibulotomy approach?

A. Carcinoma lower lip
B. Carcinoma upper lip
C. Carcinoma of mobile tongue
D. Carcinoma base of tongue
E. Cancer of the palate

22. Which one of the following cyst of the mandible is a pseudocyst?

A. Radicular cyst
B. Paradental cyst
C. Odontogenic keratocyst
D. Aneursymal bone cyst
E. Lateral periodontal cyst

23. Which one of the following cyst of the mandible is a true cyst?

A. Radicular cyst
B. Simple bone cyst
C. Static bone cyst
D. Aneursymal bone cyst
E. Focal osteoporotic bone marrow defect

24. Aneurysmal bone cyst commonly involves which part of the mandible?

A. Body
B. Ramus
C. Angle
D. Symphysis
E. Condyle

25. Which one of the following is not an odontogenic cyst?

A. Gingival cyst
B. Lateral periodontal cyst
C. Dentigerous cyst
D. Calcifying odontogenic cyst
E. Nasopalatine duct cyst

26. Eustachian tube opening is located at which one of the following site?

A. Oral cavity
B. Oropharynx
C. Nasopharynx
D. Hypopharynx
E. Larynx

27. The Eustachian tube develops from the first branchial pouch as an invagination. The narrowest portion of the Eustachian tube is located at which one of the following site?

A. Where the bony portion joins the middle ear
B. Where the bony portion joins the cartilaginous portion
C. Where the cartilaginous portion opens into the nasopharynx.
D. In the middle of the tube
E. At the site of attachment of levator

28. The opening of the Eustachian tube is controlled mainly by which one of the following muscle?

A. Tensor palati
B. Levator palati
C. Salpingopharyngeus
D. Palatopharyngeus
E. Musculus uvulae

29. The Eustachian tube at rest is in which one of the following position?

A. Open
B. Closed
C. The pharyngeal end is closed while the other one is open
D. Remains in a state of contraction
E. Any of the above

30. The bony portion of the Eustachian tube is surrounded by all of the following important structures except which one of the following?

A. Temporomandibular joint
B. Middle cranial fossa
C. Internal carotid artery
D. External carotid artery

31. Which one of the following statement regarding the role of the Eustachian tube in the hearing mechanism of the ear is correct?

A. It helps to maintain the air pressure in the middle ear
B. It helps the tympanic membrane and the ossicles to vibrate
C. It helps to protect the ear against loud and abnormal sounds
D. It protects the ear during the flight
E. All of the above

32. Which one of the following statement regarding the role of the Eustachian tube in the mechanism of swallowing is correct?

A. It remains closed at rest
B. It opens for a short while, 0.3 to 0.5 seconds during the act of swallowing
C. It opens fully once or twice in an hour
D. It does not allow upward movement of food or liquids into the ear
E. All of the above

33. The Ostmann fat pad is located in proximity to which one of the following structure?

A. Superior turbinate
B. Posterior pharyngeal wall
C. Eustachian tube
D. Tonsil
E. Passavant's ridge

34. Which one of the following is the function of the Ostmann fat pad located near the Eustachian tube?

A. Closure of the tube
B. Helps in equalising the pressure on both the sides of the tube
C. Helps in sucking function
D. Helps in gliding of parapharyngeal muscles
E. All of the above

35. An individual with a perforated tympanic membrane will experience which one of the following during flight?

A. Pain during ascent
B. Pain during descent
C. No pain during ascent or descent
D. Any of the above

36. Which one of the following should be avoided by individuals having cold and compromised Eustachian tube function during the flight to avoid pain in the ear?

A. Use cotton or the finger to plug the ear
B. Use chewing gum or chew the crystal sugar or fennel
C. Open and close the jaw as often as required and swallow the saliva
D. Valsalva procedure
E. Ear drops

37. Verruca vulgaris is caused by which one of the following?

A. Genetic predisposition
B. Trauma
C. Viral infection
D. Bacterial infection
E. Fungal infection

38. Molluscum contagiosum is caused by which one of the following?

A. Genetic predisposition
B. Trauma
C. Viral infection
D. Bacterial infection
E. Fungal infection

39. Which one of the following is characteristic of lesions of Molluscum contagiosum?

A. Confluent lesions
B. Umbilicated lesions
C. Macular lesions
D. Solitary lesions
E. Involves the palms and soles

40. Seborrheic keratosis or senile warts are characterized by which one of the following?

A. Sessile, sharply demarcated warty masses
B. Yellow, brown or black in colour with smooth or granular surface
C. Verrucous growths are frequently multiple
D. Commonly seen on the face, neck, trunk and vulva of obese and diabetic individuals
E. All of the above

41. Rhinophyma is characterised by which one of the following?

A. Proliferation of surface epidermal cells within the dermis
B. Production of keratin
C. Retention cyst following injury to the skin
D. Sebaceous glands hypertrophy
E. Benign proliferation of the eccrine ducts

42. The black head in the skin overlying a sebaceous cyst is due to which one of the following?

A. Keratin plug
B. Blood clot
C. Dust particle
D. Sebum
E. Dead cells

43. Milia are small superficial cysts arising from the pilosebaceous follicle. They contain which one of the following?

A. Keratin
B. Dust particle
C. Sebum
D. Dead cells
E. Blood clot

44. Which one of the following may develop in the skin after dermabrasion?

A. Epidermal cyst
B. Milia
C. Acne
D. Verruca vulgaris
E. Pilar cyst

45. The picket fence arrangement of nuclei in the peripheral layer around the tumour on histological examination is characteristic of which one of the following lesion?

A. Seborrheic keratosis
B. Squamous cell carcinoma
C. Basal cell carcinoma
D. Syringoma
E. Keratoacanthoma

46. The reported recurrence rate of basal cell carcinoma after five years is maximum in which one of the following site?

A. Scalp
B. Forehead
C. Nasolabial
D. Ear
E. Chin

47. The treatment of choice for basal cell carcinoma is which one of the following?

A. Surgery
B. Cryosurgery
C. Cautery and curettage
D. Radiation therapy

48. Squamous cell carcinomas are caused by which one of the following?

A. Genetic factors
B. Environmental factors, viruses
C. Ultraviolet radiation
D. Ionising radiation
E. All of the above

49. Squamous cell carcinoma can clinically manifest as which one of the following?

A. Lesion commonly seen on head and neck areas
B. Central ulceration in the nodules with bleeding, crusting and foul smell
C. Involve mucosal surfaces
D. May present as warts, eczematous lesions
E. All of the above

50. Paget disease originates on the nipple and areola. It is clinically characterized by which one of the following feature?

A. Ulceration
B. Eczema
C. Pigmentation
D. White patch
E. Exophytic growth

51. Extramammary Paget's disease is common in which one of the following site?

A. Face
B. Shoulder
C. Vulva
D. Hands
E. All of the above

52. Hutchinson's freckle is an overgrowth of which one of the following?

A. Keratinocytes
B. Melanocytes
C. Epidermal cells
D. Dermal cells
E. Piloerector apparatus

53. Which one of the following classification systems of melanoma is based on micrometer reading regarding the depth of invasion?

A. Clark's classification
B. Breslow's classification
C. TNM classification
D. Morphologic classification
E. Clinical classification

54. Tomographic gallium scans are helpful for detecting metastatic melanoma in a number of distant sites. Which one of the following site is less useful for detecting metastases by this method?

A. Intra-abdominal
B. Lymph nodes
C. Bone
D. Lung

55. Melanomas have a worse prognosis when they are located in which one of the following?

A. BANS area
B. Nose
C. Lip
D. Cheek
E. Forehead

56. Topical 5-Fluorouracil cream (5-Fu) is a chemotherapeutic agent. It acts by which one of the following mechanism?

A. Inhibiting thymidine synthesis
B. Modulation of cell differentiation
C. Nuclear cellular modifiers
D. Inhibition of cyclooxygenase pathway
E. Local stimulation of immune modifiers

57. Vitamin A helps in rejuvenating the skin by producing which one of the following?
A. Reducing stratum corneum
B. Increase in epidermal thickness
C. Increase in stratum granulosum
D. Increase in collagen synthesis and elasticity
E. All of the above

58. Cryosurgery produces its effect by excessive cooling leading to tissue necrosis and vascular stasis. The current temperature recommendations range from which one of the following for tissue destruction for all tumour regions?
A. 0°C to – 10°C
B. –10°C to – 30°C
C. –30°C to – 50°C
D. –50°C to – 60°C
E. –30°C to – 40°C

59. Radiotherapy in the treatment of skin cancer is indicated in which one of the following?
A. Cancer in burn scars
B. Radiation dermatitis
C. Lesion of palms and soles
D. Poor general health
E. All of the above

60. Marjolin's ulcer is recognised as a cancer arising from which one of the following?
A. Scar tissue
B. Burns
C. Wounds
D. All of the above

61. Marjolin's ulcer occurs in an unstable burn scar. Which one of the following is not a feature of Marjolin's ulcer?
A. Pain in the ulcer area within the scar
B. Foul smell
C. Pus discharge
D. Change in sensation of the scar
E. Lymphadenopathy

62. Marjolin's ulcer arises in burn scars. The lag time from the injury to the onset of the cancer is which one of the following?
A. More than 20 years after injury
B. More than 30 years after injury
C. More than 40 years after injury
D. More than 50 years after injury
E. 8 months to 60 years

63. Keratoacanthoma, is a tumor which is common in sun exposed areas of light skinned older individuals. It arises from which one of the following?
A. Keratinocytes
B. Melanocytes
C. Hair follicles
D. Epidermal cells
E. Merkel cell

64. Which one of the following neck incisions for radical neck dissection gives a wide exposure with lesser morbidity?
A. McFee incision
B. Posterior neck incision
C. Double opposing flaps
D. All of the above

65. The classical neck dissection removes which one of the following structures?
A. Sternocleidomastoid muscle
B. Internal jugular vein
C. Spinal accessory nerve
D. All of the above

66. In the functional neck dissection, which one of the following structure is preserved?
A. Sternocleidomastoid muscle
B. Accessory nerve
C. Internal jugular vein
D. All of the above

67. A 45-year-old man comes to the outpatient department for consultation regarding a mass in the right cheek region on the mucosal side. The mass was infiltrating and fixed to the bone. Physical examination of the neck revealed several ipsilateral lymph nodes more than 1 cm in size. It was diagnosed as a squamous cell carcinoma (photo shown). Which one of the following is the most appropriate TNM staging of this patient's tumor?
A. I
B. II
C. III
D. IV

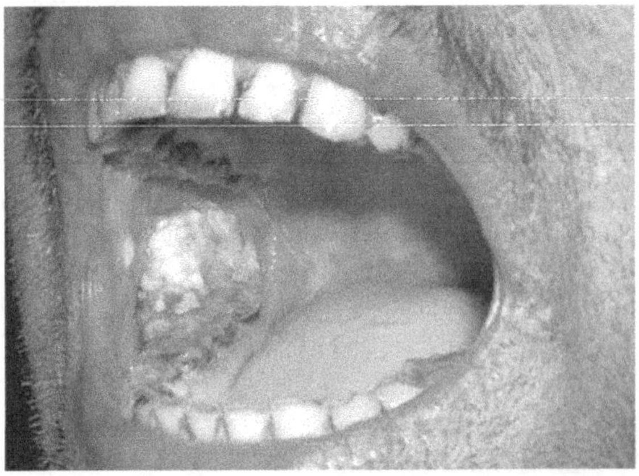

68. A 25-year-old-woman comes to the outpatient department for consultation regarding a progressively increasing mass in the midline of the chin fixed to the mandible and associated with loose teeth. On radiographs the mass is involving the whole of the mandible in the midline with a clear outline as a solitary cavity (photograph shown). The diagnosis of ameloblastoma is confirmed by biopsy. Which one of the following is the most appropriate management?

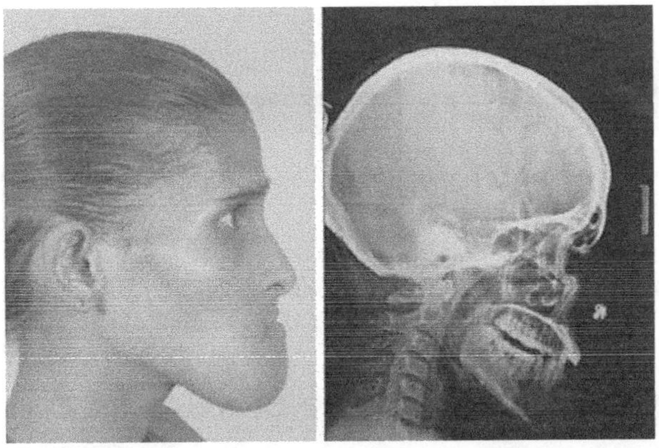

A. Radiotherapy
B. Chemotherapy
C. Enucleation
D. Curettage
E. Segmental resection

ANSWERS, EXPLANATIONS AND REFERENCES

1. The correct response is B.

Scrofula is tuberculous cervical adenitis and is typically seen in children younger than 6 years and presents as painless progressive node enlargement.

Reference:

Jervis PN, Lee JA, Bull PD. Management of non-tuberculous mycobacterial peri-sialadenitis in children: the Sheffield otolaryngology experience. Clin Otolaryngol 2001; 26: 243-248.

2. The correct response is E.

Pyogenic granulomas are characterised by all of the above. They bleed on minor touch, and are treated by cautery, excision and primary closure.

Reference:

1. *Krischner RE, Low DW. Treatment of pyogenic granuloma by shave excision and laser photocoagulation. Plast Reconstr Surg 1999; 104: 1346-1349.*
2. *Patrice SJ, Wiss K, Mulliken JB. Pyogenic granuloma (lobular capillary haemangioma): a clinicopathologic study of 178 cases. Pediatr Dermatol 1991; 8: 267-276.*

3. The correct response is C.

Proliferating capillaries in a fibromyxomatous stroma is characteristic of pyogenic granuloma. The pathognomonic lobular architecture of the lesions has given rise to the less commonly used name of lobular capillary haemangioma.

Reference:

1. *Krischner RE, Low DW. Treatment of pyogenic granuloma by shave excision and laser photocoagulation. Plast Reconstr Surg 1999; 104: 1346-1349.*
2. *Patrice SJ, Wiss K, Mulliken JB. Pyogenic granuloma (lobular capillary haemangioma): a clinicopathologic study of 178 cases. Pediatr Dermatol 1991; 8: 267-276.*

4. The correct response is C.

Dermoid cysts commonly arise in the head and neck region and are present at birth. The lateral brow is a common place for dermoid cysts originating from the zygomaticofrontal suture.

Reference:

1. *Ross JA, Swensen AR. Prenatal epidemiology of pediatric tumors, Curr Oncol Rep 2000; 2: 234-241.*
2. *Albano E, Stork LC, Greffe BS et al. Neoplastic disease. In Hay W, Groothuis J, Hayward A, Levin M, eds: Current Pediatric Diagnosis and Treatment, 13th ed. Norwalk, Ct, Appleton and Lange, 1997: 793-800.*

5. The correct response is E.

All of the above are true for haemangiomas. The term haemangioma refers to the common tumor of infancy that exhibits rapid postnatal growth and slow regression during childhood.

Reference:

1. *Folkman JB, Mulliken J, Ezekowitz RAB. Angiogenesis and hemangiomas. In Oldham K, Colombani P, Foglio R, eds: Surgery of Infants and Children: Scientific Principles and Practice. Philadelphia, Lippincott-Raven, 1997: 569-579.*
2. *Mulliken JB, Fishman SJ, Burrows PE. Vascular anomalies. Curr Prob Surg. 2000; 37: 517.*

6. The correct response is B.

Giant haemangiomas of childhood associated with thrombocytopenia, petechial haemorrhages and bleeding are together known as Kasabach-Merritt phenomenon. Sturge Weber syndrome comprises of a facial capillary malformation with ipsilateral ocular and leptomeningeal vascular anomalies. Proteus syndrome refers to a sporadic, progressive vascular, skeletal and soft tissue condition that lies at the interface of vascular anomalies and overgrowth syndromes. Mafucci syndrome denotes the coexistence of exophytic cutaneous venous malformations with bone exostoses and enchondromas.

Reference:

1. *Zukerberg LR, Nickoloff BJ, Weiss SW. Kaposiform haemangioendothelioma of infancy and childhood. An aggressive neoplasm associated with Kasabach-Merritt syndrome and lymphangiomatosis. Am J Surg Pathol 1993; 17: 321-328.*
2. *Enjolras O, Wassef M, Mazoyer E et al. Infants with Kasabach-Merritt syndrome do not have true haemangiomas. J Pediatr 1997; 130: 631-640.*

7. The correct response is A.

Sturge Weber syndrome comprises of a facial capillary malformation with ipsilateral ocular and leptomeningeal vascular anomalies. The capillary stain involves the trigeminal dermatomes. The leptomeningeal anomalies can be capillary, venous or arteriovenous malformations. Periodic ophthalmoscopic examination and tonometry are essential in observing children with Sturge-Weber syndrome.

Reference:

1. *Enjolras O, Riche MC, Merland JJ. Facial port-wine stains and Sturge-Weber syndrome. Pediatrics 1985; 76: 48-51.*
2. *Orten SS, Waner M, Flock S et al: Port wine stains. An assessment of 5 years of treatment. Arch Otolaryngol Head Neck Surg 1996; 122: 1174-1179.*

8. The correct response is C.

Haemangiomas occur most often in the craniofacial region (60%), followed by trunk (25%) and extremities. Eighty percent of cutaneous haemangiomas are single and twenty percent are multiple.

Reference:

Finn MC, Glowacki J, Mulliken JB. Congenital vascular lesions: clinical application of a new classification. J Pediatr Surg 1983; 18: 894-900.

9. The correct response is E.

All of the above are local complications which may be associated with sclerotherapy.

Reference:

Berenguer B, Burrows PE, Zurakowski D, Mulliken JB. Sclerotherapy of craniofacial venous malformations: complications and results. Plast Reconstr Surg 1999; 104: 1-11.

10. The correct response is E.

Resection is the mainstay of treatment for lymphatic malformation. It can be deferred until the infant is several months old as the older infant is better able to tolerate prolonged anaesthesia.

Reference:

1. *Padwa BL, Hayward PG, Ferraro NF et al. Cervicofacial lymphatic malformation: clinical course, surgical intervention, and pathogenesis of skeletal hypertrophy. Plast Reconstr Surg. 1995; 95: 951.*
2. *Berenguer B, Burrows PE, Zurakowski D, Mulliken JB. Sclerotherapy of craniofacial venous malformations: complications and results. Plast Reconstr Surg 1999; 104: 1-11.*

11. The correct response is E.

Digital subtraction angiography is the one that can detect aneurysmal dysplastic changes in the involved vessels. This can delineate the feeding artery, the arterio-venous malformation and the draining vessels.

Reference:

Burrows PE, Laor T, Paltiel H, Robertson RL. Diagnostic imaging in the evaluation of vascular birth-marks in pediatric dermatology. Dermatol Clin 1998; 16: 466.

12. The correct response is D.

Mafucci syndrome is associated with bone exostoses and enchondromas in combination with exophytic cutaneous venous malformations. It presents in early to middle childhood and the osseous lesions appear first in the hands, feet, long bones of the extremity, ribs, pelvis and cranium.

Reference:

1. *Lewis R, Ketcham A. Mafucci syndrome: functional and neoplastic significance. J Bone Joint Surg Am 1973; 55: 1465-1479.*
2. *Kaplan RP, Wang JT, Amron DM et al. Maffuci's syndrome: two case reports with a literature review. J Am Acad Dermatol 1993; 29: 894-899.*
3. *Lowell S, Mathay R. Head and Neck manifestations of Maffucci's syndrome. Arch Otolaryngol 1979; 105: 427.*

13. The correct response is C.

The Klippel-Trenaunay syndrome is commonly associated with skeletal hypertrophy of an extremity in combination with a slow flow capillary-lymphatic-venous malformation. It presents as a soft tissue and skeletal hypertrophy of an extremity with variation in the extent of involvement. The extremity can be slightly enlarged to a one that is grotesquely enlarged.

Reference:

Jacob AG, Driscoll DJ, Shaughnessy WJ et al. Klippel-Trenaunay syndrome: spectrum and management. Mayo Clin Proc 1998; 73: 28-36.

14. The correct response is C.

The Parkes-Weber syndrome is a complex high-flow arteriovenous malformation that involves throughout the limb with symmetric enlargement. The lower limb is more frequently involved than the upper limb. The diagnosis is confirmed by the detection of a bruit or a thrill.

Reference:

Kohout MP, Hansen M, Pribaz JJ, et al. Arteriovenous malformations of the head and neck: natural history and management. Plast Reconstr Surg. 1998; 102: 643.

15. The correct response is B.

The Wharton's duct drains the submandibular gland. It courses under the lateral floor of the mouth and exits the oral cavity just short of the midline along the root of the undersurface of the tongue.

Reference:

1. *Shah JP, Shah JP. Head and Neck Surgery andOncology. 3rd ed. Edinburgh, UK: Mosby; 2003: 732.*
2. *Shah JP, Patel SG, and the American Cancer Society. Cancer of the Head and Neck. Atlas of Clinical Oncology. Hamilton, Ont: BC Decker; 2002: ix, 484.*

16. The correct response is C.

Papillary cystadenoma lymphomatosum (Warthin's tumour) is the one neoplasm that produces the characteristic uptake of technetium in the salivary glands. The tumour consistently concentrates this isotope and gives the appearance of a "hot gland." Besides this tumour, oncocytomas are other lesions that may take up this tracer in excess of the surrounding gland.

Reference:

1. *Higashi T, Murahashi H, Ikuta H et al. Identification of Warthin's tumour with technetium-99m pertechnetate. Clin Nucl Med 1987; 12:796.*
2. *Yoo GH, Eisle DW, Askin FB et al. Warthin's tumour: a 40-year experience at the John Hopkins Hospital. Laryngoscope. 1994; 104:799.*

17. The correct response is D.

The characteristic "Swiss cheese" appearance on histological examination is seen in adenoid cystic carcinoma. This is the second most common malignant tumour of the parotid gland and has a marked affinity for perineural invasion leading to facial weakness and paralysis.

Reference:

1. *Jones AS, Hamilton JW, Rowley H et al. Adenoid cystic carcinoma of the head and neck. Clin Otolaryngol 1997; 22: 434.*
2. *Harrison LB, Sessions RB, Hong WK. Head and Neck Cancer: A Multidisciplinary Approach. 2nd ed. Philadelphia: Lippincott Williams and Wilkins; 2004: xvii, 1077.*

18. The correct response is D.

A dentigerous cyst arises at the site of an unerupted tooth within its cavity. A Gorlin cyst will have calcified material within it. Resection is the treatment of choice.

Reference:

1. *Browne RM. The pathogenesis of odontogenic cysts: a review. J Oral Pathol 1975; 4: 31.*
2. *Gorlin RJ, Pindborg JJ, Clausen FP, Vickers RA. The calcifying odontogenic cyst-a possible analogue of the cutaneous calcifying epithelioma of Malherbe. Oral Surg Oral Med Oral Pathol 1962; 15: 1235.*

19. The correct response is A.

Ameloblastomas originate from dental lamina rests, enamel organ, basal cells of the oral mucosa or the epithelial lining of a dentigerous cyst. There are three types of ameloblastoma and each of these requires a different treatment. The unicystic is treated by enucleation and curettage. The extraosseous ameloblastoma is treated by radical resection. The intraosseous ameloblastoma is also recurrent and requires a partial hemimandibulectomy. The maxillary ameloblastoma also needs radical resection.

Reference:

1. *Gardner DG, Pecak AM. The treatment of ameloblastoma based on pathologic and anatomic principles. Cancer 1980; 46: 2514.*
2. *Regezi JA, Kerr DA, Courtney RM. Odontogenic tumours: analysis of 706 cases. J Oral Surg 1978; 36: 771.*

20. The correct response is C.

Fibrous dysplasia is a developmental derangement of bone that is characterised by proliferation of fibroblasts producing a dense collagen matrix containing trabeculae of osteoid and bone in a disorganized pattern. It may be monostotic or polyostotic, which can be a part of Albright syndrome.

Reference:

1. *Greer RO Jr, Rohrer MD, Young SK. Nonodontogenic tumours, clinical evaluation and pathology. In Thawley SE, Panje WR, eds: Comprehensive management of Head and Neck tumours. Philadelphia, WB Saunders, 1987: 1510.*
2. *Harrison LB, Sessions RB, Hong WK. Head and Neck Cancer: A Multidisciplinary Approach. 2nd ed. Philadelphia: Lippincott Williams and Wilkins; 2004: xvii, 1077.*

21. The correct response is D.

The mandibulomy approach is best suited for large tumours of the posterior oral cavity or oropharynx which are not involving the mandible. Of the options listed, carcinoma of the base of the tongue would be best managed using this approach. The others can be managed by transoral resection.

Reference:

1. *Shah JP, Shah JP. Head and Neck Surgery andOncology. 3rd ed. Edinburgh, UK: Mosby; 2003: 732.*
2. *Shah JP, Patel SG, and the American Cancer Society. Cancer of the Head and Neck. Atlas of Clinical Oncology. Hamilton, Ont: BC Decker; 2002: ix, 484.*

22. The correct response is D.

A true cyst is defined as an epithelium lined pathologic space. Mandible has a much higher rate of cyst development compared with the rest of the skeleton primarily because of uniqueness of the odontogenic epithelium found within it. Pseudocysts resemble true cysts but lack an epithelial lining. Aneurysmal bone cyst is a pseudocyst which can be unilocular or multilocular having radiolucent areas surrounded by fibrous tissue. Their aetiology and pathogenesis is not clear. Pain is a presenting symptom. The swelling on the surface of the mandible can be pulsatile. Curettage and excision is the treatment of choice.

Reference:

1. *Revel MP, Vanel D, Sigal R et al. Aneurysmal bone cyst of the jaws. J Comput Assist Tomogr 1992; 16: 84-86.*
2. *Motamedi MH Yazdi E. Aneurysmal bone cyst of the jaws: Analysis of 11 cases. J Oral Maxillofac Surg 1994; 52: 471-475.*

23. The correct response is A.

Radicular cyst is a true cyst and these are the most common cysts of the jaw. These are inflammatory odontogenic cysts and are the end result of the necrosis of the dental pulp.

A true cyst is defined as an epithelium lined pathologic space. Mandible has a much higher rate of cyst development compared with the rest of the skeleton primarily because of uniqueness of the odontogenic epithelium found within it. Pseudocysts resemble true cysts but lack an epithelial lining. All the others are pseudocyts of the mandible.

Reference:

1. *Revel MP, Vanel D, Sigal R et al. Aneurysmal bone cyst of the jaws. J Comput Assist Tomogr 1992; 16: 84-86.*
2. *Motamedi MH, Yazdi E. Aneurysmal bone cyst of the jaws: Analysis of 11 cases. J Oral Maxillofac Surg 1994; 52: 471-475.*

24. The correct response is A.

The majority of aneurysmal bone cysts occur in the body (40%), 30% in the ramus, 9% at the angle, 9% at the symphysis and 2% at the condyle. Majority of them occur in patients younger than 30 years with incidence peaking in the second decade of life.

Reference:

1. *Revel MP, Vanel D, Sigal R et al. Aneurysmal bone cyst of the jaws. J Comput Assist Tomogr 1992; 16: 84-86.*
2. *Motamedi MH, Yazdi E. Aneurysmal bone cyst of the jaws: Analysis of 11 cases. J Oral Maxillofac Surg 1994; 52: 471-475.*

25. The correct response is E.

The nasopalatine duct cyst is not an odontogenic cyst. The other options are odontogenic cysts derived either from the odontogenic epithelium or from the remnants of odontogenic epithelium that remains after tooth formation is complete.

Reference:

Shear M. Cysts of the jaws: recent advances. J Oral Pathol 1985; 14: 43-59.

26. The correct response is C.

The opening of the Eustachian tube is located in the nasopharynx.

Reference:

1. *Standring S. Gray's Anatomy. The anatomical basis of clinical practice. 39th ed. Elsevier, Churchill Livingstone, 2005:655.*
2. *Cummings CW, Fredrickson JM, Harker LA, et al, eds. Otolaryngology-Head and Neck Surgery. St. Louis, Mosby, 1998.*

5

27. The correct response is B.

The narrowest portion of the tube is located at the junction of the bony and cartilaginous parts. It is 0.8–1mm in diameter. The total length of the Eustachian tube is about 37-40 mm. The base of the bony portion which opens in the middle ear is 5x3 mm, being oval in shape. The opening of the Eustachian tube in the nasopharynx is about 9 mm. This tube was described by Bartholomeo Eustachio, an anatomist in 1563. It has a bony and a cartilaginous part. Both are cone shaped with truncated apices. The cartilaginous apex lies within the bony apex. The bony part of the tube is 1/3 of the total length (12-13 mm) while the cartilaginous part is 2/3 of the length of the tube (25-27 mm).

Reference:

Robert C. O'Reilly and Isamu Sando. Anatomy and Physiology of Eustachian tube. Cumming's Otolaryngology Head and Neck Surgery. 5th ed. 2010: 1867.

28. The correct response is A.

The tensor palati is the principal dilator of the Eustachian tube. The other muscles also help in opening and closing of the tube. The Eustachian tube lies at an angle of 45° to the Frankfurt horizontal and it does not allow regurgitation of fluids into it from the nasopharynx. The adenoid pad lies between the two openings of the Eustachian tubes.

Reference:

Robert C. O'Reilly and Isamu Sando. Anatomy and Physiology of Eustachian tube. Cumming's Otolaryngology Head and Neck Surgery. 5th ed. 2010: 1870.

29. The correct response is B.

The Eustachian tube remains closed at rest due to the surface tension of the secretions within it. It however opens during swallowing, yawning, sneezing, clenching of teeth and sniffing, to equalize pressures. It also opens during ascent and descent of the flight. In case of a block in the Eustachian tube, intense pain is felt during descent of the flight. The opening of the Eustachian tube lies 10-12 mm behind and slightly below the posterior end of the inferior nasal concha. It can be cannulated by the Eustachian cannula introduced through the nose.

Reference:

Robert C. O'Reilly and Isamu Sando. Anatomy and Physiology of Eustachian tube. Cumming's Otolaryngology Head and Neck Surgery. 5th ed. 2010: 1870.

30. The correct response is D.

All the above three structures i.e. temporomandibular joint, middle cranial fossa and the internal carotid artery are within 3-5 mm of the bony portion of the tube. Care needs to be exercised during surgery within the tube for removal of blockage to save these structures.

Reference:

Robert C. O'Reilly and Isamu Sando. Anatomy and Physiology of Eustachian tube. Cumming's Otolaryngology Head and Neck Surgery. 5th ed. 2010: 1868.

31. The correct response is E.

All the above statements are correct. During flight, the Eustachian tube allows the movement of the air to the middle ear through the pharyngeal end. In case the tube is blocked, the individual feels extreme pain in the ear during the descent of the flight.

Reference:

Robert C, O'Reilly and Isamu Sando. Anatomy and Physiology of Eustachian tube. Cumming's Otolaryngology Head and Neck Surgery. 5th ed. 2010: 1870.

32. The correct response is E.

All of the above are correct. The Eustachian tube is inclined 45 degrees downwards and medially from the Frankfurt horizontal. The mucus secretions of the goblet cells produce lot of surface tension which keeps the tube closed and hence food and liquid cannot easily go into the middle ear.

Reference:

Robert C, O'Reilly and Isamu Sando. Anatomy and Physiology of Eustachian tube. Cumming's Otolaryngology Head and Neck Surgery. 5th ed. 2010: 1870.

33. The correct response is C.

The Ostmann fat pad is located in the inferolateral aspect of the Eustachian tube and is thought to be an important contributing factor in closing the tube. It is also quite likely to contribute in the protection of the Eustachian tube and the middle ear from retrograde flow of nasopharyngeal secretions.

Reference:

1. *Amoodi H, Bance M, Thamboo A. Magnetic resonance imaging illustrating change in the Ostmann fat pad with age. J Otolaryngol Head Neck Surg 2010; 39(4): 440-441.*
2. *Robert C. O' Reilly and Isamu Sando. Anatomy and Physiology of Eustachian tube. Cumming's Otolaryngology Head and Neck Surgery. 5th ed. 2010: 1870.*

34. The correct response is A.

The Ostmann fat pad is located in the inferolateral aspect of the Eustachian tube and is thought to be an important contributing factor in closing the tube. It is also quite likely to contribute in the protection of the Eustachian tube and the middle ear from retrograde flow of nasopharyngeal secretions.

Reference:

1. *Amoodi H, Bance M, Thamboo A. Magnetic resonance imaging illustrating change in the Ostmann fat pad with age. J Otolaryngol Head Neck Surg 2010; 39(4): 440-441.*
2. *Robert C. O'Reilly and Isamu Sando. Anatomy and Physiology of Eustachian tube. Cumming's Otolaryngology Head and Neck Surgery. 5th ed. 2010: 1870.*

35. The correct response is C.

The individual will feel no pain as there will be no change of air pressure between the inside of the middle ear and outside atmosphere.

Reference:

Robert C. O'Reilly and Isamu Sando. Anatomy and Physiology of Eustachian tube. Cumming's Otolaryngology Head and Neck Surgery. 5th ed. 2010: 1871.

36. The correct response is D.

The Valsalva procedure should not be done because compromised Eustachian tube function may be due to congestion and infection in the throat. In such a situation, Valsalva procedure will transmit infection in the ear.

Reference:

Robert C. O'Reilly and Isamu Sando. Anatomy and Physiology of Eustachian tube. Cumming's Otolaryngology Head and Neck Surgery. 5th ed. 2010: 1870.

37. The correct response is C.

Verruca vulgaris is caused by the human papillomavirus. Many different types of human papilloma virus have been identified by their DNA components. The rest of the options are incorrect. The lesion affects the epidermis and can present as a flat patch, outgrowth or filliform projections or as a fungating mass, if it is on the genitalia.

Reference:

Lockshin NA. Flat facial warts treated with fluorouracil. Arch Dermatol 1979; 115: 929-930.

38. The correct response is C.

Molluscum contagiosum is caused by a cytovirus and is characterised by discrete 2-5 mm umbilicated, flesh coloured papules. It spreads by autoinoculation or scratching.

Reference:

de Waard-van der Spek FB, Oranje AP, Lillieborg S et al. Treatment of molluscum contagiosum using a lidocaine/prilocaine cream (EMLA) for analgesia. J Am Acad Dermatol 1990; 23 (pt 1): 685-688.

39. The correct response is B.

Molluscum contagiosum is caused by a cytovirus and is characterised by discrete 2-5 mm umbilicated, flesh coloured papules. It spreads by autoinoculation or scratching. In addition the lesions are frequently grouped and do not involve the palms and soles.

Reference:

de Waard-van der Spek FB, Oranje AP, Lillieborg S et al. Treatment of molluscum contagiosum using a lidocaine/prilocaine cream (EMLA) for analgesia. J Am Acad Dermatol 1990; 23(pt 1): 685-688.

40. The correct response is E.

All of the above are correct for seborrheic keratosis.

Reference:

Sloan JB, Jaworsky C. Clinical misdiagnosis of squamous cell carcinoma in situ as seborrheic keratosis. A prospective study. J Dermatol Surg Oncol 1993; 19: 413-416.

41. The correct response is D.

Rhinophyma is characterised by hypertrophy of the sebaceous glands to such an extent that the nose becomes bulbous and lobulated. In addition there is fibrosis, follicular plugging and telangiectasia of the skin of the nose.

The other options are incorrect for this disease.

Reference:

Redett RJ, Manson PN, Goldberg N, et al. Methods and results of rhinophyma treatment. Plast Reconstr Surg 2001; 107: 1115-1123.

42. The correct response is A.

The black head in the skin overlying a sebaceous cyst is due to keratin plug.

Reference:

Habif TP, ed. Clinical Dermatology. 5th Ed. Philadelphia, Pa: Mosby Elsevier; 2009.

43. The correct response is A.

Milia are small superficial cysts arising from the pilosebaceous follicle containing keratin. They are commonly found on the skin and mucosa of infants. These are epidermal cysts and can be evacuated by use of the bevel of sterile needles.

Reference:

Tsuji T, Kadoya A, Tanaka R et al. Milia induced by corticosteroids. Arch Dermatol 1986; 122: 139-140.

44. The correct response is B.

Secondary milia may be seen after dermabrasion.

Milia are small superficial cysts arising from the pilosebaceous follicle containing keratin. They are commonly found on the skin and mucosa of infants. These are epidermal cysts and can be evacuated by use of the bevel of sterile needles.

Reference:

Tsuji T, Kadoya A, Tanaka R et al. Milia induced by corticosteroids. Arch Dermatol 1986; 122: 139-140.

45. The correct response is C.

The picket fence arrangement of nuclei in the peripheral layer around the tumour on histological examination is characteristic of the basal cell carcinoma. The primary cause of BCC is exposure to UV radiation. The lesions develop from the basaloid cells and can be locally invasive, but these rarely metastasize.

Reference:

1. *Hallock GG, Lutz DA. Prospective study of the accuracy of the surgeon's diagnosis in 2000 excised skin tumors. Plast Reconstr Surg 1998; 101: 1255.*
2. *Gazy S.W, Juliet G, Daniel S, Ellen G, et al. Non-melanoma skin cancers: Basal cell and Squamous cell carcinoma. Abeloff's Clinical Oncology. 2008: 1253.*
3. *Habif TP. Clinical Dermatology, 4th ed. Philadelphia, Mosby, 2004.*

46. The correct response is D.

The reported recurrence rate has been as high as 42% in the ear for basal cell carcinoma.

Reference:

1. *Silverman MK, Kopf AW, Bart RS, et al. Recurrence rate of treated basal cell carcinoma. Part 3: Surgical excision. J Dermatol Surg Oncol 1992;18:471.*
2. *Habif TP. Clinical Dermatology, 4th ed. Philadelphia, Mosby, 2004.*

47. The correct response is A.

The treatment of choice for basal cell carcinoma is surgery followed by local reconstruction as required.

Reference:

1. *Hallock GC, Lutz DA. Prospective study of the accuracy of the surgeon's diagnosis in 2000 excised skin tumours. Plast Reconstr Surg 1998; 101: 1255.*
2. *Gazy S.W, Juliet G, Daniel S, Ellen G et al. Non-melanoma skin cancers: Basal cell and Squamous cell carcinoma. Abeloff's Clinical Oncology. 2008: 1253.*

48. The correct response is E.

All of the above factors may be responsible for producing a squamous cell carcinoma.

Reference:

1. *Roth JJ, Granick MS. Squamous cell and adenexal carcinomas of the skin. Clin Plast Surg 1997; 24:687.*
2. *Gazy S.W, Juliet G, Daniel S, Ellen G et al. Non-melanoma skin cancers: Basal cell and Squamous cell carcinoma. Abeloff's Clinical Oncology. 2008: 1257.*

49. The correct response is E.

Squamous cell carcinoma have a varied presentation and can clinically manifest as all of the above.

Reference:

Gazy S.W, Juliet G, Daniel S, Ellen G, et al. Non-melanoma skin cancers: Basal cell and Squamous cell carcinoma. Abeloff's Clinical Oncology. 2009: 1257.

50. The correct response is B.

Paget's disease originates on the nipple and areola. It is clinically characterized by eczema like skin changes. On histological examination, Paget's cells are located within the epidermis. These are characteristically large cells with large nucleus and abundant cytoplasm.

Reference:

Rook A, Wilkinson DS, Ebling FJB, et al. Textbook of Dermatology, 4th ed. Oxford, Blackwell, 1986.

51. The correct response is C.

Extramammary Paget's disease besides bone is common in the vulva and male genital area where apocrine glands are found. It has a more favourable prognosis than the mammary Paget's disease.

Reference:

1. *Gunn RA, Gallagher HS. Vulvar Paget's disease. Cancer 1980; 46: 590.*
2. *Rook A, Wilkinson DS, Ebling FJB, et al. Textbook of Dermatology, 4th ed. Oxford, Blackwell, 1986.*

52. The correct response is B.

Hutchinson's freckle is a flat, brown, macular lesion that may grow at various rates and achieve different shades of pigmentation. On histological examination, this lesion appears as an overgrowth of melanocytes at the epidermis-dermis junction.

Reference:

1. *Koh HK, Michalik E, Sober AJ et al. Lentigo maligna melanoma has not better prognosis than other types of melanoma. J Clin Oncol 1984; 2: 994.*
2. *Julie RL, Leslie AF, Williams HS, Rhoda MA et al. Melanoma. Abeloff's Clinical Oncology, 4th ed. 2008:1235.*

53. The correct response is B.

The Breslow's classification is based on ocular micrometry i.e. measurement of the depth of involvement histologically that gives an idea about the depth of involvement in a case of melanoma in millimetres. Clarks's classification is based on depth of invasion in the dermis. TNM classification as proposed in 2003, by the American joint Committee on Cancer, is now being followed. The morphologic classification provides prognostic assessment of the melanoma based on the morphologic features of the primary tumour. The clinical classification is based upon the extent of clinical spread of disease.

Reference:

Breslow A. Thickness, cross-sectional areas and depth of invasion in the prognosis of cutaneous melanomas. Ann Surg 1970; 172: 902.

54. The correct response is D.

Tomographic gallium scans are helpful for detecting metastatic melanoma in a number of distant sites. They are however less useful for detecting metastases in the lung parenchyma and brain. However metastases in lymph nodes, abdominal viscera and soft tissues can be detected well by this modality.

Reference:

1. *Kirkwood JM, Myers JE, Vlock DR et al. Tomographic gallium-67 citrate scanning. Useful new surveillance for metastatic melanoma. Ann Intern Med 1982; 97: 694.*
2. *Kirkwood JM, Myers JE, Vlock DR et al. Tomographic gallium-67 citrate scanning. Useful new surveillance for metastatic melanoma. Ann Surg 1983; 198: 102.*

55. The correct response is A.

The melanomas located in thick areas of skin have a worse prognosis. These areas are collectively grouped as BANS areas which stands for upper back, upper arm, posterior neck and posterior scalp.

Reference:

1. *Briggs JC, Ibrahim NB, Hasting AG, et al. Experience of thin cutaneous melanomas (0.76 and 0.85 mm thick) in a large plastic surgery unit: a 5-to 17-year follow up. Br J Plast Surg 1984; 37: 501.*
2. *Handley WS. The pathology of melanocytic growths in relation to their operative treatment. Lecture II. Lancet. 1907; 1: 996.*

56. The correct response is A.

Topical 5-FU cream acts by inhibiting both thymidine and DNA syntheses leading to cell death. The arrest of cell growth in the S phase causes the cells to undergo apoptosis with the production of proinflammatory mediators.

Reference:

1. *Miller E. The metabolism and pharmacology of 5-fluorouracil. J Surg Oncol 1971; 3: 309-315.*
2. *Harrison LB, Sessions RB, Hong WK. Head and Neck Cancer: A Multidisciplinary Approach. 2nd ed. Philadelphia: Lippincott Williams and Wilkins; 2004: xvii, 1077.*

57. The correct response is E.

All of the above options are correct. The overall effect is that the skin looks younger. The recommended dose is 2250 units daily and is up to 4000 units for nursing mothers. Excess of Vitamin A can cause dry hair, dry skin, hepatomegaly, raised ESR, serum calcium and serum alkaline phosphatase levels. It can cause birth defects as well. Deficiency of Vit A leads to development of ocular defects (xerophthalmia).

Reference:

DiGiovanna JJ. Retinoid chemoprevention in the high-risk patient. J Am Acad Dermatol 1998; 39(pt 3): 582-85.

58. The correct response is D.

Cryosurgery produces its effect by excessive cooling leading to tissue necrosis and vascular stasis. The current temperature recommendations range from –50 degree C to – 60 degree C for all tumour regions. In general, collagen and cartilage resist freezing injuries and therefore freezing is effective in the ear and the nose.

Reference:

1. *Kuflik EG. Cryosurgery updated. J Am Acad Dermatol 1994; 31: 925-944, quiz 944-946.*
2. *Mazur P. Freezing of living cells: mechanisms and implications. Am J Physiol 1984; 247 (pt 1): C125-C142.*
3. *Zacarian SA. Cryosurgery of cutaneous carcinomas. An 18-year study of 3,022 patients with 4,228 carcinomas. J Am Acad Dermatol 1983; 9: 947-956.*

59. The correct response is D.

Poor general health, advanced age, medical conditions that preclude surgery and tumour size between 1 and 5 cm are the indications of radiotherapy for skin cancers. The rest are contraindications for radiotherapy.

Reference:

1. *Finizio L, Vidali C, Calacione R et al. What is the current role of radiation therapy in the treatment of skin carcinomas? Tumour 2002; 88: 48-52.*
2. *Westgate SJ. Radiation therapy for skin tumours. Otolaryngol Clin North Am 1993; 26: 295-309.*

60. The correct response is D.

Marjolin's ulcer is now synonymous with cancers arising in scar tissue, burns and wounds though Marjolin had first noted it in burn scars. De Costa gave the eponym Marjolin to scar cancer in 1903.

Reference:

1. *DeCosta JC. Carcinomatous changes in an area of chronic ulceration, or Marjolin's ulcer. Ann Surg 1903; 37: 496-502.*
2. *Koga Y, Sawada Y. Basal cell carcinoma developing on a burn scar. Burn 1997; 23: 75-77.*
3. *Smith J, Mello LE, Nogueira Neto NC, et al. Malignancy in chronic ulcers and scars of the leg (Marjolin's ulcer): a study of 21 patients. Skeletal Radiol 2001; 30: 331-337.*

61. The correct response is E.

All of the above may be seen in Marjolin's ulcer. The involvement of lymph glands is not a feature of Marjolin's ulcer, because it develops within the scar, which does not have lymphatics. The lesion needs to be excised and skin grafted. Peripheral and deep margins must be assessed for clearance. Amputations may have to be done in cases which recur.

Reference:

1. *Koga Y, Sawada Y. Basal cell carcinoma developing on a burn scar. Burn 1997; 23: 75-77.*
2. *Smith J, Mello LE, Nogueira Neto NC, et al. Malignancy in chronic ulcers and scars of the leg (Marjolin's ulcer): a study of 21 patients. Skeletal Radiol 2001; 30: 331-337.*

62. The correct response is E.

Marjolin's ulcers occur at any age and in all races. The lag time from the injury to the onset of the cancer varies from 8 months to 60 years. The median seems to be about 31 years. This time is inversely proportional to the age of the patient at the time of the injury. Elderly patients with burns have a short latency period before scar cancer appears.

Reference:

1. *Bartle EJ, Sun JH, Wang XW et al. Cances arising from burn scars. J Burn Care Rehabil 1990; 11: 46-49.*
2. *Mosborg DA, Crane RT, Tami TA et al. Burn scar carcinoma of the head and neck. Arch Otolaryngol Head Neck Surg 1988; 114: 1038-1040.*

63. The correct response is C.

Keratoacanthoma is a common tumour that arises from hair follicles and is common in sun exposed areas of light skinned older individuals. It clinically and microscopically resembles squamous cell carcinoma yet it can spontaneously regress after a rapid growth phase.

Reference:

1. *Beham A, Regauer S, Soyer HP, Beham-Schmid C. Keratoacanthoma: a clinically distinct variant of well differentiated squamous cell carcinoma. Adv Anat Pathol 1998; 5: 269-280.*
2. *Cribier B, Asch P, Grosshans E. Differentiating squamous cell carcinoma from keratacanthoma using histopathological criteria. Is it possible? A study of 296 cases. Dermatology 1999; 199: 208-212.*

64. The correct response is B.

The posterior neck incision allows good exposure of the neck while simultaneously preserving adequate blood supply for the skin flaps and also giving a good exposure of the neck. The McFee incision preserves the blood supply best but is more tedious to elevate. The double opposing flaps are easier to dissect and provide excellent exposure of the neck contents but the flaps are at risk of tip necrosis particularly when the neck has been irradiated. The posterior neck incision is the most advantageous and heals nicely.

Reference:

1. *Ariyan S. Functional neck dissection. Plast Reconstr Surg 1980; 65: 768.*
2. *Ariyan S, Chicarilli ZN. Cancer of the upper aerodigestive system. In McCarthy JG, ed: Plastic Surgery, Philadelphia, WB Saunders, 1990: 3412.*

65. The correct response is D.

The classical neck dissection removes the sternocleidomastoid, internal jugular vein and the spinal accessory nerve as one block dissection.

Reference:

1. *Ariyan S. Radical neck dissection. Surg Clin North Am 1986; 66: 133.*
2. *Ariyan S, Chicarilli ZN. Cancer of the upper aerodigestive system. In McCarthy JG, ed: Plastic Surgery, Philadelphia, WB Saunders, 1990: 3412.*

66. The correct response is D.

In the functional neck dissection sternocleidomastoid, accessory nerve and internal jugular vein are preserved. The technique was proposed by an Italian surgeon, Bocca and is known as Bocca's functional neck dissection.

Reference:

Bocca E, Pignataro D. A conservative technique in radical neck dissection. Ann Otol Rhinol Laryngol 1967; 76: 975.

67. The correct response is D.

This tumour belongs to stage IV due to involvement of the mandible.

According to the American Joint Committee on Cancer (AJCC) TNM staging, if a tumour invades the mandible through the cortical bone, it is, by definition, a stage IV tumour regardless of size.

Stage II and III tumours do not involve invasion of the mandible or adjacent structures. Stage IVB involves metastasis to a lymph node more than 6 cm in greatest dimension. Stage IVC involves distant metastasis.

Oral Cavity:

- T1 Tumor < 2 cm
- T2 Tumor > 2 but < 4 cm
- T3 Tumor >4 cm
- T4 Tumor invades adjacent structures such as cortical bone, tongue, skin, or soft tissues of the neck

- N1 One ipsilateral node <3 cm
- N2a One ipsilateral node >3 and <6 cm
- N2b Multiple ipsilateral nodes <6 cm
- N2c Bilateral contralateral nodes <6 cm
- N3 Any nodes >6 cm

- M0 No distal metastasis
- M1 Distal metastasis

Reference:

1. *Fleming ID, Cooper JS, Henson DE, et al. AJCC Cancer Staging Manual. Philadelphia: Lippincott-Raven; 1997.*
2. *Shockley WW, Pillsbury HC. The Neck: Diagnosis and Surgery. St. Louis: Mosby; 1994.*

68. The correct response is E.

The most appropriate management is segmental resection. The surgical management of ameloblastoma is controversial as to the specific modality of recommended surgical treatment. Radiotherapy and chemotherapy are not recommended for ameloblastomas. Surgical treatment revolves around curettage, enucleation and segmental resection. Unicystic ameloblastomas can be treated conservatively with enucleation as they appear clinically as a cyst. With peripheral involvement or in large ameloblastomas like in the given case which involves and surrounds bone and extends into the soft tissues, the treatment should be locally aggressive and hence segmental resection with reconstruction is recommended.

Reference:

1. *Chana JS, Chang YM, Wei FC, et al. Segmental mandibulectomy and immediate free fibula osteoseptocutaneous flap reconstruction with endosteal implants: an ideal treatment method for mandibular ameloblastoma. Plast Reconstr Surg. 2004; 113: 80.*
2. *Chapelle KA, Wilde PC, Brouns JJ et al. Rational approach to diagnosis and treatment of ameloblastomas and odontogenic keratocysts. Br J Oral Maxillofac Surg. 2004; 42: 381.*

6 TRUNK AND LOWER EXTREMITY

QUESTIONS

1. **Which one of the following breast implant produces a foul smell on leakage?**
   A. Silicon gel implant
   B. Trilucent implant
   C. Saline filled implant
   D. Double lumen implant
   E. Textured implant

2. **Which one of the following best measures the compliance of the soft tissue envelope of the breast for deciding implant placement?**
   A. Suprasternal notch to nipple distance
   B. Breast height
   C. Base width
   D. Pinch test
   E. Nipple to inframammary fold distance

3. **Which one of the following incisions would give the best view for the placement of a breast implant during breast augmentation?**
   A. Transaxillary
   B. Inframammary
   C. Periareolar
   D. Transumbilical

4. **Which one of the following incisions for breast augmentation may be associated with transection of the parenchymal ducts at the time of implant placement?**
   A. Transaxillary
   B. Inframammary
   C. Periareolar
   D. Transumbilical

5. **Which one of the following incisions for breast augmentation can only be used with saline implants?**
   A. Transaxillary
   B. Inframammary
   C. Periareolar
   D. Transumbilical

6. **Which one of the following organism has been implicated in the aetiology of capsular contracture following breast augmentation?**
   A. Staphylococcus aureus
   B. Staphylococcus epidermidis
   C. Staphylococcus warneri
   D. Propionibacterium acnes
   E. Pseudomonas aeruginosa

7. **Which of the following intercostal nerves should be preserved during the dissection in augmentation of the breast to preserve nipple sensation?**
   A. 3rd lateral intercostal nerve
   B. 4th lateral intercostal nerve
   C. 5th lateral intercostal nerve
   D. All of the above

8. **Which one of the following is a clear advantage of subglandular placement of breast implant over submuscular placement of implant?**
   A. Reduced incidence of capsular contracture
   B. Less degree of rippling when using saline filled implants
   C. Preferred in patients for breast reconstruction after mastectomy
   D. More natural appearance of the breast
   E. All of the above

9. Which one of the following is a clear advantage of submuscular placement of breast implant over subglandular placement of implant?

A. Muscle covers upper part of the implant and provides protection

B. Breast is laterally placed

C. Less degree of rippling when using saline filled implants

D. Wobbles like a normal breast

E. All of the above

10. Ptosis of the breast is commonly classified on the basis of position of the nipple in relation to which one of the following?

A. Mid arm level

B. Level of the inframammary crease

C. At level of the seventh rib

D. At level of the eighth rib

E. At level of the ninth rib

11. Third degree ptosis of the breast is defined by which of the following?

A. The nipple is at the level of the inframammary fold

B. The nipple is 1 to 3 cm below the inframammary fold

C. The nipple is more than 3 cm below the inframammary fold

D. The nipple is more than 5 cm below the inframammary fold and below the lower contour of the breast

E. The nipple is more than 5 cm below the inframammary fold with the majority of breast tissue below it

12. Which one of the following characteristic differentiates pseudoptosis from true ptosis of the breast?

A. The nipple is at the level of the inframammary fold

B. The nipple is 1 to 3 cm below the inframammary fold

C. The nipple is more than 3 cm below the inframammary fold

D. The nipple is more than 5 cm below the inframammary fold with the majority of breast tissue below it

E. The nipple is at the level of the inframammary fold with the majority of breast tissue below it

13. Which one of the following periareolar techniques for mastopexy correction of ptosis uses a mesh support for promoting fibrosis that serves to support the breast for a longer time?

A. Benelli periareolar mastopexy

B. Goes double skin technique

C. Lassus vertical scar technique

D. Lejour vertical scar technique

E. Chiari L short scar technique

14. Which of the following is the advantage with inverted T closure mastopexy?

A. Hidden scars

B. Upper glandular plication with suspension to pectoralis fascia improves results

C. Visualisation of the end result on the table

D. Reconstructs the lateral and medial pillars with conical gland shape

E. Uses strong subglandular sutures to reshape the gland

F. All of the above

15. Many techniques have been described for mastopexy. Which one of the following technique follows the principles of wide lower skin undermining, overcorrection of the deformity and liposuction of the breast?

A. Benelli periareolar mastopexy

B. Goes double skin technique

C. Lassus vertical scar technique

D. Lejour vertical scar technique

E. Chiari L short scar technique

16. A patient with abdominal obesity should be locally examined for presence of which of the following to avoid possible complications?

A. Hernias

B. Diastasis recti

C. Scar of previous operations

D. Lumps in the abdomen

E. All of the above

17. The normal umbilicus is located at which one of the following level?

A. In line with the superior most point of the iliac crest

B. 2 cm above the superior most point of the iliac crest

C. 2 cm below the superior most point of the iliac crest

D. Sits at the level of the natural waist

E. Sits 2 cm above the natural waist

18. Characteristic fat deposits exist in men and women due to the varying anatomy of the superficial fascial system and its zones of adherence. "Love handles" are present in which one of the following location?

A. Above the iliac crest

B. Above the umbilicus

C. Above the greater trochanter

D. Above the mons pubis

E. Above the breasts

19. Characteristic fat deposits exist in men and women due to the varying anatomy of the superficial fascial system and its zones of adherence. "Saddle bags" are present in which one of the following location?
   A. Lateral to the iliac crest
   B. Above the umbilicus
   C. Above the greater trochanter
   D. Above the mons pubis
   E. Above the breasts

20. The bicycle handle bar incision is used in which one of the following abdominoplasty procedure?
   A. Regnault abdominoplasty
   B. Grazer abdominoplasty
   C. Baroudi abdominoplasty
   D. Pitanguy abdominoplasty
   E. Gonzalez Ulloa abdominoplasty

21. Which one of the following is true regarding reverse abdominoplasty?
   A. Reverses the effects of muscular laxity
   B. Reverses the effects of skin laxity in the lower abdomen
   C. Results in inframammary scars
   D. Indicated for musculofacial defects without skin excess
   E. Indicated for abdominoplasty after massive weight loss

22. Which one of the following procedure is recommended for patients with massive weight loss?
   A. High lateral tension abdominoplasty
   B. Reverse abdominoplasty
   C. Endoscopically assisted abdominoplasty
   D. Circumferential torsoplasty
   E. Neoumbilicoplasty

23. Which of the following factor contributes to seroma formation after abdominoplasty?
   A. Raw surface exudes serum
   B. Compromised lymphatic drainage
   C. Impairment of flap adhesion to abdominal wall fascia
   D. Inadequate drainage of serum
   E. All of the above

24. Which one of the following is not a feature of a normal umbilicus?
   A. Hollow depression
   B. Base fixed to the anterior rectus sheath
   C. Side walls are sloping and may have folds
   D. Inferior hood
   E. Superior hood

25. Which one of the following is not an ingredient of the tumescent fluid for liposuction?
   A. Ringer lactate
   B. Normal saline
   C. Epinephrine
   D. Lidocaine

26. Which one of the following parameter is important during initial consultation for liposuction in evaluating prospective patients for surgery?
   A. Patient desire for surgery
   B. Psychiatric evaluation
   C. Serum cholesterol level
   D. Skin fold thickness
   E. BMI

27. The Virchow's triad related to deep venous thrombosis consists of venous stasis, intimal injury and which one of the following?
   A. Thromboembolism
   B. Paralysis
   C. Hypercoagulability
   D. Low platelet count
   E. Protein C deficiency

28. Which one of the following are the symptoms of deep vein thrombosis?
   A. Pain in the leg
   B. Swelling of the leg
   C. Chest pain
   D. Shortness of breath
   E. All of the above

29. The classic triad of fat embolism comprises of respiratory distress, cerebral dysfunction and which one of the following?
   A. Chest infiltrates
   B. Cardiac failure
   C. Petechial rashes
   D. Pulmonary oedema
   E. Fluid overload

30. Large volume liposuctions are commonly done for enhanced contouring in one sitting. It is defined as an aspirate amounting to which one of the following?
   A. More than 1 litre
   B. More than 3 litres
   C. More than 4 litres
   D. More than 5 litres
   E. More than 7 litres

31. Ageing changes in the pelvis leads to which one of the following deformity?

A. Posterior rotation of the pelvis
B. Osteoporosis of the pelvis
C. Lateral tilt of the pelvis to one side
D. Projection of the lower abdomen
E. Prominent buttocks

32. Postural changes with aging in the pelvis have been linked to which of the following factor?

A. Loss of skin elasticity
B. Osteoporosis of the pelvis
C. Relaxation of the superficial musculoaponeurotic system (SMAS)
D. Relaxation of the superficial fascial system (SFS)
E. All of the above

33. Which one of the following procedure is considered the "gold standard" tool for liposuction?

A. Suction-assisted lipoplasty (SAL)
B. Ultrasound-assisted liposuction (UAL)
C. Power-assisted liposuction (PAL)
D. Tumescent-assisted liposuction (TAL)

34. Which one of the following liposuction procedure causes the least disruption of vasculature?

A. Suction-assisted lipoplasty (SAL)
B. Ultrasound-assisted liposuction (UAL)
C. Power-assisted liposuction (PAL)
D. Tumescent-assisted liposuction (TAL)

35. Characteristic fat deposits exist in men and women due to the varying anatomy of the superficial fascial system and its zones of adherence. The "banana roll" is present in which one of the following location?

A. Lateral to the iliac crest
B. Above the umbilicus
C. Above the greater trochanter
D. Inferior to gluteal fold
E. Below the breasts

36. 'Bat wing deformity' is a condition associated with which one of the following regions?

A. Pectoral region
B. Deltoid region
C. Arm region
D. Forearm region
E. Pelvic region

37. Which one of the following areas is not favourable for liposuction?

A. Lateral side of the arm
B. Posterior side of the arm
C. Medial side of the arm
D. Anterior side of the arm

38. Which one of the following is an important landmark for planning suction assisted lipoplasty of the arm?

A. Olecranon
B. Inferior border of the arm
C. Bicipital groove
D. Posterior axillary fold
E. Anterior axillary fold

39. The breast width is a close measurement of the bra cup size. A bra of 'B cup' size corresponds to which one of the following?

A. Breast width 4 inches
B. Breast width 6 inches
C. Breast width 8 inches
D. Breast width 10 inches
E. Breast width 12 inches

40. Which one of the following has been implicated as the cause for grade III capsular contracture?

A. Silicon shell of the implant
B. Silicon bleeds from the implant
C. Talcum Powder
D. Betadine
E. Poor handling during surgery

41. Rupture of breast implant can be best diagnosed by which one of the following method?

A. Sudden onset of burning breast pain
B. Detection of a mass remote from the implant
C. Mammography
D. Ultrasonography
E. MRI

42. Which of the following is not corrected by abdominoplasty?

A. Skin wrinkling
B. Skin excess
C. Stretch marks
D. Muscle laxity
E. All of the above

43. Contour irregularities are common after liposuction. The under correction in liposuction could manifest as which of the following?

A. Residual bulge
B. Residual depression
C. Asymmetry
D. Step deformity
E. All of the above

44. Contour irregularities are common after liposuction. The late complication of over correction by liposuction could be which of the following?

A. Dimples and dents
B. Furrows and grooves
C. Craters
D. Wrinkling of skin
E. All of the above

45. "French pastry" wrinkling in patients following liposuction is due to which one of the following?

A. Use of fine cannulas
B. Corrugator effects in the fatty layer
C. Over correction
D. Excess of skin in the adjoining area

46. Penile lengthening can be achieved by which one of the following procedure?

A. Release of dartos fascia
B. Release of Buck's fascia
C. Release of tunica albuginea
D. Release of suspensory ligament

47. Girth increase in the penis can be achieved by fat injection in which one of the following?

A. Dartos fascia
B. Buck's fascia
C. Tunica albuginea
D. Below the skin
E. Intracorporal injection

48. Which one of the following muscle is unsuitable as a flap for chest wall reconstruction?

A. Pectoralis major
B. Latissimus dorsi
C. Serratus anterior
D. Rectus abdominis
E. Sternocleidomastoid

49. Which one of the following is the flap of choice for closing midline sternotomy defects?

A. Pectoralis major
B. Latissimus dorsi
C. Serratus anterior
D. Rectus abdominis
E. Sternocleidomastoid

50. Which one of the following would provide an optimal cover for the sacrococcygeal meningomyelocoele defects?

A. Latissimus dorsi
B. Gluteal flap
C. Transverse rectus abdominis myocutaneous flap
D. Vastus lateralis

51. Sternum develops from the mesoderm. It begins development at which one of the following period?

A. At six weeks
B. At ten weeks
C. At twelve weeks
D. At fourteen weeks
E. At sixteen weeks

52. Which part of the sternum is spared by the Pectus excavatum, a disorder characterised by the depression of the sternum?

A. Manubrium
B. Body of the sternum
C. Xiphoid
D. Costal cartilages

53. The pectus excavatum deformity which is characterised by the depression of the sternum is due to which one of the following?

A. Inherent weakness of the sternum
B. Osteoporosis of the sternum
C. Intrauterine compression of the sternum
D. Overgrowth of the costal cartilages
E. Breech delivery

54. The pectus severity index (PSI) is a radiological index for calculating the severity of pectus excavatum. The index is calculated by which one of the following?

A. Dividing the length of sternum by its width at the narrowest point
B. Calculating the distance from the line joining the nipples to the deepest concave point on the sternum
C. Dividing the internal transverse diameter of the thorax by the anteroposterior diameter of the thorax
D. Dividing the internal transverse diameter of the thorax by the vertebral-sternal distance at the most depressed portion of the deformity
E. Dividing the internal transverse diameter of the thorax by the vertebral-sternal distance at the level of the nipple

55. Which one of the following cardiac function anomaly may be found in patients with pectus excavatum?

A. Cardiomyopathy
B. Mitral valve prolapse
C. Congenital heart block
D. Congenital cyanotic heart disease
E. Ventricular septal defect

56. The repair in cases of pectus excavatum should be done at which one of the following age?

A. At age of 1 year
B. At school going age
C. At age of 10 years
D. At age of 16 years
E. Can be done at any time

57. The Ravitch procedure for the correction of the pectus excavatum deformity is based on which one of the following?

A. Elevation of the sternum by a strut
B. Repair using plates and screw for fixation
C. Repair using bioabsorbable mesh
D. Repair using custom silicone implants
E. Bilateral resection of costal cartilages

58. Pectus carinatum is characterized by which of the following?

A. Defect in the sternum
B. Depression of the sternum
C. Abnormal growth of the cartilage at the costochondral junction
D. Manubrium is spared in this deformity
E. All of the above

59. Cleft of the sternum is characterized by which of the following?

A. Intact sternal skin
B. Visible heart movements through the intact skin
C. Haemangiomas
D. Primary repair of defect in the neonates gives good results
E. All of the above

60. "Pentalogy of Cantrell" is a rare congenital disorder and is characterised by which of the following?

A. Cleft in the sternum
B. Defect in the anterior diaphragm
C. Defect in parietal pericardium
D. Herniation of the heart and omphalocoele
E. All of the above

61. Poland's syndrome is a disorder of which of the following?

A. Thoracic musculature
B. Thoracic cage
C. Lungs
D. Limb
E. All of the above

62. Gynecomastia in males is mainly due to which one of the following?

A. Estrogen excess
B. Lower levels of androgens
C. Hypogonadism
D. Mumps epididymo-orchitis
E. Neoplastic / HIV pathology

63. Which one of the following is considered the dominant nerve supply to the nipple of breast?

A. Second intercostal nerve
B. Third intercostal nerve
C. Fourth intercostal nerve
D. Fifth intercostal nerve
E. Sixth intercostal nerve

64. Which one of the following technique of breast reduction would be suitable for massive reductions of more than 1500 gm per side?

A. Horizontal bipedicle
B. Superior pedicle
C. Superolateral pedicle
D. Vertical bipedicle
E. Breast amputation

65. Which one of the following technique of breast reduction would not be suitable for major reductions in excess of 500 gm per side?

A. Horizontal bipedicle
B. Superior pedicle
C. Superolateral pedicle
D. Vertical bipedicle
E. Periareolar technique

66. Which one of the following technique of breast reduction would be suitable for small to moderate reductions of less than 500 gm per side?

A. Horizontal bipedicle
B. Vertical mammaplasty
C. Superolateral pedicle
D. Vertical bipedicle
E. Breast amputation

67. 'Boxy' breast deformity is common after which one of the following technique of reduction?

A. Horizontal bipedicle
B. Vertical mammaplasty
C. Inferior pedicle
D. Vertical bipedicle
E. Breast amputation

68. A densely glandular breast tissue would not be suitable for breast reduction by which of the following technique?

A. Superior pedicle
B. Vertical mammaplasty
C. Inferior pedicle
D. Vertical bipedicle
E. Central mound

69. The inferior pedicle technique for breast reduction is not suitable for which one of the following indication?

A. Preservation of nipple sensation
B. Moderate reduction
C. Suitable for small size reduction
D. Suitable for large size reduction

70. A benign breast lesion on ultrasonography is unlikely to have which one of the following characteristic feature?

A. Hyperechogenecity
B. Hypoechogenecity
C. Thin capsule
D. Ellipsoid
E. Cystic

71. Which one of the following modality has the highest diagnostic accuracy for breast imaging?

A. Mammography
B. Ultrasonography
C. MRI
D. CT

72. In a case of suspected rupture of the breast implant, which one of the following procedures would demonstrate the 'step ladder sign' suggestive of the rupture of the implant?

A. Mammography
B. Ultrasonography
C. M.R.I
D. C.T
E. Plain radiograph

73. In which one of the following mastectomies, both the pectoralis major and minor are removed?

A. Simple mastectomy
B. Subcutaneous mastectomy
C. Modified radical mastectomy
D. Halsted mastectomy

74. Postoperative radiation therapy is indicated in which of the following?

A. Ductal carcinoma- in- situ (DCIS)
B. Stage I and II disease
C. Recurrence in chest wall
D. Recurrence in scar
E. All the above

75. The proper incision for lumpectomy of breast is a curvilinear incision. A radial incision for lumpectomy is preferred for which of the following location?

A. Superior pole
B. Medial quadrant
C. Lateral quadrant
D. Keyhole area
E. Axillary tail

76. The rough texture of the areola is due to presence of which one of the following?

A. Coopers ligament
B. Sweat glands
C. Montgomery glands
D. Acne
E. Hormonal changes

77. The skate flap has been described for the reconstruction of which one of the following?

A. Breast
B. Oral commissure
C. Nipple
D. Lower lip
E. Soft tissue contour deformity

78. Which one of the following is the preferred donor site for areolar reconstruction?

A. Postauricular region
B. Groin
C. Perineum
D. Thigh
E. Supraclavicular region

79. The pattern of circulation in latissimus dorsi muscle is which one of the following?

A. Type I
B. Type II
C. Type III
D. Type IV
E. Type V

80. Which one of the following action is not performed by the latissimus dorsi muscle?

A. Adduction
B. Extension
C. Medial rotation
D. Lateral rotation
E. Secures tip of scapula against the posterior chest wall

81. A total autogenous latissimus dorsi flap can provide a maximum muscle volume of which one of the following?

A. 50 -100 cc
B. 100 - 200 cc
C. 200 - 300 cc
D. 300 - 400 cc
E. Indefinite volume

82. Morbidity associated with the use of TRAM flap includes which of the following?

A. Weakness of abdominal wall
B. Hernias
C. Scarring
D. Difficulty in performing Yogic exercises
E. All of the above

83. The free TRAM flap offers several advantages over the pedicled TRAM flap. Which of the following is a major disadvantage of a free TRAM flap?

A. Difficulty in shaping the flap to desirable contour
B. Greater incidence of abdominal wall weakness and hernia
C. Poorly suited for patients with history of smoking and diabetes
D. Potential for complete flap loss
E. All of the above

84. Tissue expansion was first reported by which one of the following?

A. Neumann
B. Radovan
C. Austad
D. Gillies
E. Millard

85. Which of the following complication may be observed following use of breast implants?

A. Infection
B. Haematoma
C. Seroma
D. Leakage
E. All of the above

86. The first inflation following insertion of the expander implant is preferably done at which one of the following time interval?

A. After one week
B. After two weeks
C. After four weeks
D. After five weeks

87. Implants placed under the pectoralis major muscle can be fully covered by which of the following in cases of doubtful skin viability?

A. Pectoralis major muscle alone
B. Pectoralis major muscle and additional cover by rectus muscle flap
C. Pectoralis major muscle and additional cover by external oblique muscle flap
D. All of the above

88. In which of the following yogic asanas, the rectus-abdominis muscle does not play an active role?

A. Agnisar
B. Kapal – Bhati
C. Bhastrika
D. Anulom – Vilom
E. Gunjan – Kriya

89. Which of the following are the indications for a bipedicled TRAM flap?

A. Large volume reconstruction
B. Patients with midline abdominal incisions
C. Smokers
D. Obesity
E. All of the above

90. The paraumbilical area and the area underlying the region of the belt is mainly supplied by which one of the following?

A. Superior epigastric vessels
B. Deep inferior epigastric vessels
C. Superficial inferior epigastric vessels
D. Circumflex iliac vessels

91. The primary blood supply to the lower abdominal skin is from which one of the following source?

A. Superior epigastric artery
B. Deep inferior epigastric artery
C. Superficial inferior epigastric artery
D. Intercostal segmental vessels
E. Terminal branches of circumflex iliac vessels

92. The vascular zones of the unipedicled TRAM flap have been divided into four areas. Which of the following is the most reliable zone of this flap?

A. Zone I
B. Zone II
C. Zone III
D. Zone IV
E. All have equal blood supply

93. The vascular zones of the unipedicled TRAM flap have been divided into four areas. Which of the following is the least reliable zone and should be discarded?

A. Zone I
B. Zone II
C. Zone III
D. Zone IV
E. All have equal blood supply

94. The inframammary crease is better preserved in which of the following TRAM flap?

A. Ipsilateral TRAM flap reconstruction
B. Contralateral TRAM flap reconstruction
C. Bipedicled TRAM
D. All of the above

95. Which of the following are the advantages with the ipsilateral pedicled TRAM flap over the contralateral TRAM flap?

A. Better flap position
B. Reduced inframammary bulging
C. Better vascular supply
D. Reduced pedicle tension
E. All of the above

96. Which one of the following vessel is preferred as a recipient vessel for a free TRAM flap in immediate breast reconstruction?

A. Internal mammary vessels
B. Thoracodorsal vessels
C. Intercostal vessels
D. Thoracoacromial vessels
E. Any of the above

97. Which of the following vessel is preferred as a recipient vessel for a free TRAM flap in delayed breast reconstruction?

A. Internal mammary vessels
B. Thoracodorsal vessels
C. Intercostal vessels
D. Thoracoacromial vessels
E. Any of the above

98. Which one of the following is the biggest disadvantage of using internal mammary vessels as recipient vessels for free TRAM flap in delayed breast reconstruction?

A. Small size of artery
B. Absence of artery in some cases
C. Abnormal course of the artery
D. Inconsistent size of the vein
E. Difficulty in accessing these vessels behind the costal cartilages

99. Which one of the following costal cartilages may have to be removed before using the internal mammary vessels for microvascular anastomosis for free TRAM breast reconstruction in situations where the size of the vein is small?

A. Second costal cartilage
B. Third costal cartilage
C. Fourth costal cartilage
D. Fifth costal cartilage
E. Sixth costal cartilage

100. Latissimus dorsi muscle is a muscle on the back of the body. It owes its name from which one of the following languages?

A. Latin
B. Greek
C. English
D. French

101. The shape of the latissimus dorsi muscle is which one of the following?

A. Rectangular
B. Square
C. Triangular
D. Flat ribbon like

102. Which one of the following is an absolute contraindication for the use of latissimus dorsi muscle flap for breast reconstruction?

A. Prior division of the thoracodorsal artery
B. Previous posterolateral thoracotomy
C. Smoker
D. Diabetes mellitus
E. All of the above

103. Which one of the following movement is not performed by the latissimus dorsi muscle?

A. Adduction
B. Extension
C. Medial rotation
D. Lateral rotation
E. Climbing

104. The piriformis muscle is an important landmark in the anatomy of superior gluteal artery system. It lies under a line running along which of the following location?
   A. Joining the posterior superior iliac spine with the coccyx
   B. Joining the posterior superior iliac spine with the greater trochanter
   C. At perpendicular to the midline of a line joining the posterior superior iliac spine with the coccyx
   D. None of the above

105. The primary advantage of a musculocutaneous perforator flap is to:
   A. Increase the skin island of the flap
   B. Increase the vascularity of the flap
   C. Increase the versatility of the flap
   D. Spare the muscle
   E. Reliability

106. Which one of the following free flaps is the flap of choice for reconstruction of the breast?
   A. TRAM flap
   B. Anterolateral thigh flap
   C. Deep inferior epigastric flap
   D. Tensor fascia lata flap
   E. Gluteal flap

107. Rubens flap for breast reconstruction is based on which one of the following vessel?
   A. Superior epigastric artery
   B. Deep inferior epigastric artery
   C. Superficial inferior epigastric artery
   D. Intercostal segmental vessels
   E. Deep circumflex iliac vessels

108. Which one of the following is an undesirable complication observed by the patient following reduction mammoplasty?
   A. Unequal reduction
   B. Fat necrosis
   C. Hypertrophic scarring
   D. Dog ear
   E. None of the above

109. The location of the nipple is important for planning breast surgery. The nipple is normally placed in the mid-clavicular line. The average distance from the manubrial notch to the nipple is which one of the following?
   A. 15 cm
   B. 18 cm
   C. 22 cm
   D. 25 cm
   E. 28 cm

110. A high riding nipple following reduction mammoplasty can be repositioned by which one of the following method?
   A. Reallocation of the nipple by readjusting the inferior pedicle
   B. By advancing it into a vertical cut below the complex and closing the gap
   C. As a full thickness graft
   D. All of the above

111. Nipple convergence and divergence is a distressing problem following reduction mammaplasty. It can be corrected by which one of the following?
   A. Reposition of its pedicle
   B. Crescent excisions
   C. Dermal pedicle
   D. All of the above

112. Reduction mammaplasties can lead to which one of the following complication?
   A. Fat necrosis
   B. Skin necrosis
   C. Calcification
   D. Fibrocystic disease
   E. All of the above

113. Which one of the following is the commonest complication seen at the recipient site of the breast implant?
   A. Infection
   B. Haematoma
   C. Seroma
   D. Local skin necrosis
   E. Valve failure

114. Which one of the following is the commonest reason for reoperation following breast implant surgery?
   A. Capsule contracture
   B. Deflation
   C. Infection
   D. Prosthesis loss
   E. All of the above

115. Which one of the following complications of breast implant surgery requires reexploration?
   A. Severe capsular contracture
   B. Asymmetry
   C. Malposition
   D. Skin necrosis
   E. All of the above

116. A case of woody hard breast where the implant cannot be felt would fit into which one of the following grades as per Baker's classification?

A. Grade 1
B. Grade 2
C. Grade 3
D. Grade 4

117. Restoration of the abdominal wall is essential to preserve the functions of the abdominal wall. Which one of the following is the technique of choice for reconstructing a defect of the abdominal wall that is less than 7 cm?

A. Local fasciocutaneous flap
B. Rectus abdominis musculocutaneous flap
C. External oblique musculocutaneous flap
D. Free anterolateral thigh flap
E. Primary closure

118. The arcuate line is an anatomic demarcation denoting the change in structural composition of the rectus sheath. It is located at which one of the following level?

A. Level of umbilicus
B. Midway between umbilicus and pubic symphysis
C. Midway between xiphisternum and umbilicus
D. Midway between xiphisternum and pubic symphysis
E. At level of superior border of iliac crest

119. The lateral margin of the rectus muscle beginning from pubic tubercle to the ninth costal cartilage is denoted by which one of the following?

A. Linea semicircularis
B. Linea semilunaris
C. Linea alba
D. Linea terminalis
E. Linea aspera

120. The arcuate line is an anatomic demarcation denoting the change in structural composition of the rectus sheath. It is also known as:

A. Linea semicircularis
B. Linea semilunaris
C. Linea alba
D. Linea terminalis
E. Linea aspera

121. Which one of the following layer carries important neurovascular structures to the glans penis?

A. Skin
B. Tunica albuginea
C. Corpus cavernosum
D. Buck's fascia
E. Dartos fascia

122. The corpora cavernosa are covered by skin, dartos muscle and fascia, Buck's fascia and tunica albuginea. The chordee tissue in hypospadias is located superficial to which one of the following layer?

A. Skin
B. Tunica albuginea
C. Corpus cavernosum
D. Buck's fascia
E. Dartos fascia

123. The exstrophy of the bladder is characterized by which one of the following features?

A. Diastasis recti
B. Epispadias
C. Bladder exstrophy
D. Cloacal exstrophy
E. All of the above

124. Chordee without hypospadias is characterized by which one of the following?

A. Ventral curvature
B. Normally placed urinary opening
C. Prepuce normally placed
D. Nesbit's dorsal plication gives good results
E. All of the above

125. Phallic reconstruction by the one stage 'Chang technique' is based on which of the following flap?

A. Ulnar artery flap
B. Radial artery flap
C. Upper lateral arm flap
D. Dorsalis pedis flap
E. Deltoid flap

126. Which one of the following is the disadvantage of phallic reconstruction by the Biemer technique?

A. Poor sensory return to the phallus
B. Neourethra is reconstructed from hairy portion
C. Small size of the phallus
D. Poorly vascularised urethra
E. All of the above

127. Peyronie's disease is characterized by the formation of fibrous nodules within which of the following layer?

A. Skin
B. Tunica albuginea
C. Corpus cavernosum
D. Buck's fascia
E. Dartos fascia

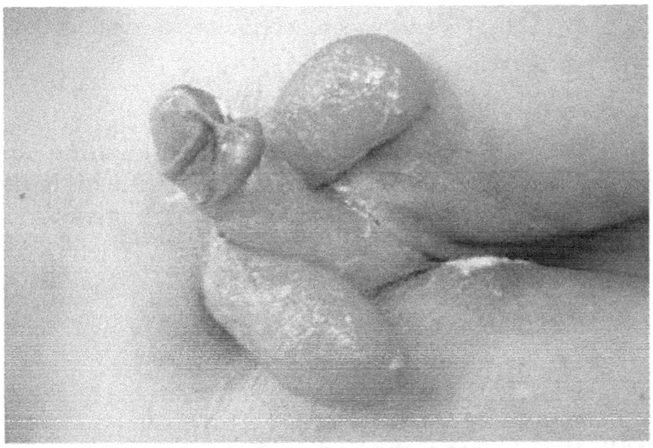

128. A 24-year-old male develops ischaemic necrosis of the scrotal skin leading to a raw area over the scrotum and the penis (picture shown). The diagnosis is consistent with Fournier's gangrene. Which one amongst the following is the commonest causative organism for this condition?

A. Gram positive organisms
B. Gram negative organisms
C. Anaerobes
D. All of the above

129. Balanitis xerotica obliterans which produces a white patch on the glans is caused by which one of the following?

A. Streptococcus pyogenes
B. Staphylococcus aureus
C. Staphylococcus epidermidis
D. Borrelia burgdorferi
E. Clostridium perfringens

130. A 23-year-old male presented to the outpatient department with a progressively enlarging swelling of the lower limb for past several years. He gives a positive history of increase in the swelling after episodes of high grade fever. Microscopic examination of aspirated fluid from the lesion led to the diagnosis of chronic filarial lymphedema along with the characteristic clinical presentation (picture shown). The disease involves the lower limb and genitals leading to a disabling and persistent lymphedema. Which of the parts of the penis escape from involvement in lymphedema?

A. Penile shaft
B. Base of penis
C. Glans and prepuce
D. All of the above

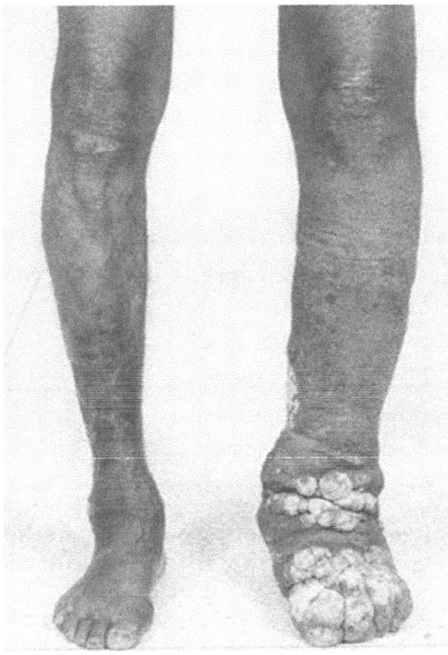

131. Which one of the following is an associated condition with hypospadias?

A. Ventral curvature
B. Misplaced urinary opening on the ventral surface of the shaft of the penis
C. Dorsal hood of skin
D. Cryptorchidism

132. Chordee in hypospadias is primarily because of which one of the following?

A. Shortening of the skin
B. Shortening of the urethra
C. Dysgenesis of corpus spongiosum
D. Spasm in the corpus cavernosum
E. Fibrous nodules in the tunica albuginea

133. Chordee is present circumferentially in which of the following location?

A. 6 O' clock position
B. All around the organ
C. Ventrally from 3 O' Clock to 9 O' Clock position
D. Dorsally from 9 O' Clock to 3 O' Clock position

134. The flip-flap procedure for hypospadias repair is preferable for which one of the following?

A. Midpenile hypospadias
B. Distal penile hypospadias
C. Penoscrotal hypospadias
D. Scrotal hypospadias
E. Perineal hypospadias

135. Horton-Devine method of hypospadias repair uses which one of the following?

A. Bucket handle prepucial flap
B. Prepucial hood
C. Inner prepucial flap
D. Outer prepucial flap

136. The MAGPI procedure is indicated for which one of the following?

A. Subcoronal hypospadias
B. Midpenile hypospadias
C. Penoscrotal hypospadias
D. Scrotal hypospadias
E. Perineal hypospadias

137. Which one of the following is the method of choice for reconstruction of the vagina for vaginal agenesis?

A. Split skin graft
B. Full thickness skin graft
C. Gracilis myocutaneous flap
D. TRAM flap
E. Loop of ileum

138. Which one of the following is the method of choice for reconstruction of the vagina following pelvic exenteration?

A. Split skin graft
B. Full thickness skin graft
C. Gracilis flap
D. Flap of colon
E. Loop of ileum

139. Which one of the following is the commonest cause for acquired vaginal defects?

A. Malignant excisions
B. Trauma
C. Infections
D. Forced manipulations

140. The modified Singapore flap is ideal for reconstruction of defects of which one of the following region?

A. Vagina
B. Groin
C. Lower abdomen
D. Sacral region
E. Lower back

141. Circumferential vaginal defects involving the entire vagina and the introitus are best managed by which one of the following flap?

A. Modified Singapore flap
B. VRAM (Vertical rectus abdominis myocutaneous) flap
C. Gracilis muscle flap
D. Sigmoid colon

142. Which one of the following represents the cut off limit of external pressure beyond which tissue perfusion would be impaired?

A. 10 mm of Hg
B. 20 mm of Hg
C. 25 mm of Hg
D. 30-32 mm of Hg
E. 40 mm of Hg

143. Which part of the body would experience maximum pressure in the supine position?

A. Occiput
B. Back of shoulder
C. Elbow
D. Buttock
E. Calf

144. Which one of the following has the highest incidence of pressure sores?

A. Sacrum
B. Ischial tuberosity
C. Greater trochanter
D. Heel
E. Malleolus

145. A pressure sore with exposed bone would be placed in which of the following grades?

A. Grade 1
B. Grade 2
C. Grade 3
D. Grade 4

146. Which one of the following flap is preferred for the management of sacral pressure sore?

A. Gluteus maximus flap
B. Tensor fascia lata flap
C. Gluteal thigh flap
D. Rhomboidal flap
E. Vastus lateralis flap

147. Which one of the following flap is likely to provide a large island of skin with maximum amount of muscle into the debrided sore and is preferred for the management of ischial pressure sore while also allowing primary closure of the donor site?

A. Inferior gluteus maximus island flap
B. Tensor fascia lata flap
C. Gluteal thigh flap
D. Rhomboidal flap
E. Vastus lateralis flap

148. Which one of the following pressure sore typically presents with minimal skin involvement and extensive bursa formation?

A. Sacral
B. Trochanteric
C. Ischial
D. Heel
E. All of the above

149. Which one of the following flap is considered the workhorse for the management of trochanteric pressure sore?

A. Inferior gluteus maximus island flap
B. Tensor fascia lata flap
C. Gluteal thigh flap
D. Rhomboidal flap
E. Vastus lateralis flap

150. The leg has four compartments having vascular supply coming from typically two angiosomes. Which of the compartment has only one source of blood supply?

A. Deep posterior
B. Lateral
C. Anterior
D. Posterior

151. Which one of the following muscle does not pass under the inguinal ligament?

A. Iliacus
B. Psoas major
C. Pectineus
D. Adductor longus
E. Sartorius

152. Which of the following is the criteria for the diagnosis of chronic osteomyelitis?

A. Exposed bone with drainage more than 6 weeks
B. Positive wound culture
C. Consistent radiographic findings
D. Bone scan consistent with chronic infection
E. All of the above

153. Leg trauma coupled with inadequate soft tissue coverage commonly would lead to which one of the following type of osteomyelitis?

A. Localized
B. Medullary
C. Diffuse
D. Superficial

154. Diabetic microangiopathy is due to increased blood viscosity leading to ischaemia. The increased blood viscosity in diabetes is attributable to which one of the following cell?

A. White blood cell
B. Red blood cell
C. Platelet
D. Macrophage
E. Monocyte

155. Which one of the following is the classical sign of lymphedema of the lower extremity?

A. Peau d'orange
B. Stemmer sign
C. Blunted appearance of digits
D. All of the above

156. Chronic ulcers above the medial malleolus in the lower third of the leg are most probably due to which one of the following?

A. Venous insufficiency
B. Arterial insufficiency
C. Diabetes
D. Vasculitis
E. Neuropathic involvement

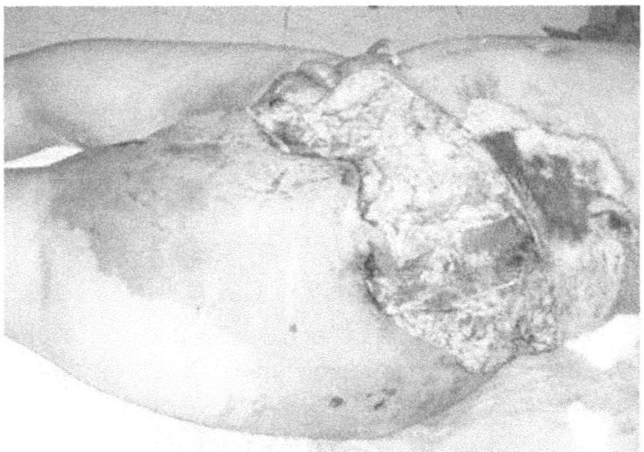

157. A 14-year-old male sustains a run over accident by a heavy vehicle over the hip region 12 hours back. He has full thickness necrosis of the skin over the iliac crest and greater trochanter region along with areas of impending ischaemia. Which one of the following would be the best management for this patient?

A. Intravenous fluids and antibiotics
B. Wait and watch approach
C. Debridement of wound
D. Wound debridement with skin grafting
E. Microvascular flap cover

ANSWERS, EXPLANATIONS AND REFERENCES

1. The correct response is B.

Soyabean oil filled implants (Trilucent) were marketed earlier for a few years between 1994–1999. Soyabean oil composed the fill material which was said to be radiolucent. These have been discontinued due to the leakage of oil, oil bleed and foul smell which led to these implants being withdrawn from the market. Gel filled implants can also have a leak, gel bleed and cause capsular contracture.

Reference:

1. *Choudhary S, Cadier MAM. Local tissue reactions to oil based breast implants bleed. Br J Plast Surg 2000; 53: 317.*
2. *Scott SL, Mardini S. Alternative filler materials and new implant designs. Clin Plast Surg 2001; 28: 435.*

2. The correct response is D.

The pinch test is a useful measurement of the compliance and elasticity of the breast skin. The skin of the superior pole of the breast is pinched between the thumb and index finger and the distance between the two is measured. A rough estimate for the amount of inherent soft tissue necessary to cover a subglandular implant is 2 cm. A pinch test result of less than 2 cm may lead to subpectoral implant placement.

Reference:

Tebbetts JB. A system for breast implant selection based on patient tissue characteristics and implant-soft tissue dynamics. Plast Reconstr Surg 2002; 109: 1396.

3. The correct response is B.

The inframammary approach provides complete visualisation of both the prepectoral and subglandular pocket and allows precise placement of all types of implants. The disadvantage however is a visible scar in the inframammary fold.

Reference:

Hidalgo DA. Breast augmentation: choosing the optimal incision, implant, and pocket plane. Plast Reconstr Surg 2000; 105: 2202.

4. The correct response is C.

The periareolar approach which is made at the areolar-cutaneous junction generally heals well. The disadvantage of this incision is a limited exposure of the surgical field along with a risk of transection of the parenchymal ducts.

Reference:

Hidalgo DA. Breast augmentation: choosing the optimal incision, implant, and pocket plane. Plast Reconstr Surg 2000; 105: 2202.

5. The correct response is D.

The transumbilical approach for breast augmentation has the advantage of having single well hidden remote incision. However it can only be used with saline implants as these can be inserted through smaller incisions (< 3 cm) as opposed to the gel implants which may require incisions upto 5.5 cm.

Reference:

Hidalgo DA. Breast augmentation: choosing the optimal incision, implant, and pocket plane. Plast Reconstr Surg 2000; 105: 2202.

6. The correct response is B.

Staphylococcus epidermidis has been implicated in causing capsular contracture. It constitutes the normal skin flora and in rabbit model inoculation with this organism has been shown to induce thicker capsules than in control animals. Numerous studies have linked subclinical infection with an increased incidence of capsular contracture.

Reference:

1. *Shah Z, Lehman JA Jr, Tan J. Does infection play a role in breast capsular contracture? Plast Reconstr Surg 1981; 68: 34.*
2. *Dobke MK, Svahn JK, Vastine VL et al. Characterisation of microbial presence at the surface of silicone mammary implants. Ann Plast Surg 1995; 34: 563.*
3. *Baker JL Jr. Classification of spherical contracture. Presented at the Aesthetic Breast Symposium, Scottsdale, Arizona, 1975.*

7. The correct response is D.

All of the above lateral intercostal nerves should be preserved during the dissection in breast augmentation to preserve the nipple sensation. These nerve branches often run with their concomitant artery and vein and often need to be stretched but should not be divided.

Reference:

Biggs TM, Yarish RS. Augmentation mammaplasty: a comparative analysis. Plast Reconstr Surg 1990; 85: 368.

8. The correct response is D.

The subglandular versus the submuscular placement of breast implant is topic of debate but there are several clear advantages with each of these. The subglandular implant gives a more natural appearance of the breast. The submuscular implant is indicated obviously in cases of breast reconstruction after mastectomy. One positive aspect of submuscular implant is that with saline filled implants, the rippling effect is decreased due to presence of the muscle between the implant and the superficial breast tissue.

Reference:

1. *Tebbetts JB. Transaxillary subpectoral augmentation mammoplasty: Long-term follow-up and refinement. Plast Reconstr Surg 1984; 74: 636.*
2. *Truppman ES, Ellenby JD. A thirteen year evaluation of subpectoral augmentation mammoplasty. In Owsley JQ, Peterson RA, eds: Symposium on Aesthetic Surgery of the Breast. St. Louis, CV Mosby, 1978.*
3. *Mahler D, Ben-Yakar J, Hauben DJ. The retropectoral root for breast augmentation. Aesthetic Plast Surg 1982; 6: 237.*

9. The correct response is C.

The subglandular versus the submuscular placement of breast implant is topic of debate but there are several clear advantages with each of these. One advantage of submuscular implant is that with saline filled implants, the rippling effect is decreased due to presence of the muscle between the implant and the superficial breast tissue. The subglandular implant gives a more natural appearance of the breast. The submuscular implant is indicated obviously in cases of breast reconstruction after mastectomy.

Reference:

1. *Tebbetts JB. Transaxillary subpectoral augmentation mammoplasty: Long-term follow-up and refinement. Plast Reconstr Surg 1984; 74: 636.*
2. *Truppman ES, Ellenby JD. A thirteen year evaluation of subpectoral augmentation mammoplasty. In Owsley JQ, Peterson RA, eds. Symposium on Aesthetic Surgery of the Breast. St. Louis, CV Mosby, 1978.*

10. The correct response is B.

The breast ptosis classification is based on the position of the nipple in relation to the inframammary crease. Minimal ptosis is when the nipple is at the level or just inferior to the crease; moderate ptosis is when the nipple is 1-3 cm below the crease and severe ptosis is when nipple is more than 3 cm below the crease.

Reference:

1. *Georgiade NG, Georgiade CGS, Riefkohl R. Esthetic breast surgery. In McCarthy JG, ed: Plastic Surgery. Philadelphia, WB Saunders, 1991: 3839.*
2. *Regnault P. Breast ptosis. Definition and treatment. Clin Plast Surg 1976; 3: 193.*

11. The correct response is C.

The Regnaults classification defines third degree of ptosis when the nipple is more than 3 cm below the inframammary crease. If the nipple is between 1-3 cm, it would be placed in second degree of ptosis. If the nipple is around 1 cm below the inframammary line it would be placed in first degree of the ptosis of the breast. Option D, E are incorrect.

Reference:

1. *Georgiade NG, Georgiade CGS, Riefkohl R. Esthetic breast surgery. In McCarthy JG, ed: Plastic Surgery. Philadelphia, WB Saunders, 1991: 3839.*
2. *Regnault P. Breast ptosis. Definition and treatment. Clin Plast Surg 1976; 3: 193.*

12. The correct response is E.

When the nipple is at or above the level of the inframammary fold with the majority of breast tissue below its line, it is classified as pseudoptosis.

Reference:

1. *Georgiade NG, Georgiade CGS, Riefkohl R. Esthetic breast surgery. In McCarthy JG, ed: Plastic Surgery. Philadelphia, WB Saunders, 1991: 3839.*
2. *Brink RR. Management of true ptosis of the breast. Plast Reconstr Surg 1993; 91: 657.*

13. The correct response is B.

Mesh is used for support in the Goes mastopexy technique. This is the double skin technique in which the basic principle involves formation of a resistant lining of the breast by the use of a layer of prosthetic mesh. This mesh provides increased support of the new breast shape during the healing and skin contraction processes.

Reference:

Goes JCS. Periareolar mastopexy and reduction with mesh support. In Spear SL, ed: Surgery of the Breast: Principles and Art. Philadelphia, Lippincott-Raven, 1998: 697.

14. The correct response is C.

The inverted scar technique is good for women having moderate to severe ptosis with a large excess of skin and a moderate amount of glandular tissue. The advantage of this technique is the ability to see the final shape of the breast while the patient is still on the operating table which allows final adjustments to the shape and symmetry of the breast.

The other options are not advantages of this technique.

Reference:

1. *McKissock PK. Reduction mammoplasty with a vertical dermal flap. Plast Reconstr Surg 1972; 49: 245.*
2. *Courtiss EH, Goldwyn RM. Reduction mammaplasty by the inferior pedicle technique. Plast Reconstr Surg 1977; 59: 500.*

15. The correct response is D.

The Lejour vertical scar with undermining technique is based on the principles of wide lower skin undermining, overcorrection of the deformity and liposuction of the breast. The detachment of the skin from the lower portion of the breast and use of strong subglandular sutures helps to reshape the gland and enhances postoperative stability. The major drawback is the amount of time it takes postoperatively before the final result can be achieved.

Reference:

1. *Lejour M. Vertical mammaplasty and liposuction of the breast. Plast Reconstr Surg 1994; 94:100.*
2. *Lejour M. Vertical mammaplasty for breast hypertrophy and ptosis. Operative Techniques Plast Surg 1996; 3: 189.*
3. *Hall-Findlay EJ. Pedicles in vertical breast reduction and mastopexy. Clin Plast Surg 2000; 29: 379.*

16. The correct response is E.

All of the above are risk factors and should be examined and taken into consideration before planning surgery

Reference:

Hansel JM, Lehman JA, Tantri MP, et al. An outcome analysis and satisfaction survey of 199 consecutive abdominoplasties. Ann Plast Surg 2001; 46: 357.

17. The correct response is A.

The normal umbilicus is located in line with the most superior point of the iliac crest in majority of patients. In relation to the natural waist, it is located below the natural waist by about 1-4 cm.

Reference:

1. *Hansel JM, Lehman JA, Tantri MP et al. An outcome analysis and satisfaction survey of 199 consecutive abdominoplasties. Ann Plast Surg 2001; 46: 357.*
2. *Moufarrege R. The Moufarrege horseshoe abdominoplasty. Aesthetic Surg J 1997; 17: 91.*
3. *Craig SB, Faller MS, Puckett CL. In search of the ideal female umbilicus. Plast Reconstr Surg 2000; 105: 389.*

18. The correct response is A.

The "Love handles" are present above the iliac crests. The other options are incorrect.

Reference:

1. *Lockwood TE. Superficial fascial system [SFS] of the trunk and extremities: a new concept. Plast Reconstr Surg 1991; 87: 1009.*
2. *Rohrich RJ, Smith PD, Marcantonio D, Kenkel JM. The zones of adherence: role in minimizing and preventing contour deformities in liposuction. Plast Reconstr Surg 2001; 107: 1562.*

19. The correct response is A.

The "saddle bags" are present lateral to the iliac crest in women and cause a fatty bulge in that area.

Reference:

Lockwood TE. Superficial fascial system [SFS] of the trunk and extremities: a new concept. Plast Reconstr Surg 1991; 87: 1009.

20. The correct response is C.

The bicycle handle bar incision is used in the Baroudi's abdominoplasty procedure. Above the pubic region, the incision is transverse, but on the sides it is raised up and this looks like a bicycle handle. The incision can be hidden under the bikini. The other options are incorrect.

Reference:

Baroudi R, Moraes M. A "bicycle-handlebar" type of incision for primary and secondary abdominoplasty. Aesthetic Plast Surg 1995; 19: 307.

21. The correct response is C.

The reverse abdominoplasty is indicated for upper epigastric laxity and results in inframammary scars. The ideal candidate for this procedure is one who has upper abdominal laxity with pre-existing epigastric scars from a prior breast reduction or lift. The other options are incorrect. Circumferential torsoplasty is recommended for patients with massive weight loss.

Reference:

Baroudi R, Keppke EM, Carvalho CG. Mammary reduction combined with reverse abdominoplasty. Ann Plast Surg 1979; 2: 368.

22. The correct response is D.

Circumferential torsoplasty is recommended for patients with massive weight loss. It involves resection of redundant tissue circumferentially and is indicated in those patients with circumferential skin excess. The reverse abdominoplasty is indicated for upper epigastric laxity and results in inframammary scars. Endoscopically assisted abdominoplasty is indicated for musculofascial defects without skin excess requiring excision. Umbilicoplasty is performed after the skin excesses are resected.

Reference:

1. *Cormenzana P, Sampron NM. Circumferential approach to contouring of the trunk. Aesthetic Surgery J 2004; 24: 13.*
2. *Aly AS, Cram AE, Heddens C. Truncal body contouring surgery in the massive weight loss patient. Clin Plast Surg 2004; 31: 611.*

23. The correct response is E.

Seroma is one of the most common postsurgical complications in abdominoplasty. The aetiology of seroma revolves around many factors including a raw surface of the flaps, compromised lymphatic drainage, impairment of flap adhesion to the abdominal wall fascia and also persistent movement of the flaps. Undrained fluid beneath the flaps also hampers flap adhesion to abdominal fascia promoting seroma formation.

Reference:

1. *Baroudi R, Ferreira CA. Seroma: how to avoid it and how to treat it. Aesthetic Surg J 1998; 18: 439.*
2. *Pitanguy I. Evaluation of body contouring surgery today: a 30-year perspective. Plast Reconstr Surg 2000; 105: 1499.*

24. The correct response is D.

The inferior hood is not a characteristic feature of the umbilicus.

Reference:

Craig SB, Faller MS, Puckett CL. In search of the ideal female umbilicus. Plast Reconstr Surg 2000; 105: 389.

25. The correct response is B.

Normal saline is not used in tumescent fluid, instead Ringer lactate 1000 cc is used.

Reference:

1. *Pitman GH, Aker JS, Tripp ZD. Tumescent liposuction: a surgeon's prospective. Clin Plast Surg 1996; 23: 633.*
2. *Illouz Y, De Villers Y. Body sculpturing by lipoplasty. Edinburgh, Churchill Livingstone, 1989.*

26. The correct response is E.

The body mass index is the single most important factor in initial evaluation for liposuction. Surgery is advised for patients having index less than 30. The other options are also important but do not contribute as the initial deciding parameters for surgery.

Reference:

Pitman GH, Fikry BA. Liposuction: safety issues in 1300 cases. Scientific presentation at Annual meeting of American Society of Aesthetic Plastic Surgery, New York, May 7; 2001.

27. The correct response is C.

Hypercoagulability along with venous stasis and injury to intimal layer constitutes the Virchow's triad. These together may produce DVT and pulmonary embolism.

Reference:

Teimourian B, Rogers WB 3rd. A national survey of complications associated with suction lipectomy: a comparative study. Plast Reconstr Surg 1989; 84: 628.

28. The correct response is E.

All of the above are the symptoms of deep vein thrombosis.

Reference:

1. *Teimourian B, Rogers WB 3rd. A national survey of complications associated with suction lipectomy: a comparative study. Plast Reconstr Surg 1989; 84: 628.*
2. *Illouz Y, De Villers Y. Body sculpturing by lipoplasty. Edinburgh, Churchill Livingstone, 1989.*

29. The correct response is C.

Petechial rash in combination with respiratory distress and cerebral dysfunction constitutes the triad of fat embolism. The other options may be a part of clinical presentation of fat embolism.

Reference:

1. *Ross R, Johnson G. Fat embolism after liposuction. Chest 1988; 93: 1294.*
2. *Illouz Y, De Villers Y. Body sculpturing by lipoplasty. Edinburgh, Churchill Livingstone, 1989.*

30. The correct response is D.

The American Society of Plastic Surgeons defines large volume liposuction as the removal of more than 5 litres of total aspirate in one setting. This distinction has been made to help make guidelines for the overall management of these patients especially with large volume liposuctions.

Reference:

1. *Illouz YG. Body contouring by lipolysis: a 5-year experience with over 3000 cases. Plast Reconstr Surg 1983; 72: 591-597.*
2. *Illouz Y, De Villers Y. Body sculpturing by lipoplasty. Edinburgh, Churchill Livingstone, 1989.*

31. The correct response is D.

Aging changes in the pelvis lead to anterior rotation of the pelvis causing a more projection of the lower abdomen with a loss of the youthful lordosis of the lower back. There is a flattening of the posterior body contour with loss of projection of the buttocks leading to flat buttocks.

The treatment consists in tightening of the rectus abdominis and superficial fascial system of the abdomen and thighs.

Reference:

1. *Lockwood T. Lower body lift. Operative Techniques Plast Reconstr Surg 1996; 3: 132–144.*
2. *Illouz Y, De Villers Y. Body sculpturing by lipoplasty. Edinburgh, Churchill Livingstone, 1989.*

32. The correct response is D.

Postural changes with aging in the pelvis have been attributed to relaxation of the musculoskeletal framework especially the superficial fascial system (SFS). This is also termed as the "body suit" of the trunk and thighs. Evidence to support such an observation stems from the fact that the lateral tension abdominoplasty has a "buttock lift" effect.

SMAS exists in the face and not in the pelvic area.

Reference:

1. *Lockwood T. Superficial fascial system (SFS) of the trunk and extremities: a new concept. Plast Reconstr Surg 1991; 87: 1009-1018.*
2. *Turek S. Orthopedics – Principles and their application, vol 2, 4th ed. Philadelphia, JB Lippincott, 1984: 1598-1600.*

33. The correct response is A.

Suction-assisted lipoplasty (SAL) has a long track record and is considered the gold standard tool for liposuction. SAL is the commonest procedure for doing liposuction.

Reference:

1. *Pitman GH, Teimourian B. Suction lipectomy: complications and results by survey. Plast Reconstr Surg 1985; 76: 65.*
2. *Illouz Y, De Villers Y. Body sculpturing by lipoplasty. Edinburgh, Churchill Livingstone, 1989.*

34. The correct response is B.

The ultrasound assisted lipoplasty (UAL) causes less disruption of vasculature as the ultrasonic energy produced in a piezoelectric crystal helps in emulsifying the fat. This fat is then suctioned with the machine. The other techniques do not give this advantage.

Reference:

1. *Kenkel JM, Robinson JB Jr, Beran SJ et al. The tissue effects of ultrasound-assisted lipoplasty. Plast Reconstr Surg 1998; 102: 213.*
2. *Pitman GH, Teimourian B. Suction lipectomy: complications and results by survey. Plast Reconstr Surg 1985; 76: 65.*

35. The correct response is D.

The banana roll is a preoperative or postoperative roll of fat inferior to the gluteal fold.

Reference:

1. *Lockwood T. Superficial fascial system (SFS) of the trunk and extremities: a new concept. Plast Reconstr Surg 1991; 87: 1009-1018.*
2. *Illouz Y, De Villers Y. Body sculpturing by lipoplasty. Edinburgh, Churchill Livingstone, 1989.*

36. The correct response is C.

The 'Bat wing deformity' is a condition where there is accumulation of fat and loose skin in the region of the upper arm. This may lead to discomfort when clothing with short sleeves. Laxity is most commonly seen in people with significant weight loss or through the aging process when fat deposits tend to diminish leading to the development of this deformity.

Reference:

1. *Vogt PA. Brachial suction-assisted lipoplasty and brachioplasty. Aesthetic Surg J 2001; 21: 164.*
2. *Illouz Y, De Villers Y. Body sculpturing by lipoplasty. Edinburgh, Churchill Livingstone, 1989.*

37. The correct response is C.

The medial side of the arm is not a favourable site for liposuction because of the presence of nerves, veins and vessels traversing this site.

Reference:

1. *Vogt PA. Brachioplasty. Aesthetic Surg Q 1995; 15: 13.*
2. *Illouz Y, De Villers Y. Body sculpturing by lipoplasty. Edinburgh, Churchill Livingstone, 1989.*

38. The correct response is C.

The bicipital groove is an important landmark for evaluation of patients for suction assisted lipoplasty of the upper arm. Many measurements of the upper arm are based on this, which is particularly helpful in grading the deformity of the upper arm.

Reference:

1. *Vogt PA. Brachioplasty. Aesthetic Surg Q 1995;15:13.*
2. *Illouz Y, De Villers Y. Body sculpturing by lipoplasty. Edinburgh, Churchill Livingstone, 1989.*

39. The correct response is C.

The breast width is a close measurement of the bra cup size. A 'B-cup' size bra corresponds to breast width of 8 inches. A-cup size corresponds to breast width 7 inches, C-cup size corresponds to 9 inches and D-cup size corresponds to 10 inches of breast width.

Reference:

Pechter EA. A new method for determining bra size and predicting postaugmentation breast size. Plast Reconstr Surg 1998; 102: 1259–1265.

40. The correct response is B.

Silicon bleeds from the implant is a chronic inflammatory stimulus for capsular contracture. The most common cause is the silicon bleed, which causes a chronic inflammatory reaction. Initially polymorphonuclear leucocytes and monocytes appear around the implant. Gradually lymphocytes, fibroblasts and myofibroblasts start producing the collagen which gets organized to form a capsule outside the implant. It takes about 4-6 weeks to develop. The thickness of the capsule may be from 0.25 mm to 4 mm. It gets lined by a synovium due to movement of the implant within the capsule.

Reference:

1. *Peters W, Smith D, Fornasier V et al. An outcome analysis of 100 women after explantation of silicone gel breast implants. Ann Plast Surg 1997; 39: 9–19.*
2. *Raso DS, Crymes LW, Metcalf JS. Histological assessment of fifty breast capsules from smooth and textured augmentation and reconstruction mammoplasty prostheses emphasis on the role of synovial metaplasia. Mod Pathol 1994; 7: 310–316.*

41. The correct response is E.

Breast implant rupture can be diagnosed by clinical examination with a suggestive history and examination findings. Imaging studies are also helpful but the only technique to reliably diagnose or exclude rupture is an MRI.

Reference:

1. *Middleton MS. Magnetic resonance evaluation of breast implants and soft tissue silicone. Top Magn Reson Imaging 1998; 9:92-137.*
2. *Mentor Corporation: Saline-filled breast implant surgery: making an informed decision [patient brochure]. Santa Barbara, Calif, 2004.*

42. The correct response is C.

Stretch marks are due to rupture of elastic fibres of the skin. These are not corrected by abdominoplasty. The rest of the options are correctable by abdominoplasty.

Reference:

Grazer FM. Body contouring. Introduction. Clin Plast Surg 1996; 23: 190–194.

43. The correct response is E.

All of the above mentioned complications can be seen in cases of post-liposuction contour undercorrection.

Reference:

1. *Illouz Y. Body Sculpturing by Lipoplasty. Edinburgh, Churchill Livingstone, 1989: 181.*
2. *Gingrass MK. Lipoplasty complications and their prevention. Clin Plast Surg 1999; 26: 341.*

44. The correct response is E.

All of the above complications can be seen in cases where overcorrection has been done.

Reference:

1. *Gingrass MK. Lipoplasty complications and their prevention. Clin Plast Surg 1999; 26: 341.*
2. *Illouz Y. Body Sculpturing by Lipoplasty. Edinburgh, Churchill Livingstone, 1989: 181.*

45. The correct response is D.

"French pastry" wrinkling in patients following liposuction is due to excess of skin in the adjoining area.

Reference:

1. *Gingrass MK. Lipoplasty complications and their prevention. Clin Plast Surg 1999; 26: 341.*
2. *Illouz Y. Body Sculpturing by Lipoplasty. Edinburgh, Churchill Livingstone, 1989: 181.*

46. The correct response is D.

Release of suspensory ligament is the one that will lead to penile lengthening. It is done close to the pubic bone. Release of the ligament frees more of the penis to be stretched by inferior displacement. The restricting bands of Scarpa's fascia also need to be incised.

Reference:

Alter GJ. Penile enhancement surgery. Techniques Urol 1998; 4: 70.

47. The correct response is A.

Girth increase in penis can be done by autologous fat injection into the dartos fascia. The fat is movable and gives a spongy texture to the penis. However less than 50% of the fat that is injected actually survives.

Reference:

1. *Ersek RA. Transplantation of purified autologous fat: a 3-year follow up is disappointing. Plast Reconstr Surg 1991; 87: 219.*
2. *Niechajev I, Sevcuk O. Long term results of fat transplantation: clinical and histologic studies. Plast Reconstr Surg 1994; 94: 496.*

48. The correct response is E.

The sternocleidomastoid muscle is not the muscle of choice for chest wall reconstruction.

Reference:

Mathes SJ, Nahai F. Reconstructive Surgery: Principles, Anatomy, and Technique. New York, Churchill Livingstone, 1997: 483.

49. The correct response is A.

The pectoralis major muscle on the thoraco-acromial pedicle can be moved medially from either side i.e. right and left to close midline sternotomy defects and is the muscle of choice for these defects.

Reference:

Hugo NE, et al. Single-stage management of 74 consecutive sternal wound complications with pectoralis major myocutaneous advancement flaps. Plast Reconstr Surg 1994; 93: 1433– 1441.

50. The correct response is B.

The gluteus maximus is the flap of choice for cover of meningomyelocoele defect. It has a reliable type III circulation with significant versatility. The gluteus offers moderate donor site morbidity without significantly impairing ambulation.

Reference:

McDonell DE, Seyfer AE. Myelomeningomyelocele. In Cohen M, ed: Mastery of Plastic Surgery. Boston, Little, Brown, 1994: 1240.

51. The correct response is A.

The sternum is a structure of mesodermal origin. It begins to form at six weeks. Its fusion is completed at ten weeks and ossification of the cartilage also begins at 5 to 6 months.

Reference:

1. *Williams PL. Gray's Anatomy. The anatomical basis of Medicine and Surgery, 38th ed. New York, Churchill Livingstone, 1995.*
2. *Netscher DT, Peterson R. Normal and abnormal development of the extremities and trunk. Clin Plast Surg 1990; 17: 13–21.*

52. The correct response is A.

The manubrium and the first and the second costal cartilages are not affected in Pectus excavatum. It affects the body of the sternum below the sternal angle of Louis and the cartilages attached to it. The most common presentation is a symmetric depression of the inferior two thirds to three fourths of the sternum with extension to the costal cartilages.

Reference:

1. *Fonkalsrud EW. Current management of pectus excavatum. World J Surg 2003; 27: 502–508.*
2. *Garcia VF, Seyfer AE, Graeber GM. Reconstruction of congenital chest-wall deformities. Surg Clin North Am 1989; 69: 1103–1118.*

53. The correct response is D.

The pectus excavatum deformity which is characterised by the depression of the sternum is due to the overgrowth of the costal cartilages which takes the growing lower part of the malleable sternum inwards. Sternum grows independently from mesodermal masses in the midline. The ribs beyond the costo-cartilaginous junction are normal.

Reference:

1. *Fonkalsrud EW. Current management of pectus excavatum. World J Surg 2003; 27: 502–508.*
2. *Garcia VF, Seyfer AE, Graeber GM. Reconstruction of congenital chest-wall deformities. Surg Clin North Am 1989; 69: 1103–1118.*

54. The correct response is D.

The pectus severity index (PSI) is a radiological index for calculating the severity of pectus excavatum. The index is calculated by dividing the internal transverse diameter of the thorax by the vertebral-sternal distance at the most depressed portion of the deformity. The normal value is approximately 2.5 cm. If the distance is 5 cm or less it is called severe. If the distance is between 5-7 cm, it is called moderate. If the distance is more than 7 cm, it is called mild deformity. The evaluation of these measurements is preferably done when the child is around six years of age by CT scan.

Reference:

Fonkalsrud EW, DeUgarte D, Choi E. Repair of pectus excavatum and carinatum deformities in 116 adults. Ann Surg 2002; 236: 304.

55. The correct response is B.

Mitral valve prolapse may be found incidentally on echocardiography in 15% of patients with pectus excavatum. No other listed anomaly exists. However the stroke volume during exercise is less. The pulmonary function tests are also reduced e. g. vital capacity, forced expiratory volume and gas diffusion studies show changes because of poor expansion of lungs.

Reference:

Shamberger RC. Cardiopulmonary effects of anterior chest wall deformities. Chest Surg Clin North Am 2000; 10: 245.

56. The correct response is D.

The operation should preferably be done around 16 years or later as operations done in childhood would interfere with the growth.

Reference:

Brodkin SH. Pectus excavatum : surgical indications and time of operation. Pediatrics 1953; 11: 582.

57. The correct response is E.

Pectus excavatum has been hypothesized to be caused by overgrowth of the costal cartilages. The Ravitch technique is based on resection of the costal cartilages.

Reference:

Davis JT, Weinstein S. Repair of the pectus deformity: results of the Ravitch approach in the current era. Ann Thorac Surg 2004; 78: 421-426.

58. The correct response is C.

Pectus carinatum is characterised by anterior displacement of the sternum due to abnormal growth of the cartilage at the costochondral junction. The entire sternum may protrude forward with the most severe protrusion over the middle and lower portions of the sternum.

Reference:

Mansour KA, Thourani VH, Odessey EA et al. Thirty-year experience with repair of pectus deformities in adults. Ann Thorac Surg 2003; 76: 391–395, discussion 395.

59. The correct response is E.

All of the above are features of cleft of the sternum. The overlying skin is intact, visible heart movements are present, haemangiomas are often associated with sternal clefts and primary repair in neonates gives good results.

Reference:

Domini M, Cupaioli M, Rossi F et al. Bifid sternum: neonatal surgical treatment. Ann Thorac Surg 2000; 69: 267–269.

60. The correct response is E.

Pentalogy of Cantrell is a rare congenital disorder and is characterised by all of the above. It is a rare condition having an incidence of 1 in 65,000 births. It is probably due to a mesodermal defect in the midline which is responsible for all the five defects.

Reference:

Cantrell JR, Haller JA, Ravitch MM. A syndrome of congenital defects involving the abdominal wall, sternum, diaphragm, pericardium and heart. Surg Gynecol Obstet 1958; 107: 602–614.

61. The correct response is E.

All of the above. The Poland's syndrome is mainly a disorder of the thoracic musculature i.e. pectoralis muscle, which is deficient or absent. Other muscles like latissimus dorsi, serratus anterior may also be deficient. The costal cartilage of the 3rd, 4th and 5th ribs may be absent. The breast may be hypoplastic. The digits of the hand on the same side may show brachydactyly and a syndactyly. The treatment consists of replacing the muscle by latissimus dorsi and use of an implant for breast reconstruction.

Reference:

Fokin AA, Robicsek F. Poland's syndrome revisited. Ann Thorac Surg 2002; 74: 2214.

62. The correct response is A.

Gynecomastia in males is mainly due to estrogen excess.

Reference:

Rohrich RJ, Ha RY, Kenkel JM, Adams WP Jr. Classification and management of gynecomastia: defining the role of ultrasound-assisted liposuction. Plast Reconstr Surg 2003; 111: 909–923, discussion 924–925.

63. The correct response is C.

The fourth intercostal nerve has been labelled as the most important nipple innervator. However, the lateral cutaneous branches of the third through fifth intercostal nerves and the anterior cutaneous branches all contribute to the nipple supply.

Reference:

1. *Courtiss EH, Goldwyn RM. Breast sensation before and after plastic surgery. Plast Reconstr Surg 1976; 58: 1.*
2. *Sarhadi NS, Dunn JS, Lee FD, Soutar DS. An anatomical study of the nerve supply of the breast, including the nipple and areola. Br J Plast Surg 1996; 49: 156.*

64. The correct response is E.

Breast amputation would be preferable for patients with gigantomastia as with massive resections relying on a pedicle is not practical. It becomes difficult to achieve a small enough pedicle to give adequate reduction volume while still keeping the nipple vascularised.

Reference:

1. *Thorek M. Plastic reconstruction of the breast and free transplantation of the nipple. J Int Coll Surg 1946; 9: 194.*
2. *Gradinger GP. Breast reduction with free nipple graft technique. In Spear SL, ed: Surgery of the breast: Principles and art. Philadelphia, Lippincott-Raven, 1998: 807-821.*
3. *Courtiss E, Goldwyn RM. Reduction mammaplasty by the inferior pedicle technique. Plast Reconstr Surg 1977; 59: 500.*

65. The correct response is E.

The periareolar techniques are not appropriate for resections exceeding 500 gm. The other options are viable

Reference:

1. *Robbins TH. A reduction mammoplasty with the areola-nipple based on an inferior dermal pedicle. Plast Reconstr Surg 1977; 59: 64.*
2. *Hester TR Jr, Bostwick J III, Miller L. Breast reduction utilizing the maximally vascularised central pedicle. Plast Reconstr Surg 1985; 76: 890.*

66. The correct response is B.

Vertical scar techniques are particularly suited for small resections and the vertical mammoplasty is preferable to other techniques as it gives the least amount of scar.

Reference:

1. *Robbins TH. A reduction mammoplasty with the areola-nipple based on an inferior dermal pedicle. Plast Reconstr Surg 1977; 59: 64.*
2. *Hester TR Jr, Bostwick J III, Miller L. Breast reduction utilizing the maximally vascularised central pedicle. Plast Reconstr Surg 1985; 76: 890.*

67. The correct response is C.

A 'Boxy' breast deformity is the result of inadequate excision of the inferomedial and inferolateral parts of the breast while closing the inframammary incision, which causes fullness in these areas seen particularly after inferior pedicle breast reduction. This fullness in the lower part gives the breast a 'boxy' appearance.

Reference:

Mandrekas AD, Zambacos GJ, Anastopoulos A, Hapsas DA. Reduction mammaplasty with the inferior pedicle technique: early and late complications in 371 patients. Br J Plast Surg 1996; 49: 442.

68. The correct response is A.

The superior pedicle technique is not suitable for densely glandular breast tissue as it is difficult to rotate on itself being stiff and unyielding.

Reference:

Robbins LB, Hoffman DK. The superior dermoglandular pedicle approach to breast reduction. Ann Plast Surg 1992; 29: 211.

69. The correct response is D.

The inferior pedicle technique is not suitable for large size reductions. The long pedicle which has a base width of 6–8 cm may not sustain blood supply to the nipple and areola complex, and may get constricted by the medial and lateral breast flaps when they are stitched to each other in the inframammary fold region.

Reference:

Ribeiro LA, Accorsi A, Buss A, Marcal-Pessoa M. Creation and evolution of 30 year of inferior pedicle in reduction mammaplasties: Plast Reconstr Surg 2002; 110: 960.

70. The correct response is B.

Hypoechogenecity is not a feature of benign tumours. It signifies malignancy.

Reference:

Flobbe K. The role of ultrasonography as an adjunct to mammography in the detection of breast cancer: a systemic review. Eur J Cancer 2002; 38: 1044–1050.

71. The correct response is C.

MRI has the highest diagnostic accuracy in breast imaging almost approaching to 100% accuracy.

Reference:

Boetes C. Breast tumours: comparative accuracy of MR imaging relative to mammography and US for demonstrating extent. Radiology 1995; 197: 33–42.

72. The correct response is B.

The 'step ladder sign' is a most useful sign detected by ultrasonography. It would detect rupture by showing a bulge outside the implant. MRI would show decreased intensity within the implant (Linguini sign) which represents the collapsed outer shell.

Reference:

O' Toole M, Caskey CI. Imaging spectrum of breast implant complications: mammography, ultrasound, and magnetic resonance imaging. Semin Ultrasound CTMR 2000; 21: 351–361.

73. The correct response is D.

In Halsted mastectomy, both the pectoralis major and minor muscles are removed. In modified radical mastectomy the pectoralis major is not removed.

Reference:

Fisher B et al. Twenty-five year follow-up of a randomized trial comparing radical mastectomy, and total mastectomy followed by irradiation. N Engl J Med 2002; 347: 567–574.

74. The correct response is E.

Postoperative radiation therapy is indicated in all the above four situations.

Reference:

Taghian AG et al. The role of radiation therapy for primary breast cancer. Surg Clin North Am 1999; 79: 1091–1109.

75. The correct response is D.

Lumpectomy incisions for the keyhole area of the breast are made in radial fashion so that adequate nipple projection can be preserved. For other areas, curvilinear incisions are preferred.

Reference:

Cox CE et al. Breast biopsy for benign disease. Operative Techniques Gen Surg 2000; 2: 86–95.

76. The correct response is C.

Areolar glands or Glands of Montgomery are *sebaceous glands* in the *areola* surrounding the *nipple*. The glands make oily secretions (lipoid fluid) to keep the areola and the nipple lubricated and protected. Volatile compounds in these secretions may also serve as an olfactory stimulus for newborn appetite.

The portions of the gland on skin's surface are called "Montgomery tubercles". The round bumps are found in the areola, and on the nipple itself.

Reference:

1. *Cohen BE et al. Nipple-areola reconstruction: satisfaction and clinical determinants. Plast Reconstr Surg 2002; 110: 141.*
2. *Moore KL, Persaud TVN. The Developing Human: Clinically Oriented Embryology, 6th ed. Philadephia, WB Saunders, 1998: 220.*

77. The correct response is C.

The skate flap has been described as a method for nipple reconstruction to match a contralateral nipple that is more than 5 mm in height. It can provide a reasonable projection even after long term follow up. The main disadvantage is the distortion of the areola.

Reference:

1. *Little JW. Nipple areola reconstruction. Adv Plast Surg 1987; 3: 43.*
2. *Cederna P et al. Modified technique for nipple reconstruction: a case series. Plast Reconstr Surg 2003; 112: 1274.*

78. The correct response is C.

A skin graft from the perineal region will give a good result in majority of the cases for areola reconstruction. Groin grafts can also be taken but will require tattoo.

Reference:

Cederna P et al. Modified technique for nipple reconstruction: a case series. Plast Reconstr Surg 2003; 112: 1274.

79. The correct response is E.

The pattern of circulation in latissimus dorsi is Type V according to the Mathes and Nahai classification. There is a single large vascular pedicle and multiple segmental pedicles. It has two large veins and a nerve.

Reference:

Mathes SJ, Nahai F. Latissimus dorsi flap. In Mathes SJ, Nahai F, eds: Reconstructive Surgery: Principles, Anatomy, and Technique, vol 1. New York, Churchill Livingstone, 1997; 565.

80. The correct response is D.

Lateral rotation is not performed by latissimus dorsi. It is an expendable muscle because function is preserved by the remaining synergistic shoulder girdle muscles. Transposition of this muscle is well tolerated.

Reference:

Fraulin FOG, Louie G, Zorrilla L et al. Functional evaluation of the shoulder following latissimus dorsi muscle transfer. Ann Plast Surg 1995; 35: 349.

81. The correct response is D.

A total autogenous latissimus dorsi flap can provide a maximum muscle volume of 300 –400 cc. However postoperative muscle atrophy may occur to the tune of 20–25% which should be taken into consideration.

Reference:

Fraulin FOG, Louie G, Zorrilla L et al. Functional evaluation of the shoulder following latissimus dorsi muscle transfer. Ann Plast Surg 1995; 35: 349.

82. The correct response is E.

All of the above complications may be associated with the TRAM flap. Patients need to be explained about all these possibilities.

Reference:

Watterson PA, Bostwick J, Hester TR et al. TRAM flap anatomy correlated with a 10-year clinical experience with 556 patients. Plast Reconstr Surg 1995; 95: 1185–1194.

83. The correct response is D.

The free TRAM flap offers otherwise several advantages over the pedicled TRAM flap. The flap can be conveniently folded into desired shape to achieve greater ptosis or projection of breast. Less muscle is required for free TRAM, hence there is reduced incidence of abdominal wall weakness and hernias.

The major disadvantage is the potential for complete flap loss.

Reference:

Feller AM, Biemer E, Steinau HU. The free TRAM flap: In Strauch B, Vasconez L, Hall-Findlay EJ, eds: Grabb's Encyclopedia of Flaps. Boston, Little, Brown, 1990: 1326.

84. The correct response is A.

Neumann, C.G. in 1957 was the one who first reported tissue expansion for coverage of a subauricular defect.

Reference:

Neumann CG. The expansion of an area of skin by progressive distension of a subcutaneous balloon. Plast Reconstr Surg 1957; 19: 124.

85. The correct response is E.

All of the above are likely following the use of breast implants.

Reference:

1. *Gutowski KA, Mesna GT, Cunningham BL. Saline-filled breast implants: a Plastic Surgery Educational Foundation Multicenter Outcome Study. Plast Reconstr Surg 1997; 100: 1019.*
2. *Zones JS. The political and social context of silicone breast implant use in the United States. J Long Term Eff Med Implants 1992; 1: 225.*

86. The correct response is B.

The first inflation following insertion of the expander implant is preferably done after two weeks. However it can be modified if the patient is receiving chemotherapy.

Reference:

Camilleri IG, Malata CM, Stavrianos S, McLean NR. A review of 120 Becker permanent tissue expander in reconstruction of the breast. Br J Plast Surg 1996; 49: 346.

87. The correct response is D.

Muscle coverage of the expander is desirable to avoid potential implant exposure if skin envelope necrosis or wound separation occurs. Pectoralis major muscle and additional cover by rectus muscle flap may be required. The lateral fascial fibres of the external oblique may also be included with the segmental rectus flap.

Reference:

Gui GP, Tan SM, Faliakou EC et al. Immediate breast reconstruction using biodimensional anatomical permanent expander implants : a perspective analysis of outcome and patient satisfaction. Plast Reconst Surg 2003; 111: 125.

88. The correct response is E.

In gunjan – kriya, the rectus abdominis does not play an active role.

Reference:

Gothe N, Pontifex MB, Hillman C et al. The acute effects of yoga on executive function. J Phys Act Health 2012; 9.

89. The correct response is E.

All of the above are the indications for a bipedicled TRAM flap.

Reference:

Suominen S, Asko-Ssljavaara S, von Smitten K. Sequelae in the abdominal wall after pedicled or free TRAM flap surgery. Ann Plast Surg 1996; 36: 629.

90. The correct response is B.

The paraumbilical area and the area underlying the region of the belt is mainly supplied by the deep inferior epigastric vessels.

Reference:

Taylor GI, Palmer JH. The vascular territories (angiosomes) of the body: experimental study and clinical applications. Br J Plast Surg 1987; 40: 113.

91. The correct response is B.

All of these sources supply the lower abdomen, but the primary supply is from the deep inferior epigastic system. The superior epigastric artery is the main source of blood supply to the TRAM flap.

Reference:

1. *Taylor GI, Palmer JH. The vascular territories (angiosomes) of the body: experimental study and clinical applications. Br J Plast Surg 1987; 40: 113.*
2. *Moon HK, Taylor GI. The vascular anatomy of rectus abdominis musculocutaneous flaps based on the deep superior epigastric system. Plast Reconstr Surg 1988; 82: 815.*

92. The correct response is A.

The vascular zones of the unipedicled TRAM flap have been divided into four areas. These zones have functional significance from a vascular standpoint. Zone I directly overlies the muscle and hence is the most reliable.

Reference:

1. *Watterson PA, Bostwick J 3rd , Hester TR Jr et al. TRAM flap anatomy correlated with a 10-year clinical experience with 556 patients. Plast Reconstr Surg 1995; 95: 1185.*
2. *Taylor GI, Palmer JH. The vascular territories (angiosomes) of the body: experimental study and clinical applications. Br J Plast Surg 1987; 40: 113.*

93. The correct response is D.

The vascular zones of the unipedicled TRAM flap have been divided into four areas. These zones have functional significance from a vascular standpoint. Zone I directly overlies the muscle and hence is the most reliable. Zone IV is farthest away from the muscle hence is discarded even in free flaps.

Reference:

1. *Watterson PA, Bostwick J 3rd , Hester TR Jr et al. TRAM flap anatomy correlated with a 10-year clinical experience with 556 patients. Plast Reconstr Surg 1995; 95: 1185.*
2. *Taylor GI, Palmer JH. The vascular territories (angiosomes) of the body: experimental study and clinical applications. Br J Plast Surg 1987; 40: 113.*

94. The correct response is A.

The inframammary crease is better preserved in ipsilateral pedicled TRAM flap owing to a direct 180 degree transposition over the costal margin. In contralateral TRAM flaps, the flap pedicle has to be tunnelled and passed over the costal margin and hence it disturbs the definition of the inframammary fold and presents as a bulge when the patients sits up.

Reference:

1. *Clugston PA, Gingrass MK, Azurin D et al. Ipsilateral pedicled TRAM flaps: the safer alternative? Plast Reconstr Surg 2000; 105: 77.*
2. *Watterson PA, Bostwick J 3rd , Hester TR Jr, et al. TRAM flap anatomy correlated with a 10-year clinical experience with 556 patients. Plast Reconstr Surg 1995; 95: 1185.*

95. The correct response is E.

All of the above are the advantages with the ipsilateral pedicled TRAM flap over the contralateral pedicled TRAM flap.

Reference:

1. *Clugston PA, Gingrass MK, Azurin D et al. Ipsilateral pedicled TRAM flaps: the safer alternative? Plast Reconstr Surg 2000; 105: 77.*
2. *Watterson PA, Bostwick J 3rd , Hester TR Jr, et al. TRAM flap anatomy correlated with a 10-year clinical experience with 556 patients. Plast Reconstr Surg 1995; 95: 1185.*

96. The correct response is B.

For immediate breast reconstruction with free flaps, the thoracodorsal vessels are the obvious choice as they are already exposed during the axillary dissection that accompanies mastectomy and hence are readily available.

Reference:

Grotting JC. Immediate breast reconstruction using the free TRAM flap. Clin Plast Surg 1994; 21: 207–221.

97. The correct response is A.

For delayed breast reconstruction with free flaps, the internal mammary vessels are the obvious choice for the recipient vessels. They are closer to the breast, are usually not scarred from previous surgery and the artery is less likely to be affected by vascular spasm. Moreover the arms of the patient can be placed at her side which is convenient to the surgeon.

Reference:

1. *Dupin CL, Allen RJ, Glass CA et al. The internal mammary artery and vein as a recipient site for free-flap breast reconstruction: a report of 110 consecutive cases. Plast Reconstr Surg 1996; 98: 685–689.*
2. *Ninkovic M, Anderl H, Hefel HA et al. Internal mammary vessels: a reliable recipient system for free flaps in breast reconstruction. Br J Plast Surg 1995; 48: 533–539.*

98. The correct response is D.

For delayed breast reconstruction with free flaps, the internal mammary vessels are the obvious choice for the recipient vessels. They are closer to the breast, are usually not scarred from previous surgery and the artery is less likely to be affected by vascular spasm. Moreover the arms of the patient can be placed at her side which is convenient to the surgeon.

The biggest disadvantage with these vessels is the inconsistent size of the vein, especially on the left side the vein may be small. The artery however is adequate for anastomosis.

Reference:

1. *Dupin CL, Allen RJ, Glass CA et al. The internal mammary artery and vein as a recipient site for free-flap breast reconstruction: a report of 110 consecutive cases. Plast Reconstr Surg 1996; 98: 685–689.*
2. *Ninkovic M, Anderl H, Hefel HA et al. Internal mammary vessels: a reliable recipient system for free flaps in breast reconstruction. Br J Plast Surg 1995; 48: 533–539.*

99. The correct response is B.

Removal of the third costal cartilage may be helpful for access to the internal mammary vessels for microvascular anastomosis for free TRAM breast reconstruction in situations where the size of the vein is small. It is better to remove the third costal cartilage, as it gives a better exposure. The artery at this level is single. It may divide below the level of the fourth costal cartilage.

Reference:

Dupin CL, Allen RJ, Glass CA, Bunch R. The internal mammary artery and vein as a recipient site for free-flap breast reconstruction: a report of 110 consecutive cases. Plast Reconstr Surg 1996; 98: 685–689.

100. The correct response is A.

Latissimus is 'Latin' in origin and means wide. Since this muscle is wide and is present on the back of the body, it is called Latissimus dorsi.

Reference:

Maxwell GP. Iginio Tansini and the origin of the latissimius dorsi musculocutaneous flap. Plast Reconstr Surg 1980; 65: 686.

101. The correct response is C.

The shape of the latissimus dorsi is triangular. Its size is 10" to 14" (25 cm to 35 cm). The tendon of its insertion is 3 cm long and thickness is 1-2 cm.

Reference:

Mathes SJ, Nahai F. Latissimus dorsi flap. In Mathes SJ, Nahai F, eds: Reconstructive Surgery: Principles, Anatomy, and Technique, vol 1. New York, Churchill Livingstone, 1997: 565.

102. The correct response is B.

A posterolateral thoracotomy with prior division of the muscle constitutes an absolute contraindication for the use of latissimus dorsi muscle. The rest options do not negate use of this muscle.

Reference:

Mathes SJ, Nahai F. Latissimus dorsi flap. In Mathes SJ, Nahai F, eds: Reconstructive Surgery: Principles, Anatomy, and Technique, vol 1. New York, Churchill Livingstone, 1997: 565.

103. The correct response is D.

The latissimus dorsi muscle does not help in lateral rotation.

Reference:

Mathes SJ, Nahai F. Latissimus dorsi flap. In Mathes SJ, Nahai F, eds: Reconstructive Surgery: Principles, Anatomy, and Technique, vol 1. New York, Churchill Livingstone, 1997: 565.

104. The correct response is C.

The piriformis is located under a line which is at a perpendicular drawn from the midpoint of the line joining the posterior superior iliac spine and the coccyx. The superior gluteal artery lies along the proximal third of this line after coming out from the greater sciatic notch. The surface landmark is helpful in locating the superior gluteal artery and superior gluteal artery flap.

Reference:

Allen RJ. The superior gluteal artery perforator flap. Clin Plast Surg 1998; 25: 293–302.

105. The correct response is D.

The primary advantage of a musculocutaneous perforator flap is to spare the muscle. The other options are not suitable.

Reference:

Angrigriani C, Grilli D, Siebert J. Latissimus dorsi musculocutaneous flap without muscle. Plast Reconstr Surg 1995; 96: 1608–1614.

106. The correct response is A.

The TRAM flap is the flap of choice for reconstruction of the breast. It serves the dual purpose of reconstructing the breast and reducing the abdominal fat. It constitutes a natural autogenous reconstruction of the breast with good long term results.

Reference:

Chang DW, Wang B, Robb GL et al. Effect of obesity on flap and donor site complications in free transverse rectus abdominis myocutaneous flap breast reconstruction. Plast Reconstr Surg 2000; 105: 1640–1648.

107. The correct response is E.

Rubens flap for breast reconstruction is based on the deep circumflex iliac vessels. It is the iliac crest flap but without the bone.

Reference:

1. *Hartrampf CR. Noel RT, Drozan L et al. Ruben's fat pad for breast reconstruction: a peri-iliac soft tissue free flap. Plast Reconstr Surg 1994; 93: 402–407.*
2. *Taylor GI, Townsend P, Corlett RT. The superiority of the deep circumflex iliac vessels as the supply for free groin flaps. Plast Reconstr Surg 1979; 64: 745–749.*

108. The correct response is A.

Unequal reduction and nipple asymmetry are the two most undesirable complications observed by the patient following reduction mammaplasty.

Reference:

Hoffman S. Reduction mammaplasty: a medicolegal hazard? Aesthetic Plast Surg 1987; 11:113.

109. The correct response is C.

The average distance of the nipple from the manubrial notch is 22 cm. The distance between the right and left nipple is also about the same.

Reference:

Elashy N. Correction of abnormally high nipples after reduction mammaplasty. Aesthetic Plast Surg 1990; 14: 21.

110. The correct response is D.

All of the above are true for repositing the high nipple.

Reference:

Elashy N. Correction of abnormally high nipples after reduction mammaplasty. Aesthetic Plast Surg 1990; 14: 21.

111. The correct response is D.

All of the above procedures may be necessary for correcting nipple convergence and divergence following reduction mammaplasty.

Reference:

Salema R, Aboudib JH, de Castro CC. Convergent nipple-areola complexes corrected by inferior curved pedicle technique. Ann Plast Surg 1987; 19: 555.

112. The correct response is E.

All of the above complications may be associated with reduction mammaplasties.

Reference:

Sarwer DB, Bartlett SP, Bucky L, et al. Bigger is not always better: body image dissatisfaction in breast reduction and breast augmentation patients. Plast Reconstr Surg 1998; 101: 1956.

113. The correct response is A.

Infection is by far the commonest complication seen in breast implants followed by implant loss which may be in some cases more common than infection.

Reference:

Gui GP, Tan SM, Faliakou EC et al. Immediate breast reconstruction using biodimensional anatomical permanent expander implants: a perspective analysis of outcome and patient satisfaction. Plast Reconstr Surg 2003; 111: 125.

114. The correct response is A.

Open capsulotomy for contracture (41% of 83 reoperations), deflation (38.6%), infection (7.2%) have been the reasons for reoperation following breast implant surgery.

Reference:

Gui GP, Tan SM, Faliakou EC et al. Immediate breast reconstruction using biodimensional anatomical permanent expander implants: a perspective analysis of outcome and patient satisfaction. Plast Reconstr Surg 2003; 111: 125.

115. The correct response is E.

All of the above may require re-exploration.

Reference:

Gabriel SE, Woods JE, O'Fallon WM et al. Complications leading to surgery after breast reconstruction. N Eng J Med 1997; 336: 677–682.

116. The correct response is D.

According to the Baker's classification for capsular contracture, in grade 1 capsular contracture the breast is soft and the implant is palpable. In Grade 2 the breast is firm and the implant is palpable. In Grade 3, the breast is moderately firm and the implant is still detectable. In Grade 4, the breast is woody hard and the implant cannot be felt. Patient complains of discomfort all the time. The result is unacceptable aesthetically and otherwise.

Reference:

Spear SL, Baker JL Jr. Classification of capsular contracture after prosthetic breast reconstruction. Plast Reconstr Surg 1995; 96: 1119–1123.

117. The correct response is E.

Primary direct and layered closure techniques are useful in closing an abdominal wall defect that is no larger than 7 cm. The other options are useful for closing bigger defects.

Reference:

Gottlieb JR, Engrav LH, Walkinshaw MD et al. Upper abdominal wall defects: immediate or staged reconstruction? Plast Reconstr Surg 1990; 86: 281.

118. The correct response is B.

The arcuate line is an anatomic demarcation denoting the change in structural composition of the rectus sheath, especially the posterior layer. It is located midway between umbilicus and pubic symphysis.

Reference:

Cunningham SC, Rosson GD, Lee RH et al. Localization of the arcuate line from surface anatomic landmarks: a cadaveric study. Ann Plast Surg 2004; 53(2): 129–31.

119. The correct response is B.

Linea semilunaris denotes the lateral margin of the rectus. It begins inferiorly at the pubic tubercle and ends superiorly at the ninth costal cartilage. Linea semicircularis is the arcuate line. The arcuate line is an anatomic demarcation denoting the change in structural composition of the rectus sheath, especially the posterior layer. It is located midway between umbilicus and pubic symphysis. Linea alba is a fibrous structure in the midline of the abdomen in humans. Linea terminalis or innominate line consists of the pectineal line, arcuate line and the sacral promontory. Linea aspera is found on the posterior aspect of the femur.

Reference:

1. *Koontz AR. Hernia in the linea semilunaris. Ann Surg 1952; 135(6): 875–878.*
2. *Cunningham SC, Rosson GD, Lee RH et al. Localization of the arcuate line from surface anatomic landmarks: a cadaveric study. Ann Plast Surg 2004; 53(2): 129–31.*

120. The correct response is A.

The arcuate line is an anatomic demarcation denoting the change in structural composition of the rectus sheath, especially the posterior layer. It is located midway between umbilicus and pubic symphysis. It is also known as linea semicircularis.

Linea semilunaris denotes the lateral margin of the rectus. It begins inferiorly at the pubic tubercle and ends superiorly at the ninth costal cartilage. Linea alba is a fibrous structure in the midline of the abdomen in humans. Linea terminalis or innominate line consists of the pectineal line, arcuate line and the sacral promontory. Linea aspera is found on the posterior aspect of the femur.

Reference:

1. *Koontz AR. Hernia in the linea semilunaris. Ann Surg 1952; 135(6): 875-878.*
2. *Cunningham SC, Rosson GD, Lee RH et al. Localization of the arcuate line from surface anatomic landmarks: a cadaveric study. Ann Plast Surg 2004; 53(2): 129–31.*

121. The correct response is D.

The Buck's fascia carries important neurovascular structures to the glans penis including the deep dorsal vein and arteries, the deep dorsal nerves of penis, the circumflex arteries and veins and the penile lymphatics.

Reference:

Quartey JKM. Microcirculation of penile and scrotal skin. Atlas Urol Clin North Am 1997; 5: 1–9.

122. The correct response is B.

The chordee in hypospadias is present superficial to the tunica albuginea. The corpora cavernosa are covered by a white fibrous capsule, the tunica albuginea which has a superficial and a deep layer. The deep layer has circular fibres which surround the corpora circumferentially. These fibres of the adjoining sides join to form a septum between the two corpora. The superficial layer surrounds both the corpora and the corpus spongiosum present on the ventral surface, renamed as Buck's fascia. The fibres in this layer are longitudinal and are rather loosely arranged. In patients with hypospadias, there is fibrosis on the ventral side of the corpora, which would not allow the corpora to get engorged. The chordee also accentuates the curvature on erection of the organ, it is therefore essential that during correction of chordee, all the fibrous tissue must be excised carefully from the ventral surface of the organ. Per-operatively, the organ can be distended with an injection of normal saline. A straight organ would confirm that the chordee has been completely excised.

Reference:

Devine CJ Jr, Blackley SK, Horton CE et al. The surgical treatment of chordee without hypospadias in men. J Urol 1991; 146: 325.

123. The correct response is E.

All of the above features can be seen in exstrophy of the bladder, though cloacal exstrophy is observed in 10% of the cases. The pubic bones are splayed. There is divarication of the recti and associated hernias.

Reference:

Muecke EC. Exstrophy, epispadias and other anomalies of the bladder. In Harrison JH, Gittes RF, Perlmutter AD et al. eds. Campbell's Urology, vol 2, 4th ed. Philadelphia, WB Saunders, 1979; 1443–1468.

124. The correct response is D.

All of the above are true for chordee without hypospadias. The prepucial skin is present all around. The condition is due to shortage in the length of the urethra. The condition could be associated with torsion of the phallus.

Reference:

Devine CJ Jr, Blackley SK, Horton CE, Gilbert DA. The surgical treatment of chordee without hypospadias in men. J Urol 1991;146: 325.

125. The correct response is B.

The Chang technique of phallic reconstruction is based on the radial artery forearm flap. A tube within a tube is formed and is used for reconstruction. The neourethra is formed from a skin island on the most ulnar aspect of the radial forearm flap and the larger radial paddle is wrapped around the neourethra to form the outer phallic shaft.

Reference:

Chang TS, Hwang YW. Forearm flap in one-stage reconstruction of the penis. Plast Reconstr Surg 1984; 74: 251.

126. The correct response is B.

Biemer modified the Chang's design by centering the neourethra skin island over the radial artery. This places the flap on the most hairy portion of the forearm which is undesirable.

Reference:

1. *Biemer E. Penile reconstruction by the radial arm flap. Clin Plast Surg 1988;15: 425.*
2. *Chang TS, Hwang YW. Forearm flap in one-stage reconstruction of the penis. Plast Reconstr Surg 1984; 74: 251.*

127. The correct response is B.

The Peyronie's disease is characterized by scarring and nodularity within the tunica albuginea. It is present on the dorsal surface and produces dorsal curvature. These plaques impede tunica expansion during erection and result in a number of deformities.

Reference:

Jordan GH. Treatment of Peyronie disease with plaque incision or excision and dermal graft. In Ehrlich RM, Alter GJ, eds: Reconstructive and Plastic Surgery of the External Genitalia. Philadelphia, WB Saunders, 1999: chapter 82.

128. The correct response is D.

Fournier's gangrene is a necrotising fasciitis that is caused by gram positive organisms, gram negative organisms and anaerobes. The anaerobic organism responsible for the Fournier's gangrene is Clostridium perfringens. The affected area is red, swollen and tender and gangrene settles quickly. Treatment consists of intravenous hydration and antibiotic therapy in preparation for surgical debridement and skin grafting later on.

Reference:

Eke N. Fournier's gangrene : a review of 1726 cases. Br J Plast Surg 2000; 87: 718.

129. The correct response is D.

Balanitis xerotica obliterans which produces a white patch on the glans is caused by a spirochete. The organism responsible for the condition is Borrelia burgdorferi. It responds to tetracyclines, penicillins and fluroquinolones.

Reference:

Akporiaye LE, Jordan GH, Devine CJ Jr. Balanitis xerotica obliterans (BXO). AUA Update Series Lesson 21, vol 16. Houston, Texas, Americal Urological Association. Office of Education. 1997.

130. The correct response is C.

The glans and prepucial skin are not involved in lymphedema.

Reference:

Hinman F. Anatomy of the external genitalia. In Ehrlich RM, Alter GJ, eds: Reconstructive and Plastic Surgery of the External Genitalia. Philadelphia, WB Saunders, 1999: 7–12.

131. The correct response is D.

Cryptorchidism is an associated condition with hypospadias found in approximately 9.3% cases. The rest are bona fide features of hypospadias including ventral curvature of penis, abnormally placed urinary opening and hooded prepuce.

Reference:

1. *Hinman F. Anatomy of the external genitalia. In Ehrlich RM, Alter GJ, eds: Reconstructive and Plastic Surgery of the External Genitalia. Philadelphia, WB Saunders, 1999: 7–12.*
2. *Khuri FJ, Hardy BE, Churchill BM. Urologic anomalies associated with hypospadias. Urol Clin North Am 1981; 8: 565–571.*

132. The correct response is C.

Chordee results from shortening of the ventral tissues of the penis, specifically it is due to fibrosis of the corpus spongiosum that would otherwise have developed into a normal urethra.

Reference:

Hogson NB. History of hypopadias repair. In Ehrlich RM, Alter GJ, eds: Reconstructive and Plastic Surgery of the External Genitalia. Philadelphia, WB Saunders, 1999: 13-17.

133. The correct response is C.

The chordee is present from 3–9 O' Clock position, on the ventral side and hence must be dissected out completely for proper straightening of the organ.

Reference:

Rowsell AR, Morgan BDG. Hypopadias and embryogenesis of the penile urethra. Br J Plast Surg 1987; 40: 201–206.

134. The correct response is B.

The flip-flap procedure is suitable for cases of distal penile hypospadias. A 'U' shaped tube is raised from the tissues proximal to the meatus to make the urethra.

Reference:

Johnson D, Coleman DJ. The selective use of a single-stage and a two-stage technique for hypopadias correction in 157 consecutive cases with the aim of normal appearance and function. Br J Plast Surg 1998; 51: 195–201.

135. The correct response is C.

The inner prepucial flap is raised on the fascial pedicle. It is tubed and is used for reconstructing the missing urethra. This flap can be used either as a complete tube or as an onlay flap or sutured to the urethral plate.

Reference:

Devine CJ, Horton CE, Gilbert DA, Winslow BH. Hypopadias. In Mustarde JC, Jackson IT, eds: Plastic Surgery in Infancy and Childhood, 3rd ed. Edinburgh, Churchill Livingstone, 1988: 493–570.

136. The correct response is A.

The MAGPI (meatoplasty and glanuloplasty) procedure is suitable for coronal hypospadias. It was reported in 1981 by Duckett.

Reference:

Duckett JW. MAGPI (meatoplasty and glanuloplasty): a procedure for subcoronal hypospadias. Urol Clin North Am 1981; 8: 513.

137. The correct response is A.

The split thickness skin graft wrapped around a conformer is a time honoured and successful modality for the treatment of vaginal agenesis. A full thickness graft may not be available in sufficient quantity. Flaps are quite bulky for vaginal reconstruction for agenesis and use of segments of gastrointestinal tract are complicated by necrosis, infection, abscess formation in addition to giving undesirable secretions in the vagina.

Reference:

1. *Lesavoy MA. Vaginal reconstruction. Urol Clin North Am 1985; 12: 369–379.*
2. *McIndoe A. The application of cavity grafting. Surgery 1937; 1: 535.*

138. The correct response is C.

The gracilis flap is the most commonly used flap after pelvic exenteration for vaginal reconstruction. This flap is able to fill the large vaginal defect after exenteration and provides adequate vaginal length and bulk to fill the empty space. Skin grafts are not suitable for this indication and segments of intestine give undesirable mucus secretions, hence are not preferred.

Reference:

1. *Wee JT, Joseph VT. A new technique for vaginal reconstruction using neurovascular pudendal thigh flaps: a preliminary report. Plast Reconstr Surg 1989; 83: 701-709.*
2. *Soper JT, Berchuck A, Creasman WT et al. Pelvic exenteration: factors associated with major surgical morbidity. Gynaecol Oncol 1989; 35: 93–98.*

139. The correct response is A.

Excision of malignant tumours is responsible for majority of acquired vaginal defects. Advanced colorectal carcinomas frequently involve the posterior vaginal wall, carcinoma of the bladder may extend into the anterior vaginal wall or primary sarcomas of the vaginal wall may all lead to extensive vaginal defects after resection.

Reference:

Martello JY, Vasconez HC. Vulvar and vaginal reconstruction after surgical treatment for gynaecologic cancer [review]. Clin Plast Surg 1995; 22: 129–140.

140. The correct response is A.

The modified Singapore (vulvoperineal or pudendal thigh) fasciocutaneous flap is ideal for defects of the anterior vaginal wall where it provides a highly vascularised and reliable thin flap that conforms well to the surface of the vaginal wall. The flap is based on the posterior labial arteries and is innervated by the posterior labial branches of the pudendal nerve as well as perineal branches of the posterior cutaneous nerve of the thigh.

Reference:

1. *Woods JE, Alter G, Meland B et al. Experience with vaginal reconstruction utilising the modified Singapore flap. Plast Reconstr Surg 1992; 90: 270–274.*
2. *Wee JT, Joseph VT. A new technique for vaginal reconstruction using neurovascular pudendal thigh flaps: a preliminary report. Plast Reconstr Surg 1989; 83: 701–709.*

141. The correct response is C.

Bilateral gracilis muscle flaps are an excellent choice for management of circumferential defects of the vagina and the introitus. The advantage is that they can provide a suitably large skin island and the accompanying soft tissue can fill up the pelvis.

Reference:

Soper JT, Rodriguez G, Berchuck A, Clarke-Pearson DL. Long and short gracilis myocutaneous flap for vulvovaginal reconstruction after radical pelvic surgery: comparison of flap-specific complications. Gynecol Oncol 1995; 56: 271–275.

142. The correct response is D.

The end capillary pressure is 30-32 mm of Hg. The blood flow in the capillaries would stop if the external pressure is prolonged and is more than this end capillary pressure. It would produce ischemia and the overlying skin will show ischemic changes and necrosis in due course of time.

Reference:

Reuler JB, Cooney TG. The pressure sore: pathophysiology and principles of management. Ann Intern Med 1981; 94: 661.

143. The correct response is A.

In the supine position, the occiput, sacrum and heels are subjected to maximum pressure of about 40-60 mm of Hg. However the incidence of pressure sores is not high because of the presence of sensations which are intact and allow the patient to turn his head to one side or the other.

Reference:

Lindan O, Greenway RM, Piazza JM. Pressure distribution on the surface of the human body: 1. Evaluation in lying and sitting positions using a "bed of springs and nails". Arch Phys Med Rehabil 1965; 46: 378.

144. The correct response is B.

The most common site of occurrence of pressure sore is the ischial tuberosity followed by the trochanter. The ischial tuberosity weathers the greatest pressure with a person in the sitting position.

Reference:

Dansereau JG, Conway H. Closure of decubiti in paraplegics. Plast Reconstr Surg 1964; 33: 474

145. The correct response is D.

The answer is Grade 4. In Grade 1, only the skin is involved. In Grade 2 skin and fat are involved. In Grade 3 the underlying muscles are involved. In Grade 4, the underlying bone gets involved. The classification was proposed by Darrell Shea, an orthopaedic surgeon, in 1975.

Reference:

Shea JD. Pressure sores: classification and management. Clin Orthop 1975; 112: 89.

146. The correct response is A.

The gluteus maximus flap is the mainstay of treatment for sacral sores through its many variants. It is locally available and has a reliable blood supply.

Reference:

1. *Evans JM, Andrews KL, Chutka DS et al. Pressure sores: prevention and management. Mayo Clin Proc 1995; 70: 789.*
2. *Parry SW, Mathes SJ. Bilateral gluteus maximus myocutaneous advancement flaps: sacral coverage for ambulatory patients. Ann Plast Surg 1982; 8: 443.*

147. The correct response is A.

The inferior gluteus maximus island flap provides a large skin island to cover any size of ischial sore while still allowing primary closure of the donor site. This flap also places the maximum amount of muscle and soft tissue bulk into the debrided sore.

The inferior gluteal thigh flap also is an option though it lacks muscle.

Reference:

Wingate GB, Friendland JA. Repair of ischial pressure ulcers with gracilis myocutaneous island flaps. Plast Reconstr Surg 1978; 62: 245.

148. The correct response is B.

The trochanteric pressure sore typically presents with minimal skin involvement and extensive bursa formation. The mobile nature of the trochanter predisposes these ulcerations to extensive undermining. These must be completely removed before the defect is covered.

Reference:

1. *Evans JM, Andrews KL, Chutka DS et al. Pressure sores: prevention and management. Mayo Clin Proc 1995; 70: 789.*
2. *Paletta CD, Freedman B, Shehadi SJ. The VY tensor fasciae latae musculocutaneous flap. Plast Reconstr Surg 1989; 83: 852.*
3. *Hauben DJ, Smith AR, Sonneveld GJ, Van der Meulen JC. The use of the vastus lateralis musculocutaneous flap for the repair of trochanteric pressure sores. Ann Plast Surg 1983; 10: 359.*

149. The correct response is B.

The tensor fascia lata flap is considered the workhorse for the management of trochanteric pressure sores. The V-Y modification provides more proximal and better vascularised tissue than in the classic design. It also provides more muscle to fill up the debrided sore.

Reference:

1. *Evans JM, Andrews KL, Chutka DS et al. Pressure sores: prevention and management. Mayo Clin Proc 1995; 70: 789.*
2. *Paletta CD, Freedman B, Shehadi SJ. The VY tensor fasciae latae musculocutaneous flap. Plast Reconstr Surg 1989; 83: 852.*
3. *Siddiqui A, Wiedrich T, Lewis VI Jr. Tensor fascia lata V-Y retroposition myocutaneous flap: clinical experience. Ann Plast Surg 1993; 31: 313.*

150. The correct response is C.

The anterior compartment of the leg is somewhat unique in having blood supply only from the anterior tibial artery. The rest of the compartments have blood supply from two angiosomes.

Reference:

Taylor GI, Pan WR. Angiosomes of the leg: anatomic study and clinical implications. Plast Reconstr Surg 1998; 102: 599–616, discussion 617–618.

151. The correct response is E.

Sartorius does not pass under the ligament. It forms the lateral boundary of the femoral triangle. The four muscles lie in the floor of the triangle. Iliacus and psoas lie in the lateral part, while the pectineus and adductor longus are in the medial part.

Reference:

Standring S. Gray's Anatomy. The Anatomical Basis of Clinical Practice. 39th ed. Elsevier, Churchill Livingstone, 2005: 1421.

152. The correct response is E.

All of the above are the criteria for the diagnosis of chronic osteomyelitis as described by May et al.

Reference:

May J, Gallico G, Lukash F. Microvascular transfer of free tissue for closure of bone wounds of the distal lower extremity. N Engl J Med 1982; 306: 253–257.

153. The correct response is D.

Leg trauma coupled with inadequate soft tissue coverage commonly would lead to superficial type of osteomyelitis. The Cierny classification of adult osteomyelitis has four categories. Medullary osteomyelitis is an endosteal disease, localised osteomyelitis is a full thickness defect in the cortical bone. Diffuse osteomyelitis is a full thickness cortical breach of the bone.

Reference:

Cierny G. Chronic osteomyelitis: results of treatment. Instr Course Lect 1990; 39: 495–508.

6

154. The correct response is B.

Diabetic microangiopathy has been linked to changes in the blood viscosity which have origin in blood cells. The red blood cell has been implicated in this scenario as it has been described to have a stiffened membrane which makes it difficult to pass through capillary leading to increase in the blood viscosity.

Reference:

1. *Schmid-Schonbein H, Wells R, Goldstone J. Influence of deformability of human red cells upon viscosity. Circ Res 1969; 25: 131.*
2. *McMillan DE, Utterback NG, LaPuma J. Reduced erythrocyte deformability in diabetes. Diabetes 1982; 31 (suppl): 64.*

155. The correct response is D.

All of the above are classical signs of lower extremity lymphedema. Peau d'orange is the result of fibrosis and Stemmer sign is inability to tent the skin over the toes.

Reference:

Rockson SG, Miller LT, Senie R et al. American Cancer Society lymphedema workshop. Workgroup III: diagnosis and management of lymphedema. Cancer 1998; 83 (suppl 12): 2882–2885.

TRUNK AND LOWER EXTREMITY

156. The correct response is A.

Chronic ulcers above the medial malleolus in the lower third of the leg are most probably due to venous insufficiency. The location of the ulcer above the malleolus is typically seen in cases of varicose veins due to the incompetency of the perforator.

Reference:

Falanga V, Eaglstein WH. The trap hypothesis of venous ulceration. Lancet 1993; 341: 1006–1008.

157. The correct response is D.

The patient has sustained a degloving injury of the skin with areas of frank and impending ischemia. The best policy of management at this time would be to perform surgical debridement of the wound followed by immediate skin grafting. Wait and watch approach would not be suitable as the raw areas if not covered by skin will become infected in due course of time. Microvascular flap is not feasible because the skin requirement is quite massive in this patient which cannot be taken care by any free flap. Also the skin graft would be sufficient for this patient as the bed would easily take a graft due to the good muscle cover in this area.

Reference:

Mathes SJ, Nahai F. Latissimus dorsi flap. In Mathes SJ, Nahai F, eds: Reconstructive Surgery: Principles, Anatomy, and Technique, vol 1. New York, Churchill Livingstone, 1997; 565.

7

UPPER LIMB

QUESTIONS

1. **Sushruta, the great Indian surgeon described nose reconstruction from cheek using the principles of patterning of the defect, preparation of the wound bed and use of local and distant flaps during which of the following period?**
   A. 1st century AD
   B. 5th century AD
   C. 6th century AD
   D. 6th century BC

2. **Nobel Prize in plastic surgery was given to Joe Murray for his work on which one of the following?**
   A. Skin transplantation
   B. Tendon transplantation
   C. Nerve transplantation
   D. Kidney transplantation
   E. Liver transplantation

3. **Which one of the following surgeons received the Knighthood honour from King George V for his exceptional service to the society?**
   A. Sir Harold Gillies
   B. R. Acland
   C. P. Kilner
   D. J. C. Mustarde
   E. I. T.Jackson

4. **Hand anatomist Kaplan's cardinal line which is helpful in localising the nerves of the hand is a line extending between which one of the following?**
   A. Apex of first web space to pisiform bone
   B. Apex of second web space to pisiform bone
   C. Apex of first web space to hook of hamate
   D. Apex of second web space to hook of hamate
   E. Ulnar border of the middle finger to the pisiform bone

5. **The intersection of the Kaplan's cardinal line and the longitudinal line from the ulnar side of the middle finger corresponds to which one of the following ?**
   A. Palmar digital nerve of first web space
   B. Palmar digital nerve of second web space
   C. Palmar digital nerve of third web space
   D. Motor branch of the median nerve
   E. Palmar digital nerve of fourth web space

6. **The intersection of the Kaplan's cardinal line and the longitudinal line from the ulnar side of the ring finger corresponds to which one of the following ?**
   A. Palmar digital nerve of first web space
   B. Palmar digital nerve of second web space
   C. Palmar digital nerve of third web space
   D. Motor branch of the ulnar nerve
   E. Palmar digital nerve of fourth web space

7. **The thumb performs many different actions that are responsible for the fine movements and coordination of the hand. How many muscles control the movement of the thumb?**
   A. Seven
   B. Eight
   C. Nine
   D. Ten
   E. Eleven

8. Digital malrotations can result from malunited fractures or due to flattening of the carpal arch. Which one of the following is the skeletal landmark for assessing finger malrotations?

A. Hook of hamate
B. Tubercle of scaphoid
C. Pisiform
D. Radial styloid
E. Ulnar styloid

9. The pulleys serve to restrain the long digital flexors. Which one of the following is the largest annular pulley?

A. A1 pulley
B. A2 pulley
C. A3 pulley
D. A4 pulley

10. Which one of the following ligament in the finger is placed on the volar side of the neurovascular bundle?

A. Grayson ligament
B. Cleland ligament
C. Pretendinous band
D. Superficial transverse ligament

11. The wrist joint has a complex multiarticulated architecture and hence fractures need to be reduced accurately to preserve maximal function. Which of the following correctly describes the articular surface of the radius?

A. It is placed at right angle to the axis of the radius
B. It is obliquely placed
C. It has a large depression for articulating with the scaphoid
D. It articulates with a total of three carpal bones
E. All of the above

12. The anatomic centre of the hand lies over which of the following?

A. Metacarpophalangeal joint of the middle finger
B. Head of the third metacarpal
C. Base of the proximal phalanx of the middle finger
D. Middle of the third metacarpal
E. Base of the third metacarpal

13. Which one of the following is the only motor which can pull the central third metacarpal into extension besides also pulling the pronated hand into extension?

A. Extensor carpi radialis longus
B. Extensor carpi radialis brevis
C. Extensor digitorum longus
D. Extensor pollicis longus
E. Extensor indicis

14. The articular surface of the radius has a slope of 22 degrees in the radial to ulnar direction and 12 degrees in the dorsal to palmar direction. To recreate this slope in fractures of the lower end of radius, the wrist is immobilized in which one of the following position?

A. Neutral position
B. Flexion and radial deviation
C. Flexion and ulnar deviation
D. In extension

15. How many carpal bones of the proximal row articulate with the radius and ulna?

A. One
B. Two
C. Three
D. Four

16. A hand which has been stabilised in a position where the collateral ligaments are lax frequently ends up with stiffness. The collateral ligaments of the metacarpophalangeal joints are lax in which one of the following position?

A. Flexion
B. Extension
C. Adduction
D. Abduction

17. The supinator muscle takes origin from which of the following areas?

A. Lateral epicondyle of the humerus
B. Radial collateral ligament of elbow joint
C. Annular ligament of superior radioulnar joint
D. Supinator crest of ulna
E. All of the above

18. There are five annular and three cruciate pulleys in the finger. The cruciate pulley is not present between which one of the following annular pulleys?

A. A1 and A2
B. A2 and A3
C. A3 and A4
D. A4 and A5

19. Name the tendon which can get damaged in Zone 1 injuries of the hand?

A. Flexor digitorum sublimis
B. Flexor digitorum profundus
C. Lumbrical tendon
D. Interossei tendon

20 **The carpal tunnel ligament overlies which one of the following zones of flexor tendon injuries of the hand?**

A. Zone I
B. Zone II
C. Zone III
D. Zone IV

21. **Zone II injuries are the ones which are difficult to manage. Which one of the following fibrous flexor pulleys lies in this zone?**

A. A5 pulley
B. A4 pulley
C. A3 pulley
D. A2 pulley
E. A1 pulley

22. **Name the thenar muscle which has two heads of origin?**

A Abductor pollicis brevis
B. Flexor pollicis brevis
C. Opponens pollicis
D. Adductor pollicis

23. **Name the hypothenar muscle which is rudimentary?**

A. Abductor digiti minimi
B. Flexor digiti minimi
C. Opponens digiti minimi
D. Palmaris brevis

24. **Which one of the following is not the primary function and characteristic of the lumbricals?**

A. Connect the flexor digitorum sublimis with the extensor tendon mechanism
B. Connect the flexor digitorum profundus tendons with the extensor tendon mechanism
C. Index and middle finger lumbricals are supplied by the median nerve
D. Help in flexion of the metacarpophalangeal joints and extension of the interphalangeal joints
E. All of the above

25. **The dorsal interossei perform which of the following function?**

A. Act as abductors of the fingers
B. Act as flexors of the metacarpophalangeal joints
C. Act as extensors of the interphalangeal joints
D. All of the above

26. **The palmar interossei perform which of the following function?**

A. Act as adductors of the fingers
B. Act as flexors of the metacarpophalangeal joints
C. Act as extensors of the interphalangeal joints
D. All of the above

27. **The side to side movements of the middle finger are controlled by which one of the following?**

A. Lumbrical
B. Interossei
C. Flexor digitorum longus
D. Flexor digitorus profundus
E. Flexor digitorum superficialis

28. **The four dorsal interossei are bipennate muscles and are abductors. Which one of the following finger has two abductors?**

A. Thumb
B. Index
C. Middle
D. Ring
E. Little finger

29. **The four palmar interossei are adductors of the fingers. Which one of the following finger is without a palmar interossei?**

A. Thumb
B. Index finger
C. Middle finger
D. Ring finger
E. Little finger

30. **Which one of the following finger does not have attachment of palmar interossei?**

A. Thumb
B. Index finger
C. Middle finger
D. Ring finger
E. Little finger

31. **The four dorsal interossei have double origin, a ventral and a dorsal component and have double nerve supply and double insertion into bone and aponeurosis. Which one of the inter-ossei has a bony attachment only and has no contribution to the aponeurosis?**

A. First dorsal interossei
B. Second dorsal interossei
C. Third dorsal interossei
D. Fourth dorsal interossei

32. Which one of the following muscle has a mobile origin and demonstrates an increase in the gap between origin and insertion on inter-phalangeal flexion?

A. Lumbrical
B. Interossei
C. Flexor digitorum longus
D. Flexor digitorus profundus
E. Flexor digitorum superficialis

33. Contracture of the intrinsic muscles of the hand may be caused by which of the following?

A. Burns
B. Trauma
C. Inflammation
D. Degenerative joint changes
E. All of the above

34. Which one of the following test best assesses the vascular status of the hand?

A. Moberg test
B. Ninhydrin test
C. Allen's test
D. Froment sign
E. Jeanne sign

35. The synovial sheath of which one of the following flexor tendon extends into the forearm through the carpal tunnel?

A. Thumb
B. Index finger
C. Middle finger
D. Ring finger
E. All of the above

36. Flexion of the interphalangeal joint of the thumb while holding a piece of paperbetween the thumb and the finger indicates the paralysis of which one of the following nerve?

A. Median
B. Ulnar
C. Radial
D. Posterior interosseous nerve

37. Suppurative tenosynovitis is a deep space infection of the fiberosseous tunnel of the flexor tendon sheath. Which of the following are the cardinal features of suppurative tenosynovitis?

A. Semiflexed posture of finger
B. Tenderness over course of tendon
C. Pain with passive motion
D. Fusiform swelling
E. All of the above

38. Finkelstein test is used for testing which one of the following tendon of the dorsal compartment?

A. First
B. Second
C. Third
D. Fourth

39. The piano key sign is observed in which one of the following condition?

A. Malunited fracture radial styloid
B. Malunited fracture metacarpal
C. Unstable radio scaphoid joint
D. Unstable distal radioulnar joint
E. Unstable triquetrum

40. The interscalene block is better suited for surgery of which one of the following region?

A. Hand surgery
B. Forearm surgery
C. Shoulder surgery
D. Neck surgery
E. Ulnar fingers and ulnar border of the hand

41. Periods of uninterrupted ischaemia may be followed by undesirable induration of the limb. This post-tourniquet syndrome is characterized by which of the following?

A. Fall in tissue pH
B. Resolves spontaneously
C. Increase in capillary permeability
D. Prolongation of clotting time
E. All of the above

42. Internal fixation of bones of the hand can be done by the following methods. Whichof these would be most appropriate for treatment of fractures of the first metacarpal?

A. Interosseous wire
B. Kirschner wire
C. Interosseous screw (Lag screw)
D. Plate and screws

43. Which one of the following is likely to result in a hook nail deformity?

A. Deep laceration of more than 50% of the nail and its bed
B. Crush injury to the nail bed and bone
C. Paronychia
D. Eponychia
E. Bony avulsion of more than 50% of nail and its bed

44. If the flexor digitorum profundus insertion is damaged and the tendon is allowed to retract, then it may lead to development of which of the following?

A. Lumbrical plus finger
B. Lumbrical minus finger
C. Quadriga effect
D. All of the above

45. Which one of the following would produce a 'Quadriga effect' in fingertip injuries?

A. Stitching of the extensor tendon to the cut end of the bone
B. Stitching of the flexor tendon to the cut end of the bone
C. Stitching of the flexor and extensor tendons over the cut end of the bone
D. All of the above

46. Kutler V-Y flaps used in finger tip recon-structions are based on which one of the following surface of the digit?

A. On the volar surface
B. On the lateral surface
C. On the dorsal surface
D. On the scar tissue
E. Are based according to the geometry of the defect

47. Moberg flap is a volar advancement flap and is best used for reconstruction of which one of the following?

A. Thumb reconstruction
B. Finger reconstruction
C. Toe reconstruction
D. Dorsal hand reconstruction
E. Web space reconstruction

48. A volar V-Y advancement flap is not suitable for which one of the following?

A. Transverse amputation of finger tip
B. Volar oblique amputation of finger tip
C. Dorsal oblique amputation of finger tip
D. Finger tip amputation with exposed bone
E. Finger tip amputation with skin defect less than 1 cm

49. Which one of the following defines the lunula correctly?

A. It is the visible part of the nail which is 2/3 of its length.
B. It is the part of the nail covered by skin, which is 1/3 of its length.
C. It is the white convex portion of the nail at its junction with the skin
D. It is the portion of the nail which requires cutting or trimming.

50. Which one of the following deformity is not related to scarring in the nail bed?

A. Ridging
B. Split nail
C. Onycholysis
D. Anonychia
E. Hooked nail

51. Ganglions on the dorsum of the fingers are located in relationship with which one of the following?

A. Metacarpophalangeal joint
B. Proximal interphalangeal joint
C. Distal interphalangeal joint
D. Midpoint of proximal phalanx between the extensor creases of metacarpophalangeal and proximal interphalangeal joint
E. Midpoint of middle phalanx between the extensor creases of proximal and distal interphalangeal joint

52. The fingers are perfused by two palmar digital arteries interconnected by three constant transverse palmar arches. These arches are present in relation with which one of the following?

A. A1 and A3 pulley
B. C1 and C3 cruciate ligament
C. A2 and A4 pulley
D. A1 and A4 pulley
E. Run at the level of the middle part of the respective phalanges

53. The digital arteries of the fingers on radial and ulnar side are not similar. The ulnar digital artery is dominant over the radial digital artery in which one of the following?

A. Ring finger
B. Small finger
C. Ring and small finger
D. Index finger and middle finger
E. Ring finger and thumb

54. Which one of the following function is not performed by the thumb?

A. Opposition
B. Pencil grip
C. Power grip
D. Key pinch
E. Hook grip

55. Which one of the following tendon is not transferred during the great toe transfer?

A. Extensor hallucis longus
B. Flexor hallucis longus
C. Extensor hallucis brevis
D. Flexor hallucis brevis

56. The term 'no-man's land in management of flexor tendon injuries was coined by which one of the following stalwarts of hand surgery?

A. Bunnell S
B. Kilner P
C. Kleinert HE
D. Kessler I

57. The pulleys help to keep the flexor tendons closely apposed to the volar surface of the phalanges enabling maximal flexion of the joints with minimal tendon excursion. The number of pulleys in the thumb are which one of the following?

A. Three
B. Five
C. Six
D. Seven
E. One

58. Five annular and three cruciate pulleys hold the flexor tendon in contact with the bones and joints. Which one of the following annular pulley forms the longest tunnel?

A. A1
B. A2
C. A3
D. A4
E. A5

59. Which one of the following pulley is likely to get damaged in fractures of the shaft of the proximal phalanx?

A. A1
B. A2
C. A3
D. A4
E. A5

60. Which one of the following pulley is likely to get damaged in fractures of the shaft of the middle phalanx?

A. A1
B. A2
C. A3
D. A4
E. A5

61. The most commonly used core suture technique is which one of the following?

A. Modified Bunnell
B. Modified Kessler
C. Tajima
D. Tsuge
E. Bevel technique

62. A two stage flexor tendon grafting is indicated in which of the following situation?

A. When the flexor tendon sheath is collapsed and scarred
B. When the flexor tendon sheath will not admit a probe (3mm-5mm)
C. When the A2 and A4 pulleys are damaged (due to multiple fractures)
D. Presence of residual joint stiffness
E. All of the above

63. The dorsal retinaculum lies over the extensor tendons in which one of the following zone?

A. Zone I
B. Zone III
C. Zone V
D. Zone VII
E. Zone IX

64. Which one of the following muscle does not take origin from the distal forearm?

A. Abductor pollicis longus
B. Extensor pollicis longus
C. Extensor pollicis brevis
D. Extensor indicis
E. Extensor digiti minimi

65. The extensor tendons pass through six dorsal compartments having different configuration of the quota of tendons within them. Which one of the following compartment has five tendons in it?

A. First compartment
B. Second compartment
C. Third compartment
D. Fourth compartment
E. Fifth compartment

66. Which of the following criteria will help you to diagnose the presence of the intrinsic muscle contracture in hand deformity?

A. The range of PIP joint flexion would be less if the MCP joint is kept in extension
B. The range of PIP joint flexion would be more if the MCP joint is kept in a flexed position
C. The PIP joint and MCP joint will both be in a position of contracture
D. All of the above

67. The functional integrity of the radial, median and ulnar nerves can be assessed by testing the movement of which of the following digit?

A. Thumb
B. Index Finger
C. Middle Finger
D. Ring Finger
E. Little Finger

68. Fist fights if untreated may result in loss of knuckle prominence due to which one of the following?

A. Fracture neck of second metacarpal
B. Fracture neck of third metacarpal
C. Fracture neck of fourth and fifth metacarpal
D. Fracture neck of first and second metacarpal

69. Stack splint is useful in the primary management of which one of the following finger deformity?

A. Swan neck deformity
B. Mallet finger deformity
C. Boutonniere deformity
D. Claw hand deformity
E. Syndactyly

70. Fracture of the thumb metacarpal base into three fragments is called which one of the following?

A. Bennett's fracture
B. Reverse Bennett's fracture
C. Rolando's fracture
D. Colle's fracture
E. Lisfranc fracture

71. Chip fractures of the base of the phalanges are caused by the ligaments and the tendons attached to them. Which of the following would produce chipping of the base of the proximal phalanx of the thumb on the radial side?

A. Extensor pollicis brevis
B. Flexor pollicis brevis
C. Abductor pollicis brevis
D. First dorsal interossei
E. All of the above

72. In a case of sprained wrist, tenderness over the snuff box is due to injury to which one of the following structure?

A. Scaphoid
B. Scapholunate ligament
C. Triangular fibrocartilage
D. Lunotriquetral ligament
E. Capitotrapezoid ligament

73. Which one of the following fracture is commonly seen in baseball players?

A. Radial styloid
B. Neck of second metacarpal
C. Hook of hamate
D. Neck of scaphoid
E. Neck of proximal phalanx of thumb

74. Tinel's sign is progressive in which one of the following injuries?

A. Neurapraxia
B. Axonotmesis
C. Neurotmesis
D. Neurotmesis with anatomic continuity
E. Neurotmesis without anatomic continuity

75. Which one of the following nerve can provide a 40 cm long nerve graft?

A. Medial cutaneous nerve of the arm and forearm
B. Lateral cutaneous nerve of the arm
C. Radial sensory nerve
D. Saphenous nerve
E. Entire medial antebrachial cutaneous nerve

76. Which one of the following is not a feature of brachial plexus injury?

A. Sensory loss over neck and shoulder region, arm and forearm region
B. Motor loss over paravertebral, parascapular, arm, forearm and hand region
C. Root pains
D. Horner's syndrome
E. Hoarseness of voice

77. Radiologically, the brachial plexus injuries are best evaluated by which one of the following modality?

A. Ultrasonography
B. Plain X-Ray
C. CT scan
D. MRI scan
E. Myelography

78. Which one of the following is not a characteristic of Horner's syndrome?

A. Enophthalmos
B. Exophthalmos
C. Miosis
D. Ptosis
E. Anhydrosis

79. Erb's palsy is due to involvement of which one of the following roots?

A. C_5 and C_6
B. C_6 and C_7
C. C_7 and C_8
D. C_8 and T_1
E. C_6, C_7 and C_8

80. Which one of the following attitudes is not a feature of Erb's palsy?

A. Shoulder (Adduction)
B. Arm (Internal rotation)
C. Elbow (Extended)
D. Forearm (Pronated)
E. Wrist (Extended)

81. A child with brachial plexus injury following childbirth is referred at the age of 1 year. Which one of the following investigations will help you to decide the plan of management?

A. X-ray
B. Muscle power testing
C. CT scan
D. MRI
E. NCV studies

82. Which one of the following muscles can be used for restoring abduction at the shoulder?

A. Trapezius
B. Supraspinatus
C. Levator Scapulae
D. All of the above

83. Which of the following muscle can be used for correcting the internal rotation of the arm in brachial plexus palsy?

A. Subscapularis
B. Pectoralis major
C. Latissimus dorsi
D. All of the above

84. Which one of the following tendon is likely to give a good result for correcting the wrist drop?

A. Flexor carpi radialis
B. Flexor carpi ulnaris
C. Flexor digitorum sublimis
D. Palmaris longus
E. Flexor digitorum profundus

85. Which one of the following structure usually escapes damage in ring avulsion injuries of the ring finger?

A. Skin
B. Subcutaneous tissue
C. Digital vessels
D. Digital nerves
E. Flexor tendon

86. A burnt hand should be kept elevated and dressed in which of the following position?

A. Wrist, MCPJ and IPJ in flexion (Coin picking position)
B. Wrist, MCPJ and IPJ in extension (Hammer throw position)
C. Wrist, IPJ in extension and MCPJ in flexion (Cricket ball holding position)
D. Any of the above

87. The compartment pressure of the limb is best tested by which one of the following?

A. Central venous pressure monitoring
B. Blood pressure monitoring
C. Doppler study
D. A needle in the compartment attached to a central venous pressure monitor

88. The mechanism of tissue injury in electrical burns is due to which of the following?

A. Thermal trauma
B. Passage of current through the skin, subcutaneous tissue, nerves, vessels and muscles which offer least resistance.
C. High levels of chemicals that develop inside the tissues namely thromboxane
D. All of the above

89. Which one of the following procedure would you choose in order to perform a five flap plasty for correcting a linear contracture?

A. Z- plasty
B. Two consecutive Z-plasties
C. Triple Z-plasty
D. Double Z-plasty with a V-Y plasty
E. Double Z-plasty with a Y-V plasty

90. Which one of the following joints after release of contracture should be placed in abduction?

A. Axilla
B. Elbow
C. Wrist
D. Proximal interphalangeal joint
E. Metacarpophalangeal joint

91. In a case having burn contractures of the axilla, elbow and wrist, which one should be released first?

A. Axilla
B. Elbow
C. Wrist
D. Elbow and wrist
E. All should be released simultaneously

92. Patients of frost bite should be treated initially by which of the following?

A. Slow thawing
B. Rapid rewarming by hot water at 40°C
C. Topical agents
D. Manual debridement of the blisters
E. All of the above

93. Acids and alkalies cause necrosis of the tissues. Which one of the following is the mechanism of action of acids?

A. Coagulation necrosis
B. Liquefaction necrosis
C. Thermal necrosis
D. Cell lysis
E. Thrombosis

94. Which one of the following is the specific antidote for hydrofluoric acid burns?

A. Dilute sodium hyposulfite
B. Milk
C. Carbolic acid sticks
D. Calcium gluconate gel
E. Kerosene

95. Which one of the following antidote would you choose for mustard gas burns?

A. Soap solution
B. Mineral oil
C. Kerosene
D. Magnesium Hydroxide
E. Calcium gluconate gel

96. Contracture is defined as a condition where there is which one of the following?

A. Limitation of active and passive range of motion across a joint
B. Fibrosis of skin or underlying musculoskeletal structures across a joint
C. Approximation of the two opposing surfaces across a joint due to fibrosis with loss of full range of active and passive motion
D. Contracture of tendon with loss of active movements
E. Contracture of joint with loss of passive movements

97. Six dorsal compartments on the extensor aspect of the hand allow twelve tendons to pass through. How many tendons are there in the fourth compartment?

A. One
B. Two
C. Three
D. Four
E. Five

98. Dupuytrens contracture is due to contracture of which one of the following?

A. Skin
B. Palmar fascia
C. Flexor tendon
D. Joint capsule
E. Volar plate

99. Which one of the following tendon may have an additional muscle belly under the extensor retinaculum?

A. Extensor digitorum longus
B. Extensor pollicis longus
C. Extensor indicis
D. Extensor digiti minimi
E. Extensor carpi radialis longus

100. Tenosynovitis of tendons lying in which one of the extensor compartments is termed as de Quervain's disease?

A. First compartment
B. Second compartment
C. Third compartment
D. Fourth compartment
E. Fifth compartment

101. A thumb drop in an elderly patient without history of trauma is due to rupture of which one of the following tendons?

A. Abductor pollicis longus
B. Extensor pollicis brevis
C. Extensor pollicis longus
D. Flexor digitorum longus
E. Flexor pollicis longus

102. In a case of trigger finger which one of the following pulleys needs to be released?

A. A1
B. A2
C. A3
D. A4
E. A5

103. Swanson's arthroplasty is indicated in the osteoarthritis of which one of the following joints?
A. Distal interphalangeal joint
B. Proximal interphalangeal joint
C. Metacarpophalangeal joint
D. Radioulnar joint
E. Carpometacarpal joint

104. Dupuytren's disease affects the palm of the hands. It commonly involves which one of the following finger?
A. Thumb
B. Index
C. Middle
D. Ring finger

105. Which one of the following method will give good long term results in the treatment of Dupuytren's disease?
A. Steroid injection
B. Enzymatic fasciotomy
C. Fasciotomy
D. Fasciectomy

106. The open method of fasciectomy in Dupuytren's disease was devised by which one of the following?
A. Dupuytren
B. McCash
C. McFarlane
D. Swanson
E. Lister

107. The Kanavel's cardinal signs of tenosynovitis of the flexor tendons of the index, middle and the ring finger include which of the following?
A. Symmetrical swelling of the finger
B. Finger in flexion
C. Pain and tenderness on movements
D. Site of maximal tenderness in the distal palm
E. All of the above

108. The structure likely to be damaged in the drainage of the thenar space infection is which one of the following?
A. Flexor pollicis longus
B. Flexor carpi radialis
C. Superficial and deep branches of the median nerve
D. Radial artery

109. Boutonniere deformity of the proximal interphalangeal joint is due to which one of the following?
A. Septic arthritis
B. Damage to the central slip of the extensor expansion
C. Damage to the collateral ligaments
D. Damage to the oblique retinacular ligament
E. Damage to the Grayson's ligament

110. Which one of the following condition in a patient with supracondylar fracture requires immediate attention?
A. Dislocated condyle
B. Damage to median nerve
C. Damage to ulnar nerve
D. Damage to brachial artery
E. Damage to radial nerve

111. An arterial aneurysm is defined when there is permanent localized arterial dilatation amounting to which one of the following?
A. More than 10% of the normal diameter
B. More than 30% of the normal diameter
C. More than 50% of the normal diameter
D. More than 70% of the normal diameter
E. Involving atleast two layers of the normal arterial wall

112. Reflex sympathetic dystrophy is characterized by which of the following?
A. Disproportionate pain
B. Loss of function
C. Vasomotor abnormalities
D. Skeletal muscle atrophy
E. All of the above

113. Vasomotor changes in reflex sympathetic dystrophy include which of the following?
A. Colour change (redness, cyanosis)
B. Temperature change (warmth, cool)
C. Sudomotor (sweating, dryness)
D. Oedema
E. All of the above

114. Dermatological changes in reflex sympathetic dystrophy include which of the following?
A. Thin / glossy atrophied skin
B. Loss of hairs
C. Hyperpigmentation
D. Ridging of nails
E. All of the above

115. Which one of the following musculoskeletal change is not observed in reflex sympathetic dystrophy?
A. Ankylosis of joints
B. Osteoporosis
C. Flexion / extension contractures
D. Sub-chondral cyst formations
E. Onion peel appearance

116. Which one of the following is not a feature of Volkmann's ischemic contracture (VIC)?

A. Paresthesia

B. Pain

C. Pulselessness

D. Pallor

E. Paralysis

117. Which one of the following is not a feature of Horner's syndrome?

A. Enophthalmos

B. Miosis

C. Mydriasis

D. Ptosis

E. Loss of sweating on one side of face

118. Which one of the following is the commonest site of aneurysm formation in the ulnar artery?

A. Proximal to Guyon canal

B. Distal to Guyon canal

C. Inside Guyon canal

D. In the forearm

119. How many nerve compression syndromes have been described in the upper extremity?

A. Five

B. Six

C. Seven

D. Eight

120. How many nerve compression syndromes have been described in the lower extremity?

A. Five

B. Six

C. Seven

D. Eight

E. Nine

121. If a patient has normal sensation in the little finger and motor weakness of the ulnar nerve, what is he likely to be suffering from?

A. Ulnar nerve compression at the elbow

B. A lipoma / tumour in the palm

C. Ulnar nerve compression in the Guyon's canal

D. Vascular injury

122. A patient has a weakness of pinch and weakness of grip strength. He is most likely to be suffering from which one of the following?

A. Ulnar nerve compression in Guyon's canal

B. Ulnar nerve compression at the elbow

C. Ulnar nerve compression at the hand

D. Ulnar nerve compression at the midforearm

123. Cubital tunnel syndrome is compression of which one of the following nerve?

A. Median

B. Ulnar

C. Radial

D. Posterior interosseous

E. Antebrachial nerve

124. The operative requirements for a peripheral nerve decompression include which of the following?

A. Tourniquet for blood less field

B. Bipolar cautery

C. Loupe magnification

D. Nerve stimulation

E. All of the above

125. Clinical presentation of weakness of the flexor pollicis longus is indicative of compression of median nerve by which one of the following?

A. High origin of pronator teres

B. Lacertus fibrosus

C. Fibrous arch related to flexor digitorum sublimis origin

D. Deep head of pronator teres

E. Ligament of Struthers

126. The complications of the ulnar nerve decompression at the elbow consist of which of the following?

A. Recurrence of compression

B. Numbness behind the scar

C. Trigger point anterior to the scar

D. Referred pain to the little finger

E. All of the above

127. A patient having loss of extension of the thumb and fingers at the metacarpophalangeal joints but having ability to extend the wrist is suffering from radial nerve compression at which one of the following site?

A. Above the elbow joint

B. At the level of the elbow joint

C. Below the level of the elbow joint

D. At the level of the arcade

128. A patient having numbness, aching and burning pain in the lateral thigh from hip to the knee is likely to be having which one of the following?

A. Disc prolapse at L2
B. Disc prolapse at L3
C. Bursitis
D. Lateral femoral cutaneous nerve entrapment

129. The tarsal tunnel syndrome should be suspected in a patient who complains of numbness and tingling in the toes. Its treatment consists of which one of the following?

A. Release of flexor retinaculum of the tarsal tunnel
B. Release of medial plantar tunnel
C. Release of lateral plantar tunnel
D. Release of four separate medial ankle tunnels in addition to the tarsal tunnel
E. All of the above

130. Morton neuroma is due to chronic compression of the plantar digital nerve between the intermetatarsal ligament and the metatarsal heads. It is commonly present in which one of the following locations?

A. Between first and second metatarsal
B. Between second and third metatarsal
C. Between third and fourth metatarsal
D. Between fourth and fifth metatarsal

131. Excision of a ganglion on the dorsum of the wrist may lead to the development of a neuroma in relation to which one of the following nerve?

A. Median B. Ulnar
C. Radial D. Posterior interosseous

132. A small pedunculated erythematous lesion of the finger tip which bleeds on touch could be which one of the following?

A. Glomus tumor
B. Pyogenic granuloma
C. Capillary haemangioma
D. Melanoma
E. Wart

133. Silk threads for the treatment of lymphoedema were used by which one of the following?

A. Silver and Puckett
B. Handley
C. Goldsmith
D. O'Brien and co-workers

134. Buried dermal flap procedure for treatment of lymphoedema was popularized by which one of the following?

A. Homans and Miller B. Thompson
C. Kondolean D. Charles

135. A 22-year-old male is brought to the emergency department 2 hours after he sustained this injury as a result of agriculture thresher machine accident. He sustained total tran-section of the thumb skeleton with a deep laceration extending across the palm of the hand. Which is the most appropriate order of management of the injured hand?

A. Artery, vein, tendon, nerve and bone
B. Artery, nerve, tendon and bone
C. Bone, tendons, nerves, arteries and veins
D. Tendons, bone, nerve, arteries and veins
E. Nerve, artery, veins, tendon and bone

136. A 25-year-old male presents to the outpatient department after having sustained a sharp cut injury over the proximal phalanx of fifth digit of right hand while using a kitchen knife 3 years back. He is now unable to flex his little finger and has difficulty in doing his daily job and also it is socially unacceptable for him to have his little finger in an extended position all the time. Physical examination revealed an injury to the long flexors of the digit. No joint stiffness was observed. At the time of surgery the finger and adjoining palm was accessed and the repair of the tendon was performed by a tendon graft attached to the base of the distal phalanx (shown in picture) for reconstruction of flexor digitorum profundus function. Which of the following would serve as a suitable source of graft in this situation?

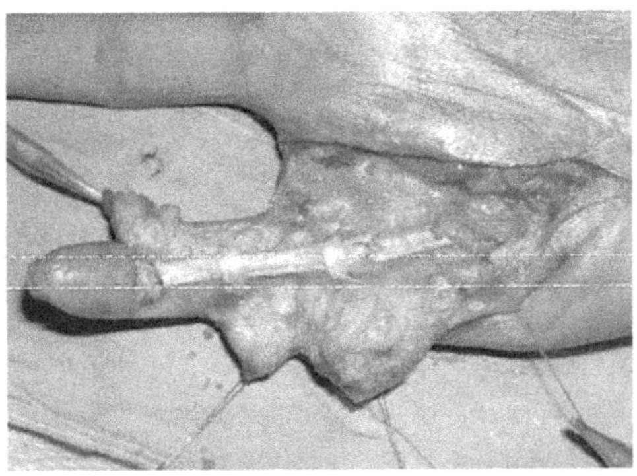

A. Fascia lata B. Temporalis fascia
C. Palmaris longus D. Flexor pollicis longus
E. Lumbrical

137. **A 20-year-old male presents to the outpatient department after having sustained a sharp cut injury over the extensor aspect of the distal phalanx one year back. He has inability to straighten the tip of the finger which has been gradually developing after this injury. The distal interphalangeal joint is in good range of motion. Which type of splint would be required for this patient?**

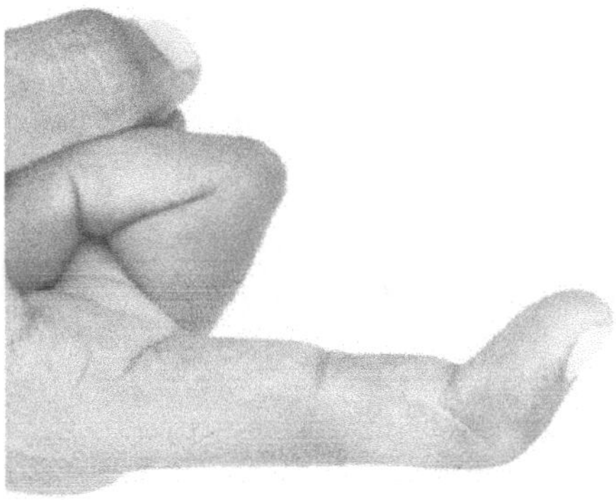

A. Finger outrigger splint
B. Buddy splint
C. Stack splint
D. Dorsal finger splint
E. Palmar finger splint

138. **A 10-year-old female presents with congenital deformity of both hands with absence of fingers (picture shown). What is the likely diagnosis for this patient?**

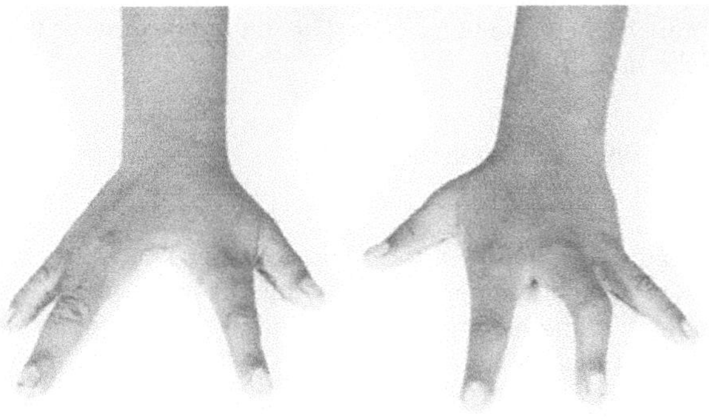

A. Radial club hand
B. Ulnar club hand
C. Cleft hand
D. Ectrodactyly
E. Symbrachydactyly

139. **Thumb polydactyly is rare and the morphologic appearance of all patients is different. The guiding principle in treatment is to construct one good thumb. The commonest variety originates at the MP joint and is which one of the following?**

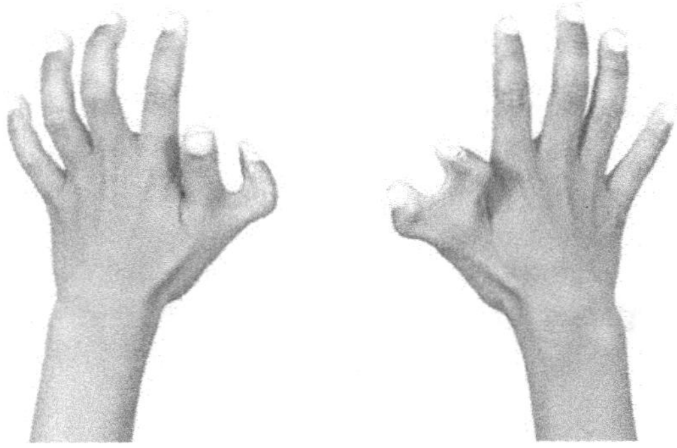

A. Type I Iowa classification
B. Type II Iowa classification
C. Type III Iowa classification
D. Type IV Iowa classification
E. Type V Iowa classification

ANSWERS, EXPLANATIONS AND REFERENCES

1. **The correct response is D.**

The period during which Sushruta performed these operations was around 600 BC.

He performed nose reconstruction using pedicled flap from the face by using the leaf of a tree as a template placed on the cheek skin. After the cheek skin was cut off he divided the pedicle in second stage to complete the reconstruction. He also described the principles of patterning of the defect, preparation of the wound bed and use of local and distant flaps.

Reference:

Puthumana PP. Through the mists of time: Sushrutha, an enigma revisited. Indian J Plast Surg 2009; 42: 226-230.

2. **The correct response is D.**

The Nobel Prize was given to Dr. J Murray for having done the first kidney transplant in 1954.

Reference:

Haeger K. The world of modern surgery. In Haeger K, ed: The Illustrated History of Surgery. Goteborg, Sweden, AB Nordbok, 1988.

3. **The correct response is A.**

It was Sir Harold Delf Gillies (1882-1960) who received the Knighthood honour in 1930, in view of his services to the victim of World War 1.

Reference:

Aram Harijan and Eric G. Halvorson: Eponymous Instruments in Plastic Surgery. Plast Reconstr Surg, 2011; 127: 460.

4. **The correct response is A.**

Kaplan's cardinal line extends from the apex of first web space to the distal edge of the pisiform bone. This line is helpful in localization of the motor branch of the median nerve. A line drawn along the ulnar side of the middle finger will join this line at a point which represents the surface landmark of the motor branch of the median nerve. The ulnar motor nerve lies on the cardinal line equidistant between the pisiform and the hook of the hamate.

Reference:

Kaplan EB. Functional and Surgical Anatomy of the Hand. Philadelphia, JB Lippincott, 1953.

5. **The correct response is D.**

Kaplan's cardinal line extends from the apex of first web space to the distal edge of the pisiform bone. This line is helpful in localization of the motor branch of the median nerve. A line drawn along the ulnar side of the middle finger will join this line at a point which represents the surface landmark of the motor branch of the median nerve. The ulnar motor nerve lies on the cardinal line equidistant between the pisiform and the hook of the hamate.

Reference:

Kaplan EB. Functional and Surgical Anatomy of the Hand. Philadelphia, JB Lippincott, 1953.

6. **The correct response is D.**

The motor branch of the ulnar nerve lies at the intersection of the Kaplan's cardinal line and another line drawn from the ulnar aspect of the ring finger'

Reference:

Kaplan EB. Functional and Surgical Anatomy of the Hand. Philadelphia, JB Lippincott, 1953.

7. **The correct response is C.**

Five intrinsic and four extrinsic muscles control the movements of the thumb. The five intrinsics are (abductor pollicis brevis, flexor pollicis brevis, opponens pollicis brevis and two heads of adductor pollicis). The four extrinsics are abductor pollicis longus, extensor pollicis brevis, extensor pollicis longus and the flexor pollicis longus.

Reference:

1. *Chase RA. Examination of the hand and relevant anatomy. In May JW Jr, Little JW, eds: The Hand. Philadelphia, WB Saunders, 1990. McCarthy J, ed: Plastic Surgery, vol 7.*
2. *Standring S. Gray's Anatomy. The Anatomical Basis of Clinical Practice. 39th ed. Elsevier Churchill Livingstone 2005: 913-921.*

8. The correct response is B.

The tubercle of scaphoid found at the distal flexion crease of the wrist joint is an important skeletal landmark. Each finger in correct alignment points to the tubercle of the scaphoid.

Reference:

1. *Chase RA. Examination of the hand and relevant anatomy. In May JW Jr, Little JW, eds: The Hand. Philadelphia, WB Saunders, 1990. McCarthy J, ed: Plastic Surgery, vol 7.*
2. *Chase RA. Atlas of hand surgery, vol 1, Philadelphia, WB Saunders, 1973.*

9. The correct response is B.

The A2 pulley is the largest pulley and extends to nearly half of the proximal phalanx.

Reference:

1. *Chase RA. Examination of the hand and relevant anatomy. In May JW Jr, Little JW, eds: The Hand. Philadelphia, WB Saunders, 1990. McCarthy J, ed: Plastic Surgery, vol 7.*
2. *Chase RA. Atlas of hand surgery, vol 1, Philadelphia, WB Saunders, 1973.*

10. The correct response is A.

The Grayson ligament is placed on the volar side of the neurovascular bundles and Cleland's ligament is located on the dorsal side of the bundle. Pretendinous band and superficial transverse ligament are proximal to the confines of the finger.

Reference:

1. *Chase RA. Examination of the hand and relevant anatomy. In May JW Jr, Little JW, eds: The Hand. Philadelphia, WB Saunders, 1990. McCarthy J, ed: Plastic Surgery, vol 7.*
2. *Chase RA. Atlas of hand surgery, vol 1, Philadelphia, WB Saunders, 1973.*

11. The correct response is B.

The articular surface is obliquely placed. It has a slope from the radial to the ulnar side which is about 22 degrees. There is also a dorsal to palmar slope of 12 degrees. The articular surface has two shallow depressions for the scaphoid and lunate.

It is important to reduce the radius in fractures of the wrist so that the slope is maintained to its normal configuration as far as possible. This would allow pain free movements at the wrist joint.

Reference:

Youm Y, McMurty RY, Flatt AE, Sprague BL. Kinematics of the wrist. An experimental study of radial-ulnar deviation and flexion-extension. J Bone Joint Surg Am 1978; 60:423.

12. The correct response is A.

The anatomic centre of the hand lies over the metacarpophalangeal joint of the middle finger.

Reference:

Youm Y, McMurty RY, Flatt AE, Sprague BL. Kinematics of the wrist. An experimental study of radial-ulnar deviation and flexion-extension. J Bone Joint Surg Am 1978; 60: 423.

13. The correct response is B.

Extensor carpi radialis brevis is attached to the base of the third metacarpal. It can independently extend a pronated hand against gravity. The extensor carpi radialis longus and the flexor carpi radialis are attached to the base of the second metacarpal bone and hence balance each other's actions. The longus is more helpful in grasping and clenching.

Reference:

Brand P, Hollister A. Clinical Mechanics of the Hand. St. Louis, Mosby-Year Book, 1999.

14. The correct response is C.

The wrist is immobilized in flexion and ulnar deviation so that the radial to ulnar and dorsal to palmar slope is recreated due to apposition of the proximal row of carpal bones against the articular surface of the radius.

Reference:

Brand P, Hollister A. Clinical Mechanics of the Hand. St. Louis, Mosby-Year Book, 1999.

15. The correct response is B.

There are four bones in the proximal row. Scaphoid and lunate articulate with the radius. The triquetrum articulates with the lunate of the proximal row of carpal bones. Pisiform is a floating bone and does not form a part of the wrist joint. The triangular fibrocartilage attached to the ulna separates it from the triquetrum.

Reference:

1. *Gilula LA. Carpal injuries: analytic approach and case exercises. Am J Radiol 1979; 133: 503.*
2. *Hentz VR, Chase RA. Hand Surgery: A Clinical Atlas. Philadelphia, WB Saunders, 2001.*

16. The correct response is B.

The collateral ligaments of MCPJ are lax in extension and allow the oedema fluid to be accommodated in the joint space. If this persists for more than 2 weeks, the joint gets fixed in extension. The ligaments later on shrink and contract. The contracted ligaments need to be released by excision, so that the joint could be flexed and start moving again. The metacarpophalangeal joint has a palmar ligament and two collateral ligaments. The palmar ligaments of the second to fifth metacarpal are connected to each other by deep transverse metacarpal ligaments. These are also connected to the palmar aponeurosis through slips. The collateral ligaments are attached to the posterior tubercle on the metacarpal head. They extend obliquely to the side of the proximal phalanx. These become lax when the finger is extended or when the joint gets swollen due to collection of oedema fluid.

Reference:

1. *Hentz VR, Chase RA. Hand Surgery: A Clinical Atlas. Philadelphia, WB Saunders, 2001.*
2. *Brand P, Hollister A. Clinical Mechanics of the Hand. St. Louis, Mosby-Year Book, 1999.*

17. The correct response is E.

The supinator takes origin from all of the above. It has two heads of origin and is inserted into the lateral surface of the upper third of radius. Heavy objects from the ground are lifted with the forearm in pronation, as the objects are lifted further up, the elbow gets flexed by the biceps brachii, which helps the supination further. The supinator is supplied by the posterior interosseous nerve (C6 and C7). The nerve also passes through it. The nerve at times may get compressed within the supinator muscle.

Reference:

1. *Hentz VR, Chase RA. Hand Surgery: A Clinical Atlas. Philadelphia, WB Saunders, 2001.*
2. *Brand P, Hollister A. Clinical Mechanics of the Hand. St. Louis, Mosby-Year Book, 1999.*

18. The correct response is A.

There is no cruciate pulley between A1 and A2 annular pulleys. A1 pulley is present at the metacarpophalangeal joint level. A3 pulley is over the proximal interphalangeal joint (PIP) and A5 pulley is over the distal interphalangeal joint (DIP). A2 pulley is the largest and is present over the proximal half of the proximal phalanx.

A4 pulley is present over the middle of the middle phalanx.The C1 cruciate pulley is present between A2 and A3. The C2 is present between A3 and A4. The C3 is present between A4 and A5.

Reference:

1. *Chase RA. Atlas of Hand Surgery. vol II. Philadelphia, WB Saunders, 1984.*
2. *Brand P, Hollister A. Clinical Mechanics of the Hand. St. Louis, Mosby-Year Book, 1999.*

19. The correct response is B.

In zone 1, the only tendon which is present and which can get damaged is the flexor digitorum profundus (FDP).

Reference:

1. *Chase RA. Atlas of Hand Surgery. vol II. Philadelphia, WB Saunders, 1984.*
2. *Brand P, Hollister A. Clinical Mechanics of the Hand. St. Louis, Mosby-Year Book, 1999.*

20. The correct response is D.

The carpal tunnel ligament overlies zone IV which is distal to the wrist crease.

Reference:

1. *Chase RA. Atlas of Hand Surgery. vol II. Philadelphia, WB Saunders, 1984.*
2. *Brand P, Hollister A. Clinical Mechanics of the Hand. St. Louis, Mosby-Year Book, 1999.*

21. The correct response is C.

The A4 pulley lies over the insertions of the flexor digitorum sublimis and hence lies in zone 2. Zone II extends from the proximal end of zone I to the proximal end of the digital fibrous flexor sheath. The A5 and C3 pulleys lie in zone 1.

Reference:

1. *Chase RA. Atlas of Hand Surgery. Vol II. Philadelphia, WB Saunders, 1984.*
2. *Brand P, Hollister A. Clinical Mechanics of the Hand. St. Louis, Mosby-Year Book, 1999.*

22. The correct response is D.

The adductor pollicis has two heads of origin. The oblique head arises from the capitate bone and base of second and third metacarpal. The transverse head arises from the distal two-thirds of the third metacarpal. It is inserted into the base of the proximal phalanx of the thumb.

Reference:

1. *Chase RA. Atlas of Hand Surgery. Vol II. Philadelphia, WB Saunders, 1984.*
2. *Brand P, Hollister A. Clinical Mechanics of the Hand. St. Louis, Mosby-Year Book, 1999.*

23. The correct response is D.

The palmaris brevis is rudimentary and is not involved in controlling the movements of the little finger.

Reference:

1. *Chase RA. Atlas of Hand Surgery. Vol II. Philadelphia, WB Saunders, 1984.*
2. *Brand P, Hollister A. Clinical Mechanics of the Hand. St. Louis, Mosby-Year Book, 1999.*

24. The correct response is A.

The lumbrical muscles are connected with the flexor digitorum profundus. They do not take origin from the flexor digitorum sublimis. The lumbricals connect the flexor digitorum profundus with the extensor apparatus. Lumbricals extend the interphalangeal joints and have weak flexion at the metacarpophalangeal joint. Lumbricals help in pulp-to-pulp pinch. In the absence of the first lumbrical, the index finger and thumb will have nail-to-nail contact and not pulp-to-pulp pinch. Lumbricals help in adjusting the effective length of the flexor digitorum profundus to control the degrees of flexion and extension required at the metacarpophalangeal, the proximal and the distal interphalangeal joints.

Reference:

1. *Chase RA. Atlas of Hand Surgery. Vol II. Philadelphia, WB Saunders, 1984.*
2. *Brand P, Hollister A. Clinical Mechanics of the Hand. St. Louis, Mosby-Year Book, 1999.*

25. The correct response is D.

The dorsal interossei perform all the above functions. They abduct the fingers. They pass volar to the metacarpophalangeal joints and hence flex these joints. They lie dorsal to the interphalangeal joints and hence extend the interphalangeal joints.

Reference:

1. *Chase RA. Atlas of Hand Surgery. Vol II. Philadelphia, WB Saunders, 1984.*
2. *Brand P, Hollister A. Clinical Mechanics of the Hand. St. Louis, Mosby-Year Book, 1999.*

26. The correct response is D.

The palmar interossei are unipennate. These are not abductors, instead these act as adductors. They also help in extension of the interphalangeal joints and flexion of the metacarpophalangeal joints.

Reference:

1. *Chase RA. Atlas of Hand Surgery. Vol II. Philadelphia, WB Saunders, 1984.*
2. *Brand P, Hollister A. Clinical Mechanics of the Hand. St. Louis, Mosby-Year Book, 1999.*

27. The correct response is B.

Side to side movements are controlled by the interossei. The middle finger has two dorsal interossei muscles on its either side. These help the middle finger to move to the right or the left side as desired. The middle finger is without any palmar interossei. On the palmar side, the transverse head of the adductor pollicis takes origin from its distal two third, and hence the middle finger is without palmar interossei as per the nature's allocation for the structural and functional management.

Reference:

1. *Chase RA. Examination of the hand and relevant anatomy. In May JW Jr, Little JW, eds: The Hand. Philadelphia, WB Saunders, 1990. McCarthy J, ed: Plastic Surgery, vol 7.*
2. *Chase RA. Atlas of hand surgery, vol 1, Philadelphia, WB Saunders, 1973.*

28. The correct response is C.

The thumb and the little finger have independent abductors. The middle finger has two abductors while the index and the ring finger have one each. The dorsal interossei are abductors of fingers.

Reference:

1. *Chase RA. Examination of the hand and relevant anatomy. In May JW Jr, Little JW, eds: The Hand. Philadelphia, WB Saunders, 1990. McCarthy J, ed: Plastic Surgery, vol 7.*
2. *Chase RA. Atlas of hand surgery, vol 1, Philadelphia, WB Saunders, 1973.*

29. The correct response is C.

The middle finger is not provided with adductors. It has two abductors instead, which move the finger towards the radial and the ulnar side. The palmar interossei are adductors (PAD).

Reference:

1. *Chase RA. Examination of the hand and relevant anatomy. In May JW Jr, Little JW, eds: The Hand. Philadelphia, WB Saunders, 1990. McCarthy J, ed: Plastic Surgery, vol 7.*
2. *Chase RA. Atlas of hand surgery, vol 1, Philadelphia, WB Saunders, 1973.*

30. The correct response is C.

The middle finger has no palmar interossei attached to it. The palmar surface of the third metacarpal gives origin to the transverse and oblique heads of the adductor pollicis. The palmar interossei do not contribute to the formation of the extensor expansion of the middle finger. The palmar interossei pass anterior to the axis of the metacarpophalangeal joints and get inserted into the triangular sheet of the extensor aponeurosis and get inserted on to the proximal, middle and distal phalanx through the extensor aponeurosis. These therefore help in flexion of the metacarpophalangeal joint (MP) and extension of the proximal interphalangeal joint (PIP) and the distal interphalangeal (DIP). The palmar interossei adduct the fingers.

Reference:

1. *Pierer V. The interossei and the lumbricals. The Hand. Edited Raoul Tubiana. 1981:244 - 254.*
2. *Chase RA. Examination of the hand and relevant anatomy. In May JW Jr, Little JW, eds: The Hand. Philadelphia, WB Saunders, 1990. McCarthy J, ed: Plastic Surgery, vol 7.*

31. The correct response is A.

The first dorsal interossei get inserted into the lateral tubercle of the proximal phalanx of the index finger. They give no contribution to the extensor aponeurosis. The aponeurosis of the index finger receives contribution of the first lumbrical muscle, which is well developed than the other lumbricals. All other interossei have a bony and an aponeurotic insertion.

The ventral portion of the dorsal interossei inserts like the palmar interossei. Its angle of approach is 20-25 degrees. It is chiefly inserted into the extensor aponeurosis. The dorsal portion is inserted mostly into the lateral tubercle of the proximal phalanx. Its angle of approach is 0-5 degrees. The dorsal interossei are abductors of the fingers and flexors of the metacarpophalangeal joint and extensors of the PIP and DIP joints. These are also responsible for rotation at the metacarpophalangeal joint. The extensor aponeurosis of the little finger is formed on the radial side by the third palmar interossei and the fourth lumbrical, while on the ulnar side it is formed by the abductor digiti minimi.

Reference:

1. *Pierer V. The interossei and the lumbricals. The Hand. Edited Raoul Tubiana. 1981:244 - 254.*
2. *Chase RA. Examination of the hand and relevant anatomy. In May JW Jr, Little JW, eds: The Hand. Philadelphia, WB Saunders, 1990. McCarthy J, ed: Plastic Surgery, vol 7.*

32. The correct response is A.

The lumbricals have a mobile origin from profundus tendon and with phalangeal flexion as the profundus moves the origin proximally the extensor expansion moves the insertion distally. They mainly help in extension of the proximal interphalangeal joints (PIP) and distal interphalangeal joints (DIP). Lumbricals because of their position, and angle of approach to the dorsal aponeurosis may at best act as starters or initiators of metacarpophalangeal flexion.

Lumbricals can also pull the FDP tendon forwards i.e. towards the metacarpophalangeal joint and thus help in reducing the flexion at the proximal and distal interphalangeal joints. This in turn would allow more extension and better pulp-to-pulp contact will not be possible, instead the finger will have nail-to-nail contact. If the MCP and PIP joints get fixed due to oedema and fibrosis, it would affect free movement of the profundus tendon and pulp-to-pulp pinch would not be possible.

Reference:

1. *Pierer V. The interossei and the lumbricals. The Hand. Edited Raoul Tubiana. 1981:244 – 254.*
2. *Chase RA. Examination of the hand and relevant anatomy. In May JW Jr, Little JW, eds: The Hand. Philadelphia, WB Saunders, 1990. McCarthy J, ed: Plastic Surgery, vol 7.*

33. The correct response is E.

All of above can lead to contracture of the intrinsic muscles of the hand.

Reference:

1. *Smith R. Intrinsic contracture . Green's Operative Hand Surgery. 4th ed: 1999:607-618.*
2. *Chase RA. Examination of the hand and relevant anatomy. In May JW Jr, Little JW, eds: The Hand. Philadelphia, WB Saunders, 1990. McCarthy J, ed: Plastic Surgery, vol 7.*

34. The correct response is C.

The Allen's test best assesses the vascular efficiency of the hand. The procedure consists of asking the patient to do the following :

1. The patient is asked to make a tight fist to squeeze out all the blood from the hand.
2. The radial or the ulnar artery is compressed at the front of the wrist.
3. Patient is asked to extend the fingers which show the blanched out appearance of the digits.
4. Pressure on radial artery is released to allow the blood to flow and flush the hand. Flush indicates normal flow and patency of the radial artery. The test is then repeated after blocking the ulnar artery.

Moberg and Ninhydrin tests are for assessing the sensory / sudomotor status of the hand. Froment's sign is a test for function of ulnar innervated adductor pollicis muscle. Jeanne sign is a "recurvatum" or hyperextension of the metacarpophalangeal joint after the patient is asked to hold a piece of paper between the thumb and the radial side of the index finger.

Reference:

1. *Chase RA. Atlas of Hand Surgery. vol I. Philadelphia, WB Saunders, 1973.*
2. *Chase RA. Examination of the hand and relevant anatomy. In May JW Jr, Little JW, eds: The Hand. Philadelphia, WB Saunders, 1990. McCarthy J, ed: Plastic Surgery, vol 7.*

35. The correct response is A

The synovial sheaths of the thumb (flexor pollicis longus) extends through the carpal tunnel into the forearm. The synovial sheaths of the index, middle and ring fingers are short and these do not communicate with the sheaths of the thumb and the little finger. Effusions and collection of pus in these sheaths have different clinical presentations.

Reference:

1. *Standring S. Gray's Anatomy. The Anatomical Basis of Clinical Practice. 39th ed. Elsevier Churchill Livingstone 2005:914.*
2. *Chase RA. Examination of the hand and relevant anatomy. In May JW Jr, Little JW, eds: The Hand. Philadelphia, WB Saunders, 1990. McCarthy J, ed: Plastic Surgery, vol 7.*

36. The correct response is B.

The ulnar nerve palsy results in weakness of the adductor pollicis muscle. To compensate for this weakness, the flexor pollicis longus flexes the interphalangeal joint to hold the piece of paper firmly. This flexion of the joint is the basis of the "Froment's sign". In some individuals this joint may go into hyperextension. It is then referred to as 'Jeanne sign'.

Reference:

1. *Chase RA. Atlas of Hand Surgery. vol I. Philadelphia, WB Saunders, 1973.*
2. *Chase RA. Examination of the hand and relevant anatomy. In May JW Jr, Littler JW, eds: The Hand, Philadelphia, WB Saunders, 1990; 4247-4248. McCarthy J, ed: Plastic Surgery; vol 7.*

37. The correct response is E.

Suppurative tenosynovitis is a deep space infection of the fiberosseous tunnel of the flexor tendon sheath usually following a puncture wound on the hand. All of the above are the cardinal signs of this infection.

Reference:

The Hand: Examination and Diagnosis. Rosemont, III, American Society for Surgery of the Hand, 2001.

38. The correct response is A

Finkelstein test is used for testing the inflammation (tendinitis) in the tendons of the 1st dorsal compartment i.e. abductor pollicis and extensor pollicis brevis.

The test consists of asking the patient to make a fist by keeping the thumb inside the fist and the wrist is passively deviated on the ulnar side. It stretches the tendons of the first dorsal compartment i.e. extensor pollicis brevis and the abductor pollicis which causes pain.

Reference:

The Hand: Examination and Diagnosis. Rosemont, III, American Society for Surgery of the Hand, 2001.

39. The correct response is D

An unstable distal radioulnar joint is forced into subluxation by steadying the pronated carpus by grasping the pisotriquetral column in one hand and depressing the ulnar head with the other. The popping down and back of the ulna is termed as piano key sign. The other options are incorrect.

Reference:

The Hand: Examination and Diagnosis. Rosemont, III, American Society for Surgery of the Hand, 2001.

40. The correct response is C

The interscalene block is the primary indication for shoulder surgery as regards dermatomal spread of local anaesthetic by this approach. The nerve function to C8 and T1 might be spared making this block unsuitable for hand and forearm surgery.

Reference:

Roch JJ, Sharrock NE, Neudachin L. Interscalene brachial plexus block for shoulder surgery: a proximal paresthesia is effective. Anesth Analg 1992; 75: 386-388.

41. The correct response is E.

All of the above are true for post-tourniquet syndrome. The tissue pH falls in cases where tourniquet is applied for a fairly long time (two to three hours or more). It is probably the most common and less appreciated complication arising from tourniquet use. It typically resolves spontaneously during a week or so but the prolonged oedema may last more.

Reference:

1. *Love BRT. The tourniquet and its complications. Proceedings and reports of universities, colleges and associations. J Bone Joint Surg Br 1979; 61: 239.*
2. *Kernerman L. The tourniquet in surgery. J Bone Joint Surg Br 1962; 44: 937-943.*
3. *Green DP. Green's Operative Surgery. 5th ed: 2005, Elsevier Churchill Livingstone.*

42. The correct response is D.

Although the fracture can be fixed by any of the above method, the plate and screw fixation would be most suitable.

Reference:

Freeland AE, Jabaley ME, Hughes JL. Stable Fixation of the Hand and Wrist. New York, Springer-Verlag, 1986:17.

43. The correct response is E.

Hook nail deformity is likely to result if more than 50% of the nail and its bed including the underlying bone is lost. Every effort should be made to preserve the underlying lost tissues and the bone by a flap and a bone graft.

Reference:

1. *Trumble T. Fingertip and nail bed injuries. In Trumble T, ed: Principles of Hand Surgery and Therapy. Philadelphia, WB Saunders, 1997:192.*
2. *Hart R, Kleinert H. Fingertip and nail bed injuries. Emerg Med Clin North Am 1993;11: 755.*

44. The correct response is A.

If the tendon of flexor digitorum profundus is transected a lumbrical plus finger will develop, which is characterized by paradoxical extension at the proximal interphalangeal joint as the finger is flexed. In this situation, the lumbrical muscle is at a disadvantage due to its laxity and an imbalance of power results in extension at the proximal interphalangeal joint.

Reference:

1. *Hart R, Kleinert H. Fingertip and nail bed injuries. Emerg Med Clin North Am 1993; 11: 755.*
2. *Trumble T. Fingertip and nail bed injuries. In Trumble T, ed: Principles of Hand Surgery and Therapy. Philadelphia, WB Saunders, 1997:192.*

45. The correct response is C.

The quadriga effect is characterized by the incomplete flexion of the other normal fingers around the affected digit. This happens if in the case of amputations, the flexor tendon is sutured to the extensor tendon across the stump of the bone.

Reference:

1. *Trumble T. Fingertip and nail bed injuries. In Trumble T, ed: Principles of Hand Surgery and Therapy. Philadelphia, WB Saunders, 1997:192.*
2. *Hart R, Kleinert H. Fingertip and nail bed injuries. Emerg Med Clin North Am 1993;11: 755.*

46. The correct response is B.

The Kutler lateral V-Y flaps are based on the lateral surface of the digit with the apex at the distal interphalangeal joint and the base is adjacent to the defect. The width of the flap is equal to half of the length of the flap.

Reference:

1. *Russell R: Fingertip injuries. In May JW Jr, Littler JW, eds: The Hand. Philadelphia, WB Saunders, 1990:4477. McCarthy J, ed: Plastic Surgery: vol 7.*
2. *Kutler W. A new method for repair of finger tip amputation. JAMA 1947; 133: 29.*

47. The correct response is A.

Moberg flap is especially indicated in cases of loss of terminal part of the thumb, where length and sensations are to be maintained. It is based on both the neurovascular pedicles and hence provides good sensation and is dependable because of its good vascularity. Flap can be advanced by 1.0-1.5 cm to cover the defect. It is specially indicated for the thumb because of presence of independent dorsal blood supply which prevents against necrosis of the dorsal skin.

Reference:

1. *Elliot D, Wilson Y. V-Y advancement of the entire volar tissue of the thumb in distal reconstruction. J Hand Surg Br 1993; 18: 399.*
2. *Moberg E. Aspects of sensation in reconstructive surgery of the extremity. J Bone Joint Surg Am 1964; 46: 817.*

48. The correct response is B.

Volar oblique amputations of the fingertip are not suitable for the volar advancement flap due to geometric considerations. The others are valid indications for this flap.

Reference:

1. *Lister G, Pederson W. Skin flaps. In Green D, Hotchkiss R, Pederson W, eds: Green's Operative Hand Surgery. New York, Churchill Livingstone, 1999: 1783.*
2. *Atasoy E, Ioakmidis E, Kasdan M et al. Reconstruction of the amputated finger tip with a triangular volar flap. J Bone Joint Surg Am 1970; 52: 921.*

49. The correct response is C.

Lunula is the visible white convex opacity of the germinal matrix of the nail at its junction with the skin (eponychium). The white colour remains after removal of the nail and is thought to be secondary to retention of the nuclei of the germinal cells to this level of the nail.

Reference:

Zook EG, Van Beek AL, Rusell RC, Beatty ME. Anatomy and physiology of the perionychium: a review of the literature and anatomic study. J Hand Surg Am 1980; 5: 528–536.

50. The correct response is E.

The hooked nail is not due to primary scarring of the nail bed. The hooked nail grows forwards but bends in a volar direction and is commonly due to loss of terminal phalanx in amputation of the tip where the stump is closed tightly.

Reference:

Kumar VP, Satku K. Treatment and prevention of "hooked nail" deformity with anatomic correlation. J Hand Surg Am 1993; 18: 617–620.

51. The correct response is C.

The ganglions are commonly seen in relation with the distal interphalangeal joints of the fingers especially between the distal interphalangeal joint extensor crease and the nail fold. They often have a communicating link with the joint space. They have a tendency to recur. Injection therapy, aspiration and excision have been tried but recurrences are known. Excision of the bony spur along with excision of the ganglion is supposed to give recurrence free results.

Reference:

Kleinert HE, Kutz JE, Fishman JH, McGraw LH. Etiology and treatment of the so-called mucous cyst of the finger. J Bone Joint Surg Am 1972; 54: 1455–1458.

52. The correct response is B.

The interconnecting transverse palmar arches are in relation with the proximal and distal cruciate C1 and C3 pulleys i.e. proximal to the proximal interphalangeal and distal interphalangeal joints. These communications lie between the flexor tendons and the bone and help in perfusing the tendons and the joints. The most distal arch lies distal to the insertion of the flexor digitorum profundus tendon.

Reference:

Foucher G, Khouri K. Digital reconstruction with island flaps. Clin Plast Surg 1997; 24: 1– 32.

53. The correct response is D.

The digital ulnar artery is larger and dominant in the index and middle fingers while the radial artery is dominant in the ring and small finger.

Reference:

Leslie BM, Ruby LK, Madell SJ et al. Digital artery diameter: an anatomical and clinical study. J Hand Surg Am 1987; 12: 740-743.

54. The correct response is E.

The function of hook grip is performed by the fingers. The other functions are performed by the thumb.

Reference:

Littler JW. On making a thumb: one hundred years of surgical effort. J Hand Surg Am 1976;1:35-51.

55. The correct response is D.

Flexor hallucis brevis is not taken during transfer of the great toe. The rest of the options are correct.

Reference:

1. *Jones NF, Gupta R. Postoperative monitoring of pediatric toe-to-hand transfers with differential pulse oximetry. J Hand Surg Am 2001; 26: 525–529.*
2. *Serafin D. The great toe flap. In Sefrfin D, ed: Atlas of Microsurgical Composite Tissue Transplantation. Philadelphia, WB Saunders, 1996: 591–606.*

56. The correct response is A.

The term 'no-man's land' was coined by Sterling Bunnell to emphasise the poor results that were obtained by flexor tendon surgery in the zone II. He recommended removal of the native tendons to enable smooth movement of the tendon after repair.

Reference:

Bunnell S. Repair of tendons in the fingers and description of two new instruments. Surg Gynecol Obstet 1918; 26: 103–108.

57. The correct response is A.

The pulleys help to keep the flexor tendons closely apposed to the volar surface of the phalanges enabling maximal flexion of the joints with minimal tendon excursion. The number of pulleys in the thumb are three. These are A1, A2 and an oblique pulley in between them. A1 lies in relation with the metacarpophalangeal and A2 in relation to the interphalangeal joint.

Reference:

1. *Doyle JR, Blythe W. Anatomy of the flexor tendon sheath and pulleys of the thumb. J Hand Surg Am 1977; 2: 149-151.*
2. *Kline SC, Moore JR. The transverse carpal ligament – an important component of the digital flexor pulley system. J Bone Joint Surg Am 1992; 74: 1478–1485.*

58. The correct response is B.

The A2 pulley lies on the proximal half of the proximal phalanx. It is the largest pulley and is about 18 mm long. A4 pulley lies over the proximal half of the middle phalanx and is another important pulley controlling the movements of the flexor tendons and prevents bow stringing. The thumb has only three pulleys (A1, A2) and an oblique pulley in between them. A1 lies in relation with the metacarpophalangeal and A2 in relation to the interphalangeal joint.

Reference:

1. *Doyle JR, Blythe W. Anatomy of the flexor tendon sheath and pulleys of the thumb. J Hand Surg Am 1977; 2: 149-151.*
2. *Kline SC, Moore JR. The transverse carpal ligament – an important component of the digital flexor pulley system. J Bone Joint Surg Am 1992; 74: 1478–1485.*

59. The correct response is B.

The pulley likely to be damaged will be A2 as it lies on the proximal phalanx.

Reference:

1. *Doyle JR, Blythe W. Anatomy of the flexor tendon sheath and pulleys of the thumb. J Hand Surg Am 1977; 2: 149-151.*
2. *Kleinert HE, Cash SI. Management of acute flexor tendon injuries in the hand. Instr Course Lect 1985; 34: 361–372.*

60. The correct response is D.

The pulley likely to get damaged will be A4 as it lies on the middle phalanx.

Reference:

1. *Doyle JR, Blythe W. Anatomy of the flexor tendon sheath and pulleys of the thumb. J Hand Surg Am 1977; 2: 149-151.*
2. *Kleinert HE, Cash SL. Management of acute flexor tendon injuries in the hand. Instr Course Lect 1985; 34: 361-372.*

61. The correct response is B.

The most commonly used core suture technique is the modified Kessler suture. The core suture is usually 3-0 or 4-0 nonabsorbable monofilament or braided polyester which is used in combination with an epitendinous suture.

Reference:

McCarthy DM, Boardman ND 3rd, Tramaglini DM et al. Clinical management of partially lacerated digital flexor tendons: a survey [corrected] of hand surgeons. J Hand Surg Am 1995; 20: 273–275.

62. The correct response is E.

All of the above indications justify a two staged flexor tendon grafting approach.

Reference:

Imbraglia JE, Hunter J, Rennie W. Secondary flexor tendon reconstruction. Hand Clin 1989; 5: 395-413.

63. The correct response is D.

The dorsal retinaculum overlies the extensor tendons in Zone VII at the level of wrist joint which separates the extensor tendons into six distal compartments.

The extensor tendons are divided into nine zones. The injuries over the DIP joint and beyond are placed in zone I. The description of the zones is as follows:

Zone I   Lies over the distal interphalangeal joint
Zone II   Lies over the middle phalanx

Zone III Lies over the PIP joints

Zone IV Lies over the proximal phalanx

Zone V Lies over the MCP joints

Zone VI Lies over the metacarpals

Zone VII Lies over the dorsal retinaculum (Wrist joint)

Zone VIII Lies over the distal forearm

Zone IX Lies over the proximal forearm.

Reference:

Littler JW. The finger extensor system. Orthop Clin North Am 1986; 17: 483–492.

64. The correct response is E.

The extensor digiti minimi takes origin in the proximal part of the forearm from the lateral epicondyle of the humerus. Two long extensors to the little finger i.e. extensor digitorum and extensor digiti minimi help in its extension more than other fingers. It helps the pianists and the computer operators. The abductor digiti minimi helps in abduction more than other fingers i.e. index, middle and the ring fingers which are abducted by the interossei muscles. Besides this, the extensor carpi ulnaris, extensor digitorum communis (four slips), extensor carpi radialis longus and extensor carpi radialis brevis also arise from the lateral epicondyle.

A total of 8 tendons control the extension of the thumb and fingers. Abduction of the thumb and the little finger is controlled by abductor pollicis longus and abductor digiti minimi respectively. The extensor and abductor digiti minimi provide extra range of movement to the little finger.

Reference:

Littler JW. The finger extensor system. Orthop Clin North Am 1986; 17: 483–492.

65. The correct response is D.

The fourth compartment has five tendons. Remember the number "221511". The tendons which pass through various compartments are:

First compartment-Abductor pollicis longus (APL), extensor pollicis brevis (EPB).

Second compartment- Extensor carpi radialis longus (ECRL), extensor carpi radialis brevis (ECRB)

Third compartment- Extensor pollicis longus (EPL)

Fourth compartment- Extensor digitorum communis (EDC) 4 tendons; extensor indicis proprius (EIP)

Fifth compartment-Extensor digiti minimi (EDM)

Sixth compartment-Extensor carpi ulnaris (ECU)

Reference:

Littler JW. The finger extensor system. Orthop Clin North Am 1986; 17: 483–492.

66. The correct response is A.

When the MCP joint is extended it would put the intrinsic on stretch and if the intrinsics have the contracture, the range of movement i.e. flexion would be less at the PIP joint. If however these joints have capsular or intra-articular fibrosis, the test will not be possible.

Reference:

Littler JW. The finger extensor system. Orthop Clin North Am 1986; 17: 483–492.

67. The correct response is A.

The thumb is the digit which can be used to evaluate all three nerves. Extension of the thumb is by radial nerve, abduction of the thumb is by median nerve and adduction of the thumb is by ulnar nerve.

Reference:

Dobyns JH. Examination of the wrist. In Berger RA, ed: Disorders of the Wrist Course Syllabus. Rosemount, Ill, American Society for Surgery of the Hand, 2001.

68. The correct response is C.

The most commonly fractured metacarpals in fist fights are the fourth and fifth which result in loss of knuckle prominence and apex dorsal angulation.

Reference:

Ford DJ, Ali MS, Steel WM. Fractures of the fifth metacarpal neck: is reduction or mobilisation necessary? J Hand Surg Br 1989; 14: 165.

69. The correct response is B.

The stack splint is useful in the management of the mallet finger deformity. It is useful both as an initial treatment for this deformity and also for postoperative management of this deformity.

Reference:

Clement R, Wray RC Jr. Mallet finger—operative and nonoperative treatment. Ann Plast Surg 1986; 16: 136.

70. The correct response is C.

The fracture of the thumb metacarpal base into three fragments is called Rolando's fracture. The three fragments are radial, ulnar and the main fragment which is the remainder of the metacarpal. The displacement is usually in the apex dorsal direction.

The Bennett's fracture is one where the base of the first metacarpal is fractured and may be dislocated. The reversed Bennett's fracture involves the base of the fifth metacarpal.

Reference:

1. *O'Brien ET. Fractures of the metacarpals and phalanges. In Green DL, ed: Operative Hand Surgery. New York, Churchill Livingstone, 1982: 703–742.*
2. *Livesley PJ. The conservative management of Bennett's fracture-dislocation: a 26 year follow up. J Hand Surg Br 1990; 15: 291.*

71. The correct response is E.

All of the above may produce chipping of the base of the proximal phalanx of the thumb on the radial side. Forceful contraction of these muscles could be responsible for chipping of the base of the phalanx. Besides these, adductor pollicis, first palmar interossei and the ulnar collateral ligaments are attached on the ulnar side of the proximal phalanx of the thumb and could be responsible for chip fractures on the ulnar side.

Reference:

1. *Green DP. Green's Operative Hand Surgery. 4th ed. Churchill Livingstone, 1999.*
2. *Peter JS. Fractures of Metacarpal and Phalanges. Green's Operative Surgery, 5th ed: 2005: 277–342.*

72. The correct response is A.

In a case of sprained wrist, tenderness over the snuff box is due to injury to scaphoid. In case of scapholunate injury, the tenderness would be felt distal to the Lister's tubercle. In case of injury to the fibrocartilage, tenderness would be felt distal to the lower end of ulna.

Reference:

Watson HK, Ashmead D, Makhlouf MV. Examination of the scaphoid. J Hand Surg Am 1988; 13:657-660.

73. The correct response is C.

Fractures of the hook of the hamate are commonly seen in baseball players. The diagnosis is difficult on plain films and a computed tomogram is required if patient has persistent pain in the region.

Reference:

Bishop AT, Beckenbaugh RD. Fracture of the hamate hook. J Hand Surg 1988; 13: 135–139.

74. The correct response is B.

The Tinel's sign is progressive in cases of axonotmesis. It is absent in neurapraxia. The Tinel's sign is present but is not progressive in neurotmesis because the nerve is totally severed inside and only has got anatomical continuity. In options D and E also the Tinel's will fail to progress.

Reference:

Mackinnon SE. New direction in peripheral nerve surgery. Ann Surg 1989; 22: 257–273.

75. The correct response is D.

The saphenous nerve can provide grafts upto 40 cm long. The sural nerve is also capable of providing a graft of similar length. The lateral cutaneous nerve of the arm can provide graft upto 10 cm long, while the medial cutaneous nerve of the arm and forearm can provide grafts upto 20 cm or more.

Reference:

1. *Seddon HJ. The use of autogenous grafts for the repair of large gaps in peripheral nerves. Br J Surg 1947; 35: 151.*
2. *Sunderland S, Ray LJ. The selection and use of autografts for bridging gaps in injured nerves. Brain 1947; 70: 75.*

76. The correct response is E.

Hoarseness of voice is not a feature of the brachial plexus injury.

Reference:

Chuang DCC. Management of traumatic brachial plexus injuries in adults. Hand Clin 1999; 15: 737.

77. The correct response is D.

The MRI scan would provide the maximum information in cases of brachial plexus injuries, whether it be fracture of cervical spine, pseudo-meningocoeles, avulsion of roots, nerve injuries or neuromas. Other modalities are also helpful but do not provide the same quantum of information as a MRI does.

Reference:

Hems TE, Birch R, Carlsted T. The role of magnetic resonance imaging in the management of traction injuries to the adult brachial plexus. J Hand Surg Br 1999; 24:550.

78. The correct response is B.

Exophthalmos is not a feature of the Horner's syndrome. The syndrome is due to sympathetic nervous system disturbance and should lead one to suspect the level of injury to be around T_1 and T_2 because of the location of the sympathetic ganglions close to that level. The syndrome is the result of paralysis of the cervical sympathetic nerves. Johann F Horner was a Swiss Ophthalmologist from 1831–1886.

Reference:

Tubiana R. Clinical examination and functional assessment of the upper limb after peripheral nerve lesions. In Tubiana R, ed: The Hand. Philadelhia, WB Saunders, 1988: 487.

79. The correct response is A.

The Erb's palsy is due to involvement of C_5 and C_6 roots. This causes weakness and paralysis in the muscles supplied by these roots. The muscles affected are deltoid, biceps, brachialis and brachioradialis. Supraspinatus, infraspinatus and supinator may also be involved. The arm hangs by the side and is medially rotated. The forearm lies extended and pronated. The arm cannot be abducted and the forearm cannot be flexed. Wilhelm Helnrich Erb was a German Neurologist from 1840-1921.

Reference:

Sandmire HF, DeMott RK. Erb's palsy: concepts of causation. Obstet Gynecol 2000; 95: 941–942.

80. The correct response is E.

The wrist is not extended in Erb's palsy, it is rather flexed and may be ulnar deviated just like a policeman asking for tips.

Reference:

Narakas AO. Obstetrical brachial plexus injuries. In Lamb DW, ed: The Paralysed Hand. Edinburgh, Churchill Livingstone, 1987: 116–135.

81. The correct response is D.

An MRI would be the most important investigation in pediatric brachial plexus injury. However, if the brachialis has not regained power, then in all probabilities, nerve surgery will not be helpful and tendon transfers would be required. The nerve surgery should preferably be done within six months of injury as surgery of nerves after this age will not give the desired result.

Reference:

Smith S. The role of neurophysiological investigation in traumatic brachial plexus lesions in adults and children. J Hand Surg Br 1996; 21: 145–147.

82. The correct response is D.

All of the above muscles given in the list can be used. The trapezius insertion can be advanced and attached to the deltoid origin or alternatively the insertion can also be advanced along with a piece of the bone from the tip of the acromion which can be fixed to the humerus with a screw. Besides this, the levator insertion on the scapula can be released and fixed to the tendon of the supraspinatus to augment the abduction at the shoulder.

Reference:

Dumont CE, Forin V, Asfazadouria H, Romana C. Function of the upper limb after surgery for obstetric brachial plexus palsy. J Bone Joint Surg Br 2001; 83: 894–900.

83. The correct response is D.

All of the above muscles can be used for correcting the internal rotation of the arm in brachial plexus palsy. The subscapularis origin from the medial border of the scapula can be released. The pectoralis major can be lengthened. The latissimus dorsi insertion can be rerouted and given fresh attachment to the rotator cuff of the shoulder joint, so that it starts working as an external rotator.

Reference:

Hentz V, Chase R. Hand Surgery: A Clinical Atlas. Philadelphia, WB Saunders, 2001: 452–457.

84. The correct response is B.

The rerouting of the tendon of the flexor carpi ulnaris to the extensor compartment, i.e. extensor carpi radialis brevis or extensor digitorum would give a good result for wrist drop.

Reference:

Zancolli EA, Zancolli ER Jr: Palliative surgical procedures in sequelae of obstetrical palsy. Hand Clin 1988; 4: 643-669.

85. The correct response is E.

The tendons, bones and joints are usually spared in ring avulsion injuries. The rest of the structures suffer avulsion injuries.

Reference:

1. *Brooks D, Schott K, Buncke GM. Functional evaluation of ring avulsion injuries. Presented at California Society of Plastic Surgery meeting, May 2000.*
2. *Hentz V, Chase R. Hand Surgery: A Clinical Atlas. Philadelphia, WB Saunders, 2001:452-457.*

86. The correct response is C.

Wrist, IPJ in extension and MCPJ in flexion (Cricket ball holding position). This position allows reduction of the oedema and prevents development of deformities and contractures.

Reference:

Greenhalgh DG. Management of acute burn injuries of the upper extremity in pediatric population. Hand Clin North Am 2000; 16: 175.

87. The correct response is D.

A needle in the compartment attached to a central venous pressure monitor is the direct method of measuring the compartment pressure. It also helps to monitor the compartment pressure. If it is more than 30 mm of Hg, fasciotomy should be done, otherwise this would interfere with capillary and venous flow and would lead to vascular damage of the muscles.

Final decision however can also be based on clinical experience of the surgeon, in cases where the patient complains of persistent pain.

Reference:

Rowland SA. Fasciotomy: the treatment of compartment syndrome. In Green DP, Hotchkiss RN, Pederson WP, eds: Green's Operative Hand Surgery. New York, Churchill Livingstone, 1999: 689-710.

88. The correct response is D.

All the factors enumerated above contribute towards the damage caused by the electrical current. The injury suffered by the muscle is the most, while the bone suffers the least because of the highest resistance.

Reference:

Neale H. Electrical injuries of the hand and upper extremity. In McCarthy JG, ed: Plastic Surgery. Philadelphia, WB Saunders, 1990: 5418–5430.

89. The correct response is D.

A double Z- plasty with a V-Y plasty would be the right approach to perform a five flap plasty for correcting linear contracture in the hand, elbow and other regions of the body.

Reference:

Strock LL, McCauley RL, Smith DJ et al: Reconstruction of the burned hand. In Herndon DN, ed: Total Burn Care. London, WB Saunders, 1996: 506–514.

90. The correct response is A

The axilla and the first web space contractures after release are placed in abduction to allow optimal function.

Reference:

Larson DL, Abston S, Evans EB, et al. Techniques of decreasing scar formation and contractures in the burned patient. J Trauma 1971; 11: 807–823.

91. The correct response is A.

The contracture of axilla should be released first so that the patient is able to get back his shoulder movements. The other ones can be released at a later date.

Reference:

Kurtzman LC, Stern PJ. Upper extremity burn contractures. Hand Clin 1990; 6: 261–279.

92. The correct response is B.

Patients of frost bite should be treated initially by rapid re-warming. Slow thawing is not recommended and topical agents / manual debridement of the blister should be undertaken after rewarming has been done.

Reference:

Robson MC, Heggers JP. Evaluation of hand frost bite blister fluid as a clue to pathogenesis. J Hand Surg 1981; 6:43-47.

93. The correct response is A.

The acids produce coagulation necrosis of tissues. Alkali produce liquefaction necrosis.

Reference:

Reilly DA, Garner WL. Management of chemical injuries to the upper extremity. Hand Clin 2000; 16:215-224.

94. The correct response is D.

Calcium gluconate is the specific antidote for the hydrofluoric acid burns.

Reference:

Reilly DA, Garner WL. Management of chemical injuries to the upper extremity. Hand Clin 2000;16:215-224.

95. The correct response is C.

Kerosene is the specific antidote for mustard gas burns. Calcium gluconate injection is the treatment of choice for hydrofluoric acid burns.

Reference:

Chick LR, Borah G. Calcium carbonate gel therapy for hydrofluoric acid burns of the hand. Plast Reconstr Surg 1990; 86: 935–940.

96. The correct response is C.

Contracture is defined as a condition where there is approximation of the two apposing surfaces across a joint with loss of full range of both active and passive motion.

Reference:

Lister G. The Hand: Diagnosis and Indications, 3rd ed. New York, Churchill Livingstone, 1993: 191–198.

97. The correct response is E.

In the fourth compartment there are five tendons i.e. extensor digitorum (four slips) and extensor indicis (one). The first and second compartment have two tendons each i.e. abductor pollicis longus and extensor pollicis brevis in the first compartment. Extensor carpi radialis longus and brevis are in the second compartment. The third compartment has extensor pollicis longus, while the fifth has extensor digiti minimi and the sixth has extensor carpi ulnaris.

Reference:

Wolfe SW. Tenosynovitis. In Green DP, Hotchkiss RN, Pederson WC, eds: Green's Operative Hand Surgery, 4th ed. New York, Churchill Livingstone, 1999: 2036.

98. The correct response is B.

Dupuytren's contracture is due to contracture of the palmar fascia.

Reference:

Lister G. The Hand: Diagnosis and Indications, 3rd ed. New York, Churchill Livingstone, 1993: 191–198.

99. The correct response is C.

The extensor indicis is a long slender muscle which takes origin from the posterior surface of ulna and the adjacent interosseous membrane. It continues as a long slender muscle into the index finger. This fact is helpful in identification of this tendon. It lies in the fourth dorsal compartment. It gets attached to the dorsal digital expansion along with the extensor digitorum. It is tested by asking the patient to extend the index finger while all other fingers remained fully flexed at the metacarpophalangeal joint.

Reference:

Lister G. The Hand: Diagnosis and Indications, 3rd ed. New York, Churchill Livingstone, 1993: 191–198.

100. The correct response is A.

Tenosynovitis of the abductor pollicis longus and extensor pollicis brevis lying in the first dorsal compartment is called de-Quervain disease. Fritz de Quervain was a Swiss surgeon, and described the condition in 1895.

Reference:

1. *Minamikawa Y, Peimer CA, Cox WL, et al. de Quervain's syndrome: surgical and anatomical studies of the fibroosseous canal. Orthopedic 1991;14:545-549.*
2. *Ilgen R, Shortkroff S. On a form of chronic tendovaginitis by Dr. Fritz de Quervain in 1a Chaux-de-Fonds. Am J Orthop 1997; 26: 641–644.*

101. The correct response is C.

The thumb drop or loss of extension is due to rupture of the extensor pollicis longus (third dorsal compartment) at the level of the Lister's tubercle. It is present on the dorsal aspect of the lower end of radius. There is friction against the tubercle which weakens the tendon. Rheumatoid arthritis is responsible for changes in the Lister's tubercle, besides other changes in bones and joints.

Reference:

Sheon RP. Repetitive strain injury: diagnostic and treatment tips on six common problems. Postgrad Med 1997; 102: 72-85.

102. The correct response is A.

It is the A1 pulley which is released as it is the one that is responsible commonly for the snapping. It is present over the metacarpophalangeal joint.

Reference:

Bonnici AV, Spencer JD. A survey of trigger finger in adults. J Hand Surg Br 1988; 13: 202.

103. The correct response is C.

Swanson's arthroplasty gives good results in cases of osteoarthritis of the metacarpophalangeal joint.

Reference:

1. *Swanson AB. Silicone rubber implants for replacements of arthritic or destroyed joint in the hand. Surg Clin North Am 1968; 48: 1113–1127.*
2. *Pellegrini VDJ, Burton RI. Surgical management of basal joint arthritis of the thumb. Part I. Long term results of silicone implant arthroplasty. J Hand Surg Am 1986; 11: 309–324.*

104. The correct response is D.

The little and ring fingers are commonly involved in Dupuytren's disease. They clinically present with flexion deformity of the metacarpophalangeal and the proximal interphalangeal joints. The deformity is caused by the myofibroblast, which contracts and produces flexion deformities and nodules in the skin.

Reference:

Tubiana R. Anatomy. In Tubiana R, Leclercq C, Hurst L, et al, eds: Dupuytren's Disease. London, Martin Dunitz, 2000: 321.

105. The correct response is D.

Radical excision of the involved fibrous tissues gives good long lasting results. Dupuytren Baron Guillaume was a French surgeon from 1777-1835.

Reference:

Tubiana R. Surgical treatment of Dupuytren's contracture: technique of fasciotomy and fasciectomy. In Hueston JT, Tubiana R, eds: Dupuytren's Disease. Edinburgh, Churchill Livingstone, 1974: 85–92.

106. The correct response is B.

McCash was the one who devised the open method of treatment.

Reference:

McCash CR. The open palm technique in Dupuytren's contracture. Br J Plast Surg 1964; 17: 271–280.

107. The correct response is E.

The site of maximal tenderness is in the distal palm cul-de-sac of the flexor sheath. In the case of the thumb and the little finger, the maximum tenderness is in the proximal palm, because the tendon sheath extends down in the palm to lie in the carpal tunnel and beyond it into the front of the wrist.

Reference:

Nevaiser RJ. Acute infections. In Green DP, Hotchkiss RN, Pederson WC, eds: Operative Hand Surgery, 4th ed. New York, Churchill Livingstone, 1999: 1033–1047.

108. The correct response is C.

The structures likely to be damaged are the superficial and the deep motor branches of the median nerve. All other structures mentioned above are not likely to be damaged inadvertently, because they are placed at a deeper level.

Reference:

Nevaiser RJ. Acute infections. In Green DP, Hotchkiss RN, Pederson WC, eds: Operative Hand Surgery, 4th ed. New York, Churchill Livingstone, 1999: 1033–1047.

109. The correct response is B.

Boutonniere deformity of the proximal interphalangeal joint is due to damage to the central slip of the extensor expansion. The pus in the joint leaks out dorsally due to delay in treatment and causes necrosis of the central slip of the extensor expansion attached to the base of middle phalanx leading to loss of extension. The flexor power can no longer be kept in balance and hence the proximal interphalangeal joint develops flexion deformity called the Boutonniere deformity.

Reference:

Murray TM. Septic arthritis of the hand and wrist. Hand Clin 1998; 14: 579–587.

110. The correct response is D.

Supracondylar fractures lead to displaced fragments which can impale the brachial artery leading to major limb ischaemia which requires urgent intervention. Damage to nerves also may occur which should also be handled along with arterial injury.

Reference:

Raskin KB. Acute vascular injuries of the upper extremity. Hand Clin 1993; 9: 115–130.

111. The correct response is C.

A true aneurysm has all the three vessel walls in it and it is defined as permanent localized arterial dilatation amounting to more than 50% or greater increase above the normal diameter of the affected artery.

Reference:

Clagett GP. Upper extremity aneurysms. In Rutherford RB: Vascular Surgery, 4th ed. Philadelphia, WB Saunders, 1995: 1112–1123.

112. The correct response is E.

All of the options are true for reflex sympathetic dystrophy.

Reference:

Merritt WH. Reflex sympathetic dystrophy. In Achauer BM, ed: Plastic Surgery: Introduction, Operations, and Outcomes, vol 4. St. Louis, Mosby, 2000: 2337.

113. The correct response is E.

All of the features described are seen in reflex sympathetic dystrophy.

Reference:

1. *Lankford LL. Reflex sympathetic dystrophy. In Green DP, ed: Operative Hand Surgery, vol III. New York, Churchill Livingstone, 1997: 627–660.*
2. *Andrew KL, Poehling GG, Smith BP, Smith TL. Complex regional pain syndrome. Green-Operative Hand Surgery, 5th ed. 2005: 2015–2044.*

114. The correct response is A.

All of the features described are seen in reflex sympathetic dystrophy.

Reference:

Lankford LL. Reflex sympathetic dystrophy. In Green DP, ed: Operative Hand Surgery, vol III. New York, Churchill Livingstone, 1997: 627–660.

115. The correct response is E.

The onion peel appearance is not a feature of reflex sympathetic dystrophy. The other options are correct.

Reference:

Van der Laan L, Goris RJ. Reflex sympathetic dystrophy: an exaggerated regional inflammatory response? Hand Clin 1997;13: 373–385.

116. The correct response is E.

Paralysis is not a feature of VIC. The ischaemic contracture can however lead to paresis later on in due course of time. Richard von Volkmann was a General surgeon from 1830-1889.

Reference:

Lankford LL. Reflex sympathetic dystrophy. In Green DP, ed: Operative Hand Surgery, vol III. New York, Churchill Livingstone, 1997: 627–660.

117. The correct response is C.

Mydriasis is not a feature of Horner's syndrome. The rest of the options are correct.

Reference:

Lankford LL. Reflex sympathetic dystrophy. In Green DP, ed: Operative Hand Surgery, vol III. New York, Churchill Livingstone, 1997: 627–660.

118. The correct response is C.

The ulnar artery in the Guyon's canal is exposed to external occupational and recreational trauma and for this reason the Guyon's canal is the most common site for arterial thrombosis and aneurysm formation.

Reference:

1. *Raskin KB. Acute vascular injuries of the upper extremity. Hand Clin 1993; 9: 115–130.*
2. *Clagett GP. Upper extremity aneurysms. In Rutherford RB: Vascular Surgery, 4th ed. Philadelphia, WB Saunders, 1995: 1112–1123.*

119. The correct response is D.

A total of eight nerve compression syndromes are known to exist in the upper extremity:

(a) Due to compression of the median nerve:
   i. Carpal tunnel syndrome
   ii. Pronator syndrome
   iii. Anterior interrosseous nerve syndrome

(b) Due to compression of ulnar nerve:
   i. Guyon canal syndrome wrist
   ii. Cubital tunnel syndrome elbow

(c) Due to compression of radial nerve
   i. Radial sensory nerve entrapment forearm
   ii. Posterior interrosseous nerve forearm
   iii. Radial tunnel syndrome elbow

   (Felix J.C. Guyon was a French surgeon from 1831-1920)

Reference:

Rydevik B, Brown MD, Lundborg G. Pathoanatomy and pathophysiology of nerve root compression. Spine 1984; 9: 2.

120. The correct response is C.

Seven nerve compression syndromes have been described in the lower extremity.

1. Adductor canal syndrome in the medial thigh is due to compression of the saphenous nerve.
2. Fibular tunnel syndrome is due to compression of the common peroneal nerve on the lateral side of the upper end of fibula.
3. Anterolateral compartment syndrome is due to compression of the superficial peroneal nerve on the lateral side during crossing of the legs. The superficial peroneal nerve pierces the deep fascia about 15-16 cm above the lateral malleolus and then lies in the subcutaneous plane.
4. Deep peroneal nerve entrapment due to compression occurs on the dorsum of the foot producing abnormal sensations in the first and second toes.
5. Tarsal tunnel syndrome occurs at the medial ankle due to compression of tibial nerve as it travels through the tarsal tunnel.
6. Heel pain syndrome is due to compression of the medial calcaneal nerve in the region of the heel.
7. Morton neuroma at the ball of the foot is due to compression of the common plantar digital nerve in the web space between the third and fourth metatarsal bones.

Reference:

Dellon AL. Management of peripheral nerve problems in the upper and lower extremities using quantitative sensory testing. Hand Clin 1999; 15: 697.

121. The correct response is B.

If a patient has normal sensations in the little finger and motor weakness of the ulnar nerve, the lesion is likely to be distal to the Guyon's canal. This lesion, most of the time is a lipoma inside the palm.

Reference:

Dellon AL. Management of peripheral nerve problems in the upper and lower extremities using quantitative sensory testing. Hand Clin 1999; 15: 697.

122. The correct response is B.

Ulnar nerve compression at the elbow will produce weakness of the flexor carpi ulnaris and the flexor digitorum profundus of the ring and little fingers and hence would weaken the grip strength, and also weakness of the pinch. On the other hand ulnar nerve compression at the wrist (Guyon's canal) will produce motor weakness of the intrinsic muscles, especially adductor paralysis, which would affect the pinch mechanism but not the grip strength.

Reference:

Dellon AL. Management of peripheral nerve problems in the upper and lower extremities using quantitative sensory testing. Hand Clin 1999; 15: 697.

123. The correct response is B.

Cubital tunnel syndrome is compression of the ulnar nerve in the postcondylar groove at the elbow. Clumsiness is the commonest symptom consisting of complaints of dropping things and weakness of the little and ring fingers.

Reference:

1. *Dellon AL. Management of peripheral nerve problems in the upper and lower extremities using quantitative sensory testing. Hand Clin 1999; 15: 697.*
2. *Greenwald D, Moffitt W, Cooper A. Effective surgical treatment of cubital tunnel syndrome based on provocative clinical testing without electrodiagnostics. Plast Reconstr Surg 1999; 104: 210.*

124. The correct response is E.

All of the above are true. The surgery should be done under tourniquet. Use of bipolar cautery, loupe magnification and nerve stimulator are helpful aids.

Reference:

Jiranec W, Seiler WA, Dellon AL. Teaching the technique for microsurgical intraneural neurolysis. J Reconstr Microsurg 1987; 3: 137.

125. The correct response is D.

Clinical presentation of weakness of the flexor pollicis longus is indicative of compression of median nerve by deep head of pronator teres.

Reference:

Dellon AL, Mackinnon SE. Musculoaponeurotic variations along the course of the median nerve in the proximal forearm. J Hand Surg Br 1987; 12: 359.

126. The correct response is E.

All of the options are true. The nerve after decompression may get surrounded by scar tissue. There is invariably damage to the posterior branch of the medial ante-brachial cutaneous nerve which gets divided during the release, resulting into numbness behind the scar and neuroma anterior to the scar. Incomplete decompression may be responsible for referred pain to the little finger.

Reference:

Mackinnon SE. Injury to the medial antebrachial cutaneous nerve during cubital tunnelsurgery. J Hand Surg Br 1985; 10: 33.

127. The correct response is D.

The compression is at the level of the arcade of Frohse, which is due to a fascial band over the supinator muscle.

Reference:

1. *Eversmann WW Jr. Entrapment and compression neuropathies. In Green DP, ed: Operative Hand Surgery, 2nd ed. New York, Churchill Livingstone, 1988: 1423.*
2. *Green DP. Radial nerve palsy. Green's Operative Hand Surgery 5th ed. 2005: 1113–1129.*

128. The correct response is D.

The lateral femoral cutaneous nerve syndrome is due to entrapment of the nerve in the inguinal ligament. The nerve could pass through the ligament, or under it. It could be ensheathed in the sartorius muscle. Exploration, identification and release of the nerve provides relief.

Reference:

Aszmann OC, Dellon ES, Dellon AL. The anatomic course of the lateral femoral cutaneous nerve and its susceptibility to compression and injury. Plast Reconstr Surg 1997; 100: 600.

129. The correct response is D.

The treatment of tarsal tunnel syndrome consists of release of four separate medial ankle tunnels in addition to the tarsal tunnel. Releasing any one of the tunnel would not lead to amelioration of the symptoms as it is a group of four tunnels i.e. medial plantar tunnel, lateral planter tunnel, calcaneal tunnel and the tarsal tunnel under cover of the flexor retinaculum. All the nerves need to be released.

Reference:

Dellon AL. Surgical approach to the Tarsal Tunnel: Release of the Four Medial Ankle Tunnels [CD-ROM]. Baltimore, Md, Institute for Peripheral Nerve Surgery, 1998.

130. The correct response is C.

It is usually present between the third and fourth metatarsal. It is approached from the dorsal side through the web space. Intermetatarsal ligament is excised and metatarsal heads are separated. Neuroma is identified and a neurectomy of the nerve is done.

Thomas G. Morton was a US surgeon from 1835-1903.

Reference:

Keh RA, Odom R, Ballew KK et al. Long-term follow-up of Morton's neuroma. J Foot Surg 1992; 31: 93.

131. The correct response is C.

The superficial sensory branch of the radial nerve may get damaged in the process of removal of the ganglion and produce a painful neuroma.

Reference:

Herndon JH, Eaton RG, Littler JW. Management of painful neuromas in the hand. J Bone Joint Surg Am 1976; 58: 369.

132. The correct response is B.

The lesion most likely is a pyogenic granuloma which are small, erythematous, pedunculated lesions on fingertips which frequently readily bleed on touch.

Reference:

Weiss SW, Goldblum JR. Benign tumors and tumor-like lesions of blood vessels. In Weiss SW, Goldblum JR, eds: Enzinger and Weiss's Soft Tissue Tumors, 4th ed. St. Louis, Mosby, 2001: 837–890.

133. The correct response is B.

Handley used silk threads while Silver and Puckett used teflon and nylon threads. Goldsmith used omentum and O'Brien et al used lympho-venous anastomosis for treatment of lymphoedema. None of the procedure however gives lasting results.

Reference:

Silver D, Pukett CL. Lymphangioplasty: a ten year evaluation. Surgery 1976; 80: 748.

7

134. The correct response is B.

Thompson was the one who popularized the buried dermal flap procedure in 1970 for lymphedema. The de-epithelialisation of the flap is usually done with the dermatome and this flap is folded in to establish contact with the deep muscle and fascia. A significant reduction of the lymphedematous tissue is simultaneously done.

Reference:

1. *Thompson N. Buried dermal flap operation for chronic lymphedema of the extremities. Plast Reconstr Surg 1970; 45: 541.*
2. *Puckett CL. Lymphedema in the upper extremity. In May JW Jr, Littler JW eds: The Hand. Philadelphia, WB Saunders, 1990: 5023. McCarthy J, ed: Plastic Surgery; vol 8.*

135. The correct response is C.

The most appropriate method and order of repair is bone, tendons, nerves arteries and veins. Bony stabilisation precedes soft tissue repairs like vessel and nerve repair in such cases. Bony stability can be achieved by crossed K wires. The heavier structures like the tendons should be repaired first followed by microsurgery for vessels and nerves. Arterial repair usually precedes venous repair, because the venous engorgement helps with identification of the best veins for anastomosis or grafting. The timing of the repairs often depends on tourniquet time but may be done either before the arterial repairs or after the venous repairs.

Reference:

1. *Neumeister MW, Brown RE. Mutilating hand injuries: principles and management. Hand Clin. 2003; 19:1.*
2. *Wilhelmi BJ, Lee WP, Pagensteert GI, et al. Replantation in the mutilated hand. Hand Clin. 2003; 19:89.*

136. The correct response is C.

The palmaris longus tendon serves as the best source of graft for tendon reconstruction. It is locally available and its presence can also be assessed preoperatively. Fascia lata can also be used as a graft but requires a distant site. Temporalis fascia is too thin to be used as a tendon graft. The flexor pollicis muscle and lumbricals are not expendable muscles and hence are unsuitable for tendon grafting.

Reference:

1. *Neumeister MW, Brown RE. Mutilating hand injuries: principles and management. Hand Clin. 2003; 19:1.*
2. *Hentz V, Chase R. Hand Surgery: A Clinical Atlas. Philadelphia, WB Saunders, 2001: 452–457.*

137. The correct response is C.

The patient has sustained injury to the extensor of the distal interphalangeal joint which is the cause of flexion of the finger tip due to unopposed action of the flexor digitorum profundus. This condition is called as mallet finger. The type of splint recommended for mallet finger is a stack splint which helps to maintain the finger tip in extension.

Reference:

1. *Brand P, Hollister A. Clinical Mechanics of the Hand. St. Louis, Mosby-Year Book, 1999.*
2. *Hentz V, Chase R. Hand Surgery. A Clinical Atlas. Philadelphia, WB Saunders, 2001: 452–457.*

138. The correct response is C.

The clinical picture is consistent with the diagnosis of cleft hand. This is due to type I failure of formation leading to longitudinal arrest. The central ray of the hand is affected and usually appears without proximal deficiencies of nerves, vessels, tendons and muscles. The cleft is 'V' shaped which helps to recognise this deformity and also to differentiate it from symbrachydacytyly where the cleft is 'U' shaped.

Reference:

1. *Miura T, Suzuki M. Clinical differences between typical and atypical cleft hand. J Hand Surg Br 1984; 9: 98-02.*
2. *Nutt J, Flatt A. Congenital central hand deficit. Hand Surg 1981; 6: 48-60.*

139. The correct response is D.

The largest single group of thumb polydactyly occurs at or proximal to the MP joint. It falls in Iowa type IV classification. One or both of the thumbs may have an extra phalanx. The triphalangeal rays can be either balanced when both the partners have extra bones or unbalanced when only one side is abnormal.

Reference:

1. *Barsky A. Congenital anomalies of the thumb. Clin Orthop 1959; 15: 96-110.*
2. *Wood V. Treatment of the triphalangeal thumb. Clin Orthop 1976; 120: 188-200.*

8

RECENT ADVANCES

QUESTIONS

1. **The logo of a sheep for the American Plastic surgery research council was selected in 1995 because of which of the following consideration?**
   A. Sheep is docile and helpful
   B. Sheep is often used as an experimental animal
   C. Sheep has been used for autografting and allografting
   D. None of the above

2. **The process of establishment of blood supply in the grafted skin is termed which one of the following?**
   A. Neovascularization
   B. Angiogenesis
   C. Vasculogenesis
   D. Inosculation

3. **Peripheral nerves are prone to compression at multiple places. Which one of the following nerve has the least number of possible sites for developing a compression neuropathy?**
   A. Radial
   B. Median
   C. Ulnar
   D. Greater occipital
   E. Sural

4. **Which one of the following method is most suitable for reconstructing a nipple for achieving an optimal result?**
   A. Spiral flap
   B. Top hat flap
   C. Double opposing flap
   D. Diamond shaped flap
   E. C-V flap

5. **The frontal branch of facial nerve in high SMAS facelift surgery is not liable to injury in which one of the following location?**
   A. Above the zygomatic arch
   B. 1.5 cm below the zygomatic arch
   C. Near the parotid gland
   D. At lower border of the zygomatic arch
   E. Pre-auricular region

6. **The frontal branch of the facial nerve has which one of the following relationship with the zygomatic arch?**
   A. It lies above the periosteum of the arch
   B. It lies below the periosteum of the arch
   C. It lies deep to the arch
   D. It passes through the zygomatic arch

7. **The preferred position of the scar following use of latissimus dorsi flap in breast reconstruction is which one of the following?**
   A. Vertical
   B. Oblique
   C. Upper transverse
   D. Middle transverse
   E. Lower transverse

8. Which one of the following is not a long-term abdominal consequence following use of TRAM flap?
A. Abdominal weakness and bulge
B. Hernia
C. Reduced abdominal strength
D. Reduced exercise tolerance and respiratory efficiency
E. Vertical scarring

9. Which one of the following is a more common site for the origin of migraine?
A. Frontal area
B. Occipital area
C. Temporal area
D. Nasal area
E. Parietal area

10. Absent columella in bilateral clefts can be reconstructed by which one of the following?
A. V-Y plasty
B. Z plasty
C. Prolabial flap
D. Conchal chondrocutaneous graft
E. Abbe flap

11. Cervical liposuction is done for removal of fat in the submental region. The submental fat is present in which one of the following location?
A. Superficial to the platysma muscle
B. Deep to the platysma muscle
C. Both above and below the plastysma muscle
D. In the midline of the neck between the digastric muscle

12. The vascularity of which one of the following zones is doubtful when a medial perforator based on deep inferior epigastric artery flap (DIEP) is used for breast reconstruction?
A. Zone I
B. Zone II
C. Zone III
D. Zone IV
E. Zone V

13. Extensive haemangiomas of the face in infants involving the eyelid and causing visual obstruction can be best treated by which one of the following modality?
A. Oral corticosteroid
B. Oral antibiotic
C. Laser
D. Cryotherapy
E. Surgery

14. Which one of the following is not a feature of the simple type of Poland's syndrome?
A. Absence of pectoralis major muscle
B. Non-muscular anterior axillary fold
C. Deformed hemithorax
D. Displaced smaller breast and nipple-areola complex
E. Abnormal chest hairs

15. Which one of the following is not a feature of the complex form of Poland's syndrome?
A. Absence of pectoralis major muscle
B. Non-muscular anterior axillary fold
C. Axillary web
D. Bony cage deformity
E. Simple syndactyly

16. Which one of the following is not an indication for the inferiorly based peroneus brevis muscle flap?
A. Post-traumatic defects around the ankle
B. Exposed tibia in the middle third of leg
C. Loss of great toe
D. Comminuted fractures of calcaneum
E. Loss of heel pad

17. Gummy smile is a condition when more than 2 mm of the gums get exposed during smiling. It can be treated by which one of the following method?
A. LeFort I osteotomy
B. Resection of the levator labii superioris
C. Frenectomy
D. All of the above

18. Which one of the following is not a characteristic feature of a youthful neck?
A. Well defined mandibular border with cervico-mental angle of 105°–120°
B. Well defined sternocleidomastoid muscles
C. Well defined thyroid bulge
D. Well defined subhyoid depression
E. Well defined digastric muscle belly

19. Which one of the following is not a characteristic feature of an aged neck?
A. Ill defined mandibular border with jowls
B. Obtuse cervicomental angle
C. Loose hanging skin folds
D. Prominent anterior belly of digastric muscles
E. Well defined thyroid bulge

20. **The nasion is a point where the nose begins. Which one of the following describes its relationship with the nasofrontal suture?**
    A. It overlies the nasofrontal suture
    B. It is above the level of the nasofrontal suture
    C. It is below the level of the nasofrontal suture
    D. It is 1.5 cm below the level of the nasofrontal suture

21. **The superficial musculoaponeurotic system (SMAS) is a recognized entity. The muscle fibers in this layer come from which one of the following structure?**
    A. Platysma
    B. Temporalis muscle
    C. Transverse nuchae muscle
    D. Frontalis muscle
    E. Corrugator muscle

22. **A tear trough depression is present below the medial canthus in facial aging. It is bounded by all the following muscles except which one of the following?**
    A. Orbicularis oculi
    B. Levator labii superioris
    C. Levator labii superioris alaequae nasi
    D. Zygomaticus minor muscle

23. **It is a well known fact that wounds in the foetus heal without scarring. Which one of the following statements about fetal wound healing is not true?**
    A. Presence of type III collagen in abundance
    B. High levels of hyaluronic acid
    C. Platelet aggregation is low
    D. Excess of inflammatory cells
    E. Excess of progenitor cells

24. **Which one of the following statements about fetal fibroblasts is true?**
    A. Fetal fibroblasts synthesize less type III and IV collagen
    B. Fetal fibroblasts do not proliferate and synthesize collagen simultaneously
    C. Fetal fibroblasts have less affinity for hyaluronic acid
    D. Fetal wounds are devoid of myofibroblasts

25. **The first full face allotransplant was performed by plastic surgeons belonging to which one of the following country?**
    A. France
    B. USA
    C. UK
    D. Germany
    E. Australia

26. **The first full face transplant patient died within two months of surgery due to which one of the following complication?**
    A. Cardiac arrest
    B. Infection
    C. Respiratory failure
    D. Renal failure
    E. Graft versus host disease

27. **The face of the donor of the first full face allotransplant was restored with all due respects by which one of the following method?**
    A. Alginate mould
    B. Resin mould
    C. Simple mask
    D. Acrylic mould
    E. Wax mould

28. **The temporomandibular joint injuries in children are commonly intracapsular in nature due to which one of the following factor?**
    A. Severity of injury
    B. Anatomical considerations
    C. Nature of injury
    D. Presence of osteopenia
    E. Age of child

29. **The stem cell isolation from the aspirated fat for use in plastic surgery involves many steps including putting them in the water bath at 37-° C, centrifugation, mixing with 1mg/ml of collagenase and diluting with 1:1 with Trypan blue stain. The stem cell count would be maximum in which one of the following layer of the processed fat sample?**
    A. Upper layer
    B. Middle layer
    C. Bottom layer
    D. Uniformly distributed

30. **Flap monitoring is an essential postoperative part of plastic surgery. Which one of the following flap monitoring method is the most reliable?**
    A. Colour of flap
    B. Colour sonography
    C. Infrared spectroscopy
    D. Laser doppler flowmetry

31. **Aging in skin depends on many factors. Which one of the following skin types is likely to show aging earlier than the others?**
    A. Individuals with oily skin
    B. Individuals with dry skin
    C. Pigmented skin
    D. Non pigmented skin

32. The lower eyelid has three fat compartments, which are medial, central and lateral. Which one of the following structure separates the central from the lateral compartment?

A. Inferior oblique muscle
B. Lockwood's ligament
C. Inferior rectus
D. Whitnall's ligament

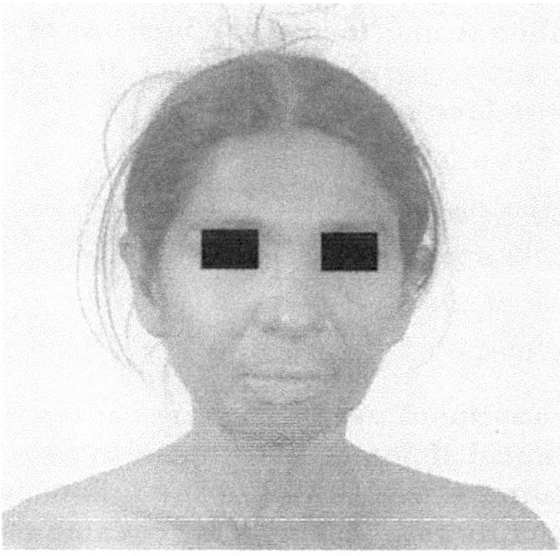

33. A 26-year-old female presents with recurrent cervical contracture of 3 years duration. Which one of the following would be the best method of treating this contracture?

A. Dynamic splinting
B. Meshed split thickness graft
C. Thick split thickness graft
D. Full thickness graft
E. Supraclavicular flap

34. The short scar periareolar inferior pedicle reduction (SPAIR) mammaplasty has proven to be a reliable and versatile method of breast reduction. This technique bases the blood supply to the nipple and areola on an inferior pedicle using which one of the following skin resection pattern ?

A. Inverted 'T' resection
B. Vertical resection
C. Circular resection
D. Circumvertical resection
E. Horizontal resection

35. Liposuction derived stem cells have recently been shown to be capable of differentiating into bone. The introduction of a three dimensional scaffold significantly enhances gene markers of angiogenesis and osteogenesis. Which one of the following is primarily responsible for promoting angiogenesis in three dimensional scaffolds at early time points and then also enhances bone formation by stimulating chemotactic migration and proliferation of primary human osteoblasts ?

A. JNK2
B. TIMP3
C. VEGF
D. TXNIP
E. CBFA-1

36. Reconstruction of large full thickness defects of the upper eyelid is challenging. Which one of the following reconstructive procedure does not block the visual axis and is preferred for patients who are monocular ?

A. Cutler-Beard flap
B. Mustarde flap
C. Hughes flap
D. Orbicularis oris myocutaneous advancement flap
E. Landolt procedure

37. Tobacco has many carcinogenic compounds and is the leading preventable cause of squamous cell carcinoma of the head and neck. In addition active smoking adversely affects wound healing and end organ oxygen delivery. Smokers however do not report accurately on their smoking habits. In head and neck reconstruction which one of the following is a reliable preoperative indicator of cigarette smoking?

A. Self reported smoking status
B. Serum aldehyde oxidase concentration
C. Serum cotinine concentration
D. Serum nicotine concentration
E. Kaplan Feinstein comorbidity scale

38. Transplantation of tissues between identical twins continues to be an important surgical treatment modality. The principles of transplantation have been applied to a variety of circumstances for reconstruction. Which of the following organs and tissues have been successfully transplanted between identical twins?

A. Full thickness skin graft
B. Small bowel
C. Prepuce mucosal graft
D. Ovarian cortical tissue
E. All of the above

39. Perforator based island flaps are widely used to reconstruct skin defects. Many methods are available to map the location and blood flow of a perforator. Which one of the following modality is most effective for detecting the distribution of flap blood flow both intraoperatively and postoperatively?

A. Magnetic resonance angiography
B. Computed tomographic angiography
C. Recovery enhanced thermography
D. Indocyanine green angiography
E. Ultrasonic doppler flowmetry

40. Fat necrosis is a common complication arising after autologous breast reconstruction. This is seen after all types of autologous reconstruction including pedicled and free flaps. Which one of the following is a safe and effective treatment for fat necrosis?

A. Wait and watch approach
B. Infrared therapy
C. Standard liposuction
D. Ultrasound-Assisted liposuction
E. Direct excision

41. The lateral vertical ligament of 'Wuringer' is related to surgery of which one of the following?

A. Face
B. Breast
C. Neck
D. Hand
E. Pelvis

42. Fractures of the palate are frequently associated with LeFort maxillary fractures in midfacial trauma. These occur in patients who have sustained high energy accidents and their presence poses diagnostic and therapeutic challenges and may result in malunion and occlusal problems. Which one of the following modality is a cost effective and less time-consuming method of treating palatal fractures while achieving anatomical occlusion with good bony union?

A. Kirschner wire fixation
B. Interosseous wiring
C. Acrylic palatal splints
D. Intermolar wiring
E. Open reduction and internal fixation

43. The term 'iTAMe' refers to intraoperative total active movement examination and is related to surgery of which one of the following?

A. Eye ball
B. Maxilla
C. Mandible
D. Tendon
E. All of the above

44. A major limitation in implant-based breast reconstruction is capsular contracture especially if irradiation is to be given. The reported incidence of identifiable capsular contracture in breast reconstruction patients is very high underlining the need of research to identify likely causes of contracture in this setting. Which one of the following serves as the best animal model to study silicone gel-related capsular contracture?

A. Rabbit
B. Monkey
C. Mice
D. Pig
E. All of the above

45. Scar formation after surgery is a major concern to both patients and surgeons. Studies have focussed on understanding and replicating the scar-free healing seen in foetuses. Which one of the following currently represents the first of a new drug that can reduce scarring?

A. Triamcinolone acetonide
B. Bleomycin
C. Placentrex
D. Avotermin
E. Topical Tamoxifen

46. Recreational use of cocaine causes a wide range of nasal defects that contribute to a stigmatic deformity. Which one of the following is the first structure to be involved by cocaine abuse?

A. Tip of nose
B. Nasal septum
C. Nasal mucosa
D. Ala
E. Columella

47. Capsular contracture remains a major problem in patients with breast reconstruction using implants who undergo irradiation. Recent studies have suggested the role of transforming growth factors in contracture formation. Which one of the following is likely to result in interruption of irradiation induced capsular contracture?

A. Blocking of Smad 3 signalling
B. Using slit beam irradiation
C. Using thick capsule
D. Using fractionated irradiation
E. All of the above

48. Gelsolin amyloidosis is a dominantly inherited syndrome in which the collection of amyloid occurs in the tissues of the body. Which one of the following is a manifestation of this disease that presents a patient to the plastic surgeon?

A. Facial hyperpigmentation
B. Excessive facial hairs
C. Facial sweating
D. Facial nerve paralysis
E. Facial erythema

49. Transoral robotic surgery is now being increasingly used for treatment of head and neck cancers. Which one of the following is a common indication of this modality?

A. Performing microvascular anastomoses

B. Dissection of free flaps

C. Resection and insetting of flaps in deep seated oral lesions

D. Osteosynthesis of craniofacial skeleton

E. Performing various ostetomies in the craniofacial skeleton

50. Human adipose-derived stromal cells (ASCs) are able to repair calvarial defects in experimental animals. This response is mediated by expression of BMP and platelet rich plasma. Which one of the following type of calvarial defect is likely to be healed by human ASCs?

A. Clean cut calvarial defect

B. Calvarial defect with irregular margins

C. Acute calvarial defect

D. Chronic calvarial defect with good skin cover

E. All of the above

51. Healing of skin incisions is important in plastic surgery and this is dependent to some extent on the type of device used for making the incision. The currently available devices for skin incision differ as regards the acute thermal injury depth, inflammation and the amount of scarring produced in the skin. Which one of the following produces the least amount of thermal injury depth, inflammatory response and scar width in healing skin?

A. Bard Parker scalpel blade

B. PlasmaBlade

C. Valleylab electrosurgical pencil

D. All of the above

ANSWERS, EXPLANATIONS AND REFERENCES

1. The correct response is C.

The logo of a sheep was selected because the sheep was used for autografting of skin within an hour by Baronio of Italy in 1804 and the graft survived. The research was however used in clinical practice quite some years later. The logo was proposed by Dr. Richard Stark.

Reference:

Glotzbach JP, Levi B, Wong VW. Basic science of vascular biology. Plast Reconstr Surg 2010; 125 (6): 1528–1538.

2. The correct response is D.

The process of establishment of the blood supply into a piece of grafted skin from the host bed i.e. joining of vascular network is called inosculation. The process does not include growth of new blood vessels. Neovascularization is defined as formation of new blood vessels. It can be either angiogenesis or vasculogenesis. Angiogenesis as defined as proliferation of mature local endothelium to form new blood vessels e.g. in cases of vascular delay of flaps, wound healing where new blood vessels sprout to form granulation tissues. vasculogenesis involves recruitment of bone marrow derived cells to ischemic areas to help in the formation of new blood vessels e.g. occlusive limb ischemia, myocardial ischemia, transfer of free tissue flaps etc.

Reference:

Glotzbach JP, Levi B, Wong VW. Basic science of vascular biology. Plast Reconstr Surg 2010; 125 (6): 1528–1538.

3. The correct response is B

Median nerve is the one that has the least number of possible sites for developing a compression neuropathy. It has five sites of compression, while the other nerves have six.

Reference:

Jainis JE. Anatomy of greater occipital nerve. Plast Reconstr Surg 2010; 126 (5): 1563–1572.

4. The correct response is D.

The diamond shaped flap is easy to design and would give a good result.

Reference:

Malcolm L, Liu TS. The diamond double opposing V-Y flap- A reliable simple and versatile technique for nipple reconstruction: Plast Reconstr Surg. 2010; 125: 1643–1648.

5. The correct response is A.

The frontal branch of the facial nerve is not liable to injury above the zygomatic arch, because it is protected by a layer of fascia (parotid temporal fascia), which is a continuation of the parotid-masseteric fascia. The parotid–temporal fascia has previously been described as superficial temporal fascia. It lies deep to the SMAS layer and frontal branch of the facial nerve lies deep to the temporal–parietal fascia. Therefore the nerve is not likely to be damaged in upper high-SMAS facelift surgery, where SMAS is excised above the zygomatic arch.

The nerve lies superficial to the periosteum of the zygomatic arch. It pierces the temporo- parietal fascia and then travels with the anterior branch of superficial temporal artery towards the forehead.

Reference:

Trussler AP, Stephan P, Hatef D et al. The frontal branch of facial nerve across the zygomatic arch: Anatomical Relevance of the High-SMAS technique. Plast Reconstr Surg 2010; 125: 1221–1229.

6. The correct response is A.

The frontal branch of the facial nerve lies above the periosteum of the zygomatic arch. At the upper border of the zygomatic arch, it is protected by a layer of a fascia and is hence not liable to injury at this location.

Reference:

Trussler AP, Stephan P, Hatef D et al. The frontal branch of facial nerve across the zygomatic arch: Anatomical Relevance of the High-SMAS technique. Plast Reconstr Surg 2010; 125: 1221–1229.

7. The correct response is E.

The majority of women prefer the lower transverse scar. It can be easily hidden in the dress or swim-wear. The appearance of the scar is also satisfactory.

Reference:

Kendall RR, Donold P, Chevray PM. Evaluation of outcomes in breast reconstructions combining lower abdominal free flaps and permanent implants. Plast Reconstr Surg, 2010; 126: 349–366.

8. The correct response is E.

Vertical scarring is not a feature following the use of TRAM flap.

Reference:

Derrick C, Charles Y et al. Inclusion of mesh in donor-site repair of free and muscle-sparing free TRAM flaps yields rates of abdominal complications comparable to those of DIEP flap reconstruction. Plast Reconstr Surg 2010; 126: 367–374.

9. The correct response is C.

The temporal area is a common site of origin of the migraine headache. It is due to the zygomatico-temporal nerve getting compressed at its exit from the temporal muscle. The frontal migraine is due to entrapment of the supraorbital and supratrochlear nerves in the corrugator muscle. The occipital headache is due to entrapment of the greater, lesser and/ or the third occipital nerves.

Reference:

Janis JE, Daniel A, Hatef HT et al. The zygomatico-temporal branch of trigeminal nerve: Part II. Anatomical variations. Plast Reconstr Surg 2010; 126: 435–442.

10. The correct response is C.

The prolabial flap is helpful in reconstructing the absent columella and also provides the desired color match. Conchal chondrocutaneous graft can also be used but the color match of the conchal skin would not be as good.

Reference:

Cheon YW, Park BY. Long term evaluation of elongating columella using conchal composite graft in bilateral secondary cleft lip nose deformity. Plast Reconstr Surg 2010; 126: 543–553.

11. The correct response is C.

The fat is present below the skin and subcutaneous tissue both in the superficial and the deeper plane of the platysma. The subplatysmal fat has a central, medial and lateral distribution. The lateral fat is superficial to submandibular salivary gland and the digastric muscle. Liposuction is done for the fat superficial to the platysma muscle.

Reference:

Rohrich RJ, Pessa JE. The subplatysmal supramylohoid fat. Plast Reconstr Surg 2010; 126: 589–595.

12. The correct response is D.

The largest perforator of the deep inferior epigastric artery (DIEP) is near the umbilicus. It is about 2 mm in diameter. The vascularity in zone I and zone II i.e paramedian area is good. The vascularity in zone III on the same side allows it to partially survive. The vascularity of the zone IV which is on the other side (contralateral) is not good, being farthest away from the perforator.

Reference:

Bailey SH, Michel SC, Wong C et al. The single dominant medial row perforator DIEP flap in breast reconstruction. The three dimensional perforasome and clinical results. Plast Reconstr Surg 2010; 126: 739–751.

13. The correct response is A.

Oral corticosteroids are helpful for reduction of swelling and volume of extensive haemangiomas. If oral corticosteroids 2 mg/kg/day do not produce the desired clinical improvement in 2-3 months, then oral b-blockers should be used. Propanolol in the dose of 2 mg/kg/day of body weight in divided doses can be given under medical guidance and evaluation of the cardio respiratory system. Residual lesion can be tackled with pulsed dye laser therapy.

Reference:

Arneja JS, Pegg N, Tor A et al. Management of complicated facial haemangiomas with B- blocker (Propanolol) therapy. Plast Reconstr Surg 2010; 126: 889–895.

14. The correct response is C.

The hemithorax may be smaller but is not deformed.

Reference:

Seyfer AE, Fox JP, Hamilton CG. Poland syndrome: Evaluation and treatment of the chest wall in 63 patients. Plast Reconstr Surg 2010; 126: 902–911.

15. The correct response is E.

Simple syndactyly is a feature of simple type of Poland's syndrome. In the complex type of Poland syndrome, the entire upper extremity is smaller and is associated with brachydactyly.

Reference:

Seyfer AE, Fox JP, Hamilton CG. Poland syndrome: Evaluation and treatment of the chest wall in 63 patients. Plast Reconstr Surg 2010; 126: 902–911.

16. The correct response is C.

The inferiorly based peroneus brevis flap can not be used for defects of the great toe. Proximally based peroneus brevis flap can be used for repairing defects of the tendoachilles. The other options are valid indications for the use of this flap.

Reference:

Schmidt AB, Giessler FA. The muscular and the new osteomuscular composite peroneus brevis flap: Experiences from 109 cases. Plast Reconstr Surg 2010; 126: 924–932.

17. The correct response is D.

All of the above are modalities for the treatment of gummy smile.

Reference:

Ishida LH, Ishida LC, Ishida J et al. Myotomy of levator labii superioris muscle and lip repositioning: A combined approach for the correction of gummy smile. Plast Reconstr Surg 2010; 126: 1014–1019.

18. The correct response is E.

The digastric muscle belly lies hidden in the submental region. The prominence is not related to the appearance of a youthful neck.

Reference:

Guyuron B, Sadek EY, Ahmadian R. A 26-year experience with vest-over-pants technique of platysmarrhaphy. Plast Reconstr Surg 2010; 126: 1027–1036.

19. The correct response is E.

The thyroid cartilage loses its prominence due to laxity of the neck skin and excessive fat on the supraplatysmal region. The treatment consists of removal of excess fat through a submental incision. The platysma muscle is either approximated in the midline or if possible it is double breasted. The excess skin is removed. This can be combined with a facelift procedure.

Reference:

Guyuron B, Sadek EY, Ahmadian R. A 26-year experience with vest-over-pants technique of platysmarrhaphy. Plast Reconstr Surg, 2010; 126: 1027–1036.

20. The correct response is B.

The nasion is above the level of the nasofrontal suture. The nasofrontal suture is 1.3 mm ± 0.6 mm below the nasion.

Reference:

Tsai FC, Liao CK, Fong TH et al. Analysis of nasal periosteum and nasofrontal suture with clinical implications for dorsal nasal augmentation. Plast Reconstr Surg 2010; 126: 1037–1047.

21. The correct response is C.

The muscle fibers in the SMAS come from the transverse nuchae muscle.

Reference:

Lei T, Cui L, Zhang YZ et al. Anatomy of the transversus nuchae muscle and its relationship with the superficial musculoaponeurotic system. Plast Reconstr Surg 2010; 126: 1058–1062.

22. The correct response is D.

The zygomaticus minor muscle lies laterally and does not contribute to the formation of tear trough depression. It helps in forming the nasolabial fold.

Reference:

Friedland JA, Lalonde DH, Rohrich RJ. An evidence based approach to blepharoplasty. Plast Reconstr Surg 2010; 126: 2222–2229.

23. The correct response is D.

The inflammatory cells in foetal wounds are few. The progenitor cells are in excess. They migrate to the site of injury and help in scar-less healing.

Reference:

Larson BJ, Longaker MT, Lorenz MP. Scar-less fetal wound healing: A basic science review. Plast Reconstr Surg 2010; 126: 1172–1180.

24. The correct response is D.

Fetal wounds are devoid of myofibroblasts. On the other hand the adult wounds have demonstrable myofibroblasts in the 1st week of wounding. The number of myofibroblast increases manifold in the second and third week of wounding.

Reference:

Larson BJ, Longaker MT, Lorenz MP. Scar-less fetal wound healing: A basic science review. Plast Reconstr Surg 2010; 126: 1172–1180.

25. The correct response is A.

It was the French who are credited with performing the first full face allotransplant. A total of 33 fresh cadavers were studied to evaluate the difficulties in procurement of the eyelid musculature, temporomandibular joint, ears, facial nerve, trigeminal nerve, lip, nose, scalp and to evaluate whether one or both external carotid arteries are needed for adequate supply of blood. Thyrolinguofacial trunks were used for venous anastomosis.

Reference:

Meningaud JP, Benjoar MD, Hivelin M et al. Procurement of total human face graft for allotransplantation: A preclinical study and the first clinical case. Plast Reconstr Surg, 2010; 126: 1881–1190.

26. The correct response is B.

The patient developed infection due to Pseudomonas on the fifteenth day and swelling of the face and hands which required sequential debridement. He could not cope up and died within two months.

Reference:

Meningaud JP, Benjoar MD, Hivelin M et al. Procurement of total human face graft for allotransplantation: A preclinical study and the first clinical case. Plast Reconstr Surg 2010; 126: 1881–1190.

27. The correct response is B.

An alginate impression was taken beforehand and a resin mould was prepared to respectfully restore the face of donor.

Reference:

Meningaud JP, Benjoar MD, Hivelin M et al. Procurement of total human face graft for allotransplantation: A preclinical study and the first clinical case. Plast Reconstr Surg 2010; 126: 1881–1190.

28. The correct response is B.

In children the neck of the mandible is broad, hence the force of the injury gets transmitted up to the condyle which gets fractured leading to intracapsular injuries. On the other hand the neck of the mandible in adults is narrow and easily gets fractured by the transmitted force causing extracapsular fracture.

Reference:

Allori AC, Chang CC, Farina R et al. Current concepts in pediatric temporomandibular joint disorders: Part I. Etiology, Epidemiology and Classification. Plast Reconstr Surg 2010; 126: 1263–1275.

29. The correct response is C.

The number of stem cells would be maximum in the bottom layer.

Reference:

Crawford JL, Hubbard BA, Colbert SH et al. Fine tuning lipoaspirate viability for fat grafting. Plast Reconstr Surg 2010; 126: 1342–1348.

30. The correct response is D.

Laser doppler flowmetry is a non-invasive method. It allows continuous monitoring. Light is passed into flap. The scattered light is collected by the same probe to detect the blood flow.

Reference:

Smit JM, Zeebregts CJ, Acosta A et al. Advancement in free flap monitoring in the last decade: A critical review. Plast Reconstr Surg 2010; 125: 177–183.

31. The correct response is B.

Individuals with dry skin will show early aging. Individuals with oily skin have more of sebaceous glands. These glands produce Vit E. Alpha-tocopherol and gamma-tocopherol. These are antioxidants and help protect the skin and delay the aging process.

Reference:

Graf J. Antioxidants and skin care: the essentials. Plast Reconstr Surg 2010; 125: 378–383.

32. The correct response is B.

The arcuate expansion of the Lockwood's ligament separates the central from the lateral compartment. The medial and the central compartments are separated by the inferior oblique muscle. The upper eyelid has two compartments, nasal and central.

Reference:

Pacella SJ, Nahai FR. Transconjunctival blepharoplasty for upper and lower eyelids. Plast Reconstr Surg 2010; 125: 384-–92.

33. The correct response is E

A local flap is always preferred over a graft for treating contractures and specifically recurrent contractures. Out of the options given, the supraclavicular artery flap is the method of choice for reconstructing cervical contractures. The supraclavicular area is also unburnt in this case and hence is suitable for resurfacing.

Dynamic splinting is helpful for incipient contracture or after surgical release of contracture to maintain the result. A meshed split thickness skin graft is liable to contracture and meshing also gives an unacceptable result cosmetically. The meshed pattern is permanently retained and has an unattractive "reptilian" appearance. Thick split-thickness skin grafts contract less and provide a more durable skin coverage but do not possess elastic properties. Full thickness skin grafts are more reliable for cervicofacial burn reconstruction. These are elastic, contract less and have a "matte finish" like normal skin. These however are limited in quantity and require a well-vascularised bed. Regional flaps are the best options in terms of their elasticity and texture match and therefore constitute an excellent option for reconstruction of cervical contractures.

The supraclavicular artery flap is based on transverse cervical artery. It is about 6–7 cm wide and about 10 cm long. It can be easily raised & donor site closed primarily.

Reference:

Chiu ES, Perry H L, Friend Lander PL. Supraclavicular artery island flap for head & neck oncologic reconstruction. Plast Reconstr Surg 2009; 124: 115–123.

34. The correct response is C

The short scar periareolar inferior pedicle reduction (SPAIR) mammaplasty has proven to be a reliable and versatile method of breast reduction. This technique bases the blood supply to the nipple and areola on an inferior pedicle using a circumvertical skin resection pattern to manage the redundant skin envelope.

The areola is placed under maximal stretch and an areolar diameter ~ 44 mm is drawn and incised. The outer periareolar incision is then incised and the intervening skin is deepithelialized. Medial and superior flaps are then developed. The inferior pedicle is resuspended superiorly to the pectoralis major fascia as needed to lift and reposition the pedicle.

Reference:

1. *Hammond D. Short scar periareolar inferior pedicle reduction (SPAIR) mammaplasty. Plast Reconstr Surg 1999; 103: 890.*
2. *Hammond D. Short scar periareolar inferior pedicle reduction (SPAIR) mammaplasty. Oper Tech Plast Reconstr Surg 1999; 6: 106.*

35. The correct response is C

Liposuction derived stem cells have recently been shown to be capable of differentiating into bone. The introduction of a three dimensional scaffold significantly enhances gene markers of angiogenesis and osteogenesis. VEGF (Vascular endothelial growth factor) promotes angiogenesis in three dimensional scaffolds at early time points and then also enhances bone formation by stimulating chemotactic migration and proliferation of primary human osteoblasts.

A VEGF scaffold has been created which has demonstrated increased blood vessel density at 2 weeks and later at 12 weeks. JNK2 is a signal transduction protein for osteogenic differentiation, TIMP3 is gene for extracellular matrix remodelling, TXNIP is gene for hypoxia and CBFA-1 is a terminal osteogenic gene transcription factor.

Reference:

1. *Mayr-Wohlfart U, Waltenberger J, Hausser H et al. Vascular endothelial growth factor stimulates chemotactic migration of primary human osteoblasts. Bone 2002; 30: 472.*
2. *Huang CK, Huang W, Zuk P et al. Genetic markers of Osteogenesis and Angiogenesis are altered in processed lipoaspirate cells when cultured on three-dimensional scaffolds. Plast Reconstr Surg 2008; 121: 411.*

36. The correct response is D

Upper eyelid reconstruction is unique and challenging. There are particular requirements for this procedure to restore good function and cosmesis. It is important to create a mobile upper lid with good height and contour. Good eyelid closure is necessary to prevent exposure keratopathy. A number of procedures are available to repair large to total upper eyelid defects. These techniques include composite eyelid grafts, Cutler-Beard flap from the lower eyelid, the Mustarde flap, the Hughes or Landolt procedure, inferiorly based tarsoconjunctival flap and the orbicularis oculi myocutaneous advancement flap.

Of these the orbicularis oculi advancement flap is single staged and does not block the visual axis for monocular patients and thereby reduces the recovery time for the patient. The rest are two staged procedures which occlude the visual axis.

Reference:

1. *Demir Z, Yuce S, Karamursel et al. Orbicularis oculi myocutaneous advancement flap for upper eyelid reconstruction. Plast Reconstr Surg 2008; 121: 443.*
2. *Yoshimura Y, Nakajima T, Yoneda K. Reconstruction of the entire upper eyelid area with a subcutaneous pedicle flap based on the orbicularis oculi muscle. Plast Reconstr Surg 1991; 88: 136.*

37. The correct response is C

Tobacco has many carcinogenic compounds and is the leading preventable cause of squamous cell carcinoma of the head and neck. In addition active smoking adversely affects wound healing and end organ oxygen delivery. Smokers however do not report accurately on their smoking habits. In head and neck reconstruction, serum cotinine concentration greater than 10 ng/ml predicts an increased risk of wound complications in head and neck reconstruction.

Patients often do not report correctly on their smoking status. Therefore self reported questionnaires are unreliable. There are no means by which serum nicotine concentrations can be accurately and reliably measured beyond several hours of smoking because the half life of nicotine is only 0.05 to 2 hours. Nicotine is hepatically metabolized by the cytochrome P450 system in a two step process (CYP2A6 and aldehyde oxidase) to cotinine. The half-life of cotinine is 18 to 24 hours which makes it a more reliable marker of recent nicotine exposure. A serum cotinine concentration greater than 50 ng /ml represents active smoking.

The Kaplan Feinstein comorbidity scale reflects the presence of comorbid disease which is an independent predictor of survival in squamous cell carcinoma of the head and neck.

Reference:

1. *Marin VP, Pytynia KB, Langstein HN et al. Serum cotinine concentration and wound complications in Head and Neck Reconstruction. Plast Reconstr Surg 2008; 121: 451.*
2. *Seccareccia F, Zuccaro P, Pacifici R et al. Serum cotinine as a marker of environmental tobacco smoke exposure in epidemiological studies: The experience of the MATISS project. Eur J Epidemio 2003; 18: 487.*

38. The correct response is E

The first successful kidney transplant was performed by a plastic surgeon, Dr. Joseph Murray on a 24-year-old man with chronic glomerulonephritis who agreed to undergo a kidney transplant with the donor kidney from his identical twin brother. Since then transplantation between identical twins has continued to be used in plastic surgery.

Many organs and tissues have been successfully transplanted since then including small bowel, haematopoietic cells, ovarian cortical tissue, liver, pancreas, full thickness skin grafts, prepuce and bladder grafts for hypospadias repair and lately perforator flaps for breast reconstruction.

Reference:

1. *Allen Jr RJ, LoTempio MM, Craigie JE et al. Transplantation in identical twins: Another option for Breast Reconstruction. Plast Reconstr Surg 2008; 122: 1019.*
2. *Kortholm B. Transplantation between monozygotic twins. Scand J Plast Reconstr Surg 1968; 2: 64.*

39. Ans. D

Perforator based island flaps are widely used to reconstruct skin defects. Many methods are available to map the location and blood flow of a perforator. Indocyanine green angiography is effective for detecting the distribution of flap blood flow both intraoperatively and postoperatively. It is performed using Diagnogreen and a near-infrared video camera system. The location of the skin defect is determined and marked with a felt-tipped pen. When the target region comes in the territory of the femoral artery or brachial artery, 1 to 2 ml of an indocyanine green solution is administered intra-arterially.

Reference:

1. *Azuma R, Morimoto Y, Masumoto K et al. Detection of skin perforators by Indocyanine Green Fluorescence Nearly Infrared Angiography. Plast Reconstr Surg 2008; 122 (4): 1062–1067.*
2. *Eren S, Rubben A, Krein R et al. Assessment of microcirculation of an axial flap using indocyanine green fluorescence angiography. Plast Reconstr Surg 1995; 96: 1636.*

40. The correct response is D

Fat necrosis is a common complication arising after autologous breast reconstruction. This is seen after all types of autologous reconstruction including pedicled and free flaps. Fat necrosis is defined as an area of hardness within the adipose tissue, usually at the periphery of the flap, consisting of devitalized tissue caused by insufficient perfusion.

Ultrasound-Assisted liposuction is a safe, effective and reproducible modality for treatment of fat necrosis with stable long-term results. Direct surgical excision of the area of fat necrosis may require extensive dissection and lead to undesirable contour deformity. Standard liposuction is difficult because of the firm and fibrous nature of the necrotic tissue.

Reference:

1. *Hassa A, Curtis MS, Colakoglu S et al. Early results using Ultrasound-Assisted Liposuction as a Treatment for Fat Necrosis in Breast Reconstruction. Plast Reconstr Surg 2010; 126: 762–768.*
2. *Caterson SA, Tobias AM, Slavin SA et al. Ultrasound assisted liposuction as a treatment of fat necrosis after deep inferior epigastric perforator flap breast reconstruction: A case report. Ann Plast Surg 2008; 60: 614–616.*

41. The correct response is B

Nipple necrosis is a potential postoperative complication of breast surgery. There exists a great variation in the blood supply to the nipple and therefore it is advisable to include as many arteries in the pedicle as is possible.

The Wuringer ligament is a ligamentous suspension of the mammary gland. The lateral Wuringer ligament contains perforators and branches of the lateral thoracic artery. During mastopexy, the transected lateral vertical ligament of Wuringer is a useful guide for preserving the horizontal septum when breast tissue is removed.

Reference:

1. *Van Deventer PV, Graewe FR. Enhancing pedicle safety in Mastopexy and Breast Reduction Procedures: The Posteroinferomedial pedicle, Retaining the Medial Vertical Ligament of Wuringer. Plast Reconstr Surg 2010; 126: 786–793.*
2. *Wuringer E, Mader N, Posch E et al. Nerve and vessel supplying ligamentous suspension of the mammary gland. Plast Reconstr Surg 1988; 101: 1486–1493.*

42. The correct response is D

Palatal fractures are frequently associated with LeFort maxillary fractures in facial trauma. These present problems in diagnosis and if left untreated lead to malunion and malocclusion.

A number of surgical techniques have been described for the treatment of palatal fractures including 'K' wire fixation, interosseous wiring, acrylic palatal splints and lastly open reduction and internal fixation.

Intermolar wiring allows a simple, yet cost effective and time efficient method of treating palatal fractures. An arch bar is initially applied on the maxilla. A 24-gauge wire is then extended between the right and the left first or second molars to form a loop. The maxilla is then brought into occlusion with the mandible followed by tightening of this wire.

Open reduction and internal fixation has been advocated by many authors. The advantages of this technique are direct visualization of the fracture site, reduced length of intermaxillary fixation and avoidance of palatal splinting. However it is not easy to be certain whether accurate alignment and anatomical reduction has been achieved. There are other risks of developing malocclusion and hardware exposure. For these reasons, open reduction and internal fixation is considered to be a difficult and time consuming procedure for the treatment of palate fractures.

Maxilla with a palate fracture is unstable from side to side. Hence intermolar wiring provides the necessary stability and helps to push back the posterior fragments. Although it is less rigid than the plate and screw fixation, this technique provides stable fixation without the risk of hardware exposure.

Reference:

1. *Chen CH, Wang TY, Tsay PK et al. A 162-Case Review of palate fracture: Management strategy from a 10-Year experience. Plast Reconstr Surg 2008; 121: 2008.*
2. *Hendrickson M, Clark N, Manson PN et al. Palatal fractures: Classification, patterns, and treatment with rigid internal fixation. Plast Reconstr Surg 1998; 101: 319.*

43. Ans. D

Wide-awake flexor tendon repair in tourniquet-free unsedated patients permits intraoperative Total Active Movement examination (iTAMe) of the freshly repaired flexor tendons. This technique permits the intraoperative observation of tendon repair gapping induced by active movement when the core suture has been tied loosely. This allows the gap to be repaired at the time of surgery and this greatly reduces postoperative tendon repair rupture rates.

Wide-awake flexor tendon repair is performed without tourniquet and sedation by using pure locally injected lidocaine with epinephrine anaesthesia. During surgery these non-sedated cooperative patients are able to totally actively flex and extend their fingers while the surgeon examines the tendon repair site so that adjustments can be made before the skin is closed.

Primary repair of flexor tendons using pure local anaesthesia allows more advantages. Firstly it enables the surgeon to make intraoperative adjustments such as dividing pulleys and trimming or adding sutures to the repair so that the freshly repaired tendons glide through the sheath and pulleys for a full range of intraoperative active movement. Secondly the surgeon is much more confident of initiating a true active movement protocol postoperatively if he or she has seen the patient move the finger through full flexion and extension with no gapping during surgery. Thirdly the surgeon gets more than a full hour of uninterrupted time to talk to the non-sedated patient during the operation to assess the patient.

Reference:

1. *Higgins A, Lalonde DH, Bell M et al. Avoiding flexor tendon repair rupture with intraoperative total active movement examination. Plast Reconstr Surg 2010; 126: 941–945.*
2. *Lalonde DH. Wide-awake flexor tendon repair. Plast Reconstr Surg 2009; 123: 623–625.*

44. The correct response is C

Capsule contracture remains a major problem in patients with prosthetic implants of the breast especially if they have to go undergo irradiation. Research into this area has been limited due to non-availability of appropriate animal models.

Mice serves as an ideal animal model in this setting to study the effects of irradiation leading to capsular contracture. This model is the first of its kind to evaluate radiation to induce and live scan micro-computed tomography to evaluate the capsular contracture.

Rabbits and other animals have been used to study capsule contracture but fibrin glue was used to induce the contracture. However the use of fibrin glue to provoke capsular formation and contracture does not accurately replicate clinical conditions for prosthetic implantation.

The mouse is the only animal in which transgenic and knockout strains can be created.

Reference:

1. *Katzel EB, Koltz PF, Tierney R et al. A novel animal model for studying silicone gel-related capsular contracture. Plast Reconstr Surg 2010; 126: 1483–1491.*
2. *Ajmal N, Riordan CL, Cardwell N et al. Chemically assisted capsulectomy in the rabbit model: A new approach. Plast Reconstr Surg 2003; 112: 1449–1454.*

45. The correct response is D

Avotermin is the first of a new class of regenerative medicines that can reduce scarring when administered once or twice to the approximated wound margins of acute skin incisions.

Studies of the scar-free healing in fetuses have revealed that the transforming growth factor

(TGF) family of proteins plays a key role in scar formation. It has been shown that TGF-b3 is present at high levels in foetal skin wounds and low levels in adult wounds. Many reports have implicated that high levels of TGF-b3 promote scar-free healing in embryos.

Avotermin is human recombinant active TGF-b3 which is a prophylactic medicine under investigation for the improvement of scarring. This drug at 200 ng / 100 m/ linear centimeter wound margin, administered once or twice, produces significantly improved scar appearance. To date Avotermin is the only pharmacological agent to have shown improvement in scarring when compared to controls in a double-blind, randomized controlled clinical trial.

Reference:

1. Bush J, Duncan JAL, Bond JS et al. *Scar-improving efficacy of Avotermin administered into the wound margins of skin incisions as evaluated by a randomized, double blind, placebo controlled, phase II clinial trial. Plast Reconstr Surg 2010; 126: 1604–1615.*
2. O'Kane S, Ferguson MWJ. *Transforming growth factor betas and wound healing. Int J Biochem Cell Biol 1997; 29: 63–78.*

46. The correct response is C

Cocaine abuse leads to a host of nasal deformities. Cocaine can be administered through a variety of routes, but the intranasal route is the most common.

The nasal mucosa bears the brunt of the harmful effects of the cocaine. The intense vasoconstrictive effects of cocaine lead to varying degrees of damage to the nasal tract leading to mucosal ulceration, destruction of the septal cartilage and in extreme cases, destruction of the nasal and maxillary bones. Repeated constriction of the blood vessels of the nasal mucosa leads to soft-tissue and osteocartilaginous necrosis. The exposed septum also becomes infected and if left untreated, the ensuing chondritis causes a septal perforation. This perforation keeps on increasing in size with repeated cocaine insufflations.

Extensive septal defects often lead to external deformities, including a foreshortened nose with exposure of the nostrils and deviation of the nose to the patient's dominant hand use side. The contraction of the nasal lining further compounds the deformity leading to pulling of the nasal tip to one side. The collapse of septal cartilage alters the dorsal alignment of the upper lateral cartilages and septum with the nasal bones which leads to the appearance of a bony hump.

Surgical correction of this deformity is gratifying but it must be ensured that the patient has been cocaine-free for several years and committed to remaining free of cocaine use permanently. Surgical correction involves the use of established principles of rhinoplasty involving adequate dissection of the soft tissues and cephalic release and caudal advancement of the nasal lining. The costal cartilage is required to elongate the nasal frame.

Reference:

1. Guyuron B, Afooz PN. *Correction of Cocaine-Related nasal defects. Plast Reconstr Surg 2008; 121: 1015–1023.*
2. Slavin SA, Goldwyn RM. *The cocaine user: The potential problem patient for rhinoplasty. Plast Reconstr Surg 1990; 86: 436.*

47. The correct response is A

Contracture of the capsule remains a major problem following breast implantation in patients who undergo irradiation. Studies have suggested that these radiation injuries are a cascading process of cytokine activation with transforming growth factor TGF-b acting as the master switch.

The *TGF-b* signals through phosphorylation of Smad3, therefore to abate *TGF-b* induced capsular contracture, interruption of Smad3 is an important step.

Reference:

1. Katzel EB, Koltz PF, Tierney R et al. *The impact of Smad3 loss of function on TGF-b signaling and radiation-induced capsular contracture. Plast Reconstr Surg 2011; 127: 2263–2269.*
2. Brown KA, Pietenpol JA, Moses HL. *A tale of two proteins: Differential roles and regulation of Smad2 and Smad3 in TGF-beta signaling. J Cell Biochem 2007; 101: 9–33.*

48. The correct response is D

Gelsolin amyloidosis is also known as Meretoja's disease which is characterized by systemic amyloid deposition leading to early aging, bilateral progressive facial paralysis and corneal lattice dystrophy.

The first symptoms of this progressive disease appear in the third decade of life. In addition to degradation of the facial expressions due to progressive facial paralysis and looseness of skin, other problems include dryness and ulceration of the eyes along with loss of hair and dry itching skin.

The normal function of gelsolin protein is to prevent the toxic effects of actin and to allow the rapid migration of cells involved in wound healing, haemostasis and inflammation. The degradation products of gelsolin, build up in the tissues as amyloid which adheres to basement membranes, arterioles and nerves causing disturbance in their structure and function.

Operative treatment of gelsolin amyloidosis is symptomatic. Relentless disease progression makes the treatment challenging and necessitates frequent procedures. It is planned individually to meet the needs of the patient to relieve the most disturbing functional deficits.

Reference:

1. *Pihlamaa T, Rautio J, Kiuru-Enari S et al. Gelsolin amyloidosis as a cause of early aging and progressive bilateral facial paralysis. Plast Reconstr Surg 2011; 127: 2342–2351.*
2. *Rintala AE, Alanko A, Makinen J et al . Primary hereditary systemic amyloidosis (Meretoja's syndrome): Clinical features and treatment by plastic surgery. Scand J Plast Reconstr Surg Hand Surg 1988; 22: 141–145.*

49. The correct response is C

Transoral robotic surgery refers to the latest use of the da Vinci robot to resect deep seated tissues of the oral cavity in the area of the laryngopharynx, base of tongue and tonsillar region. It obviates the need of performing mandibulotomies or extensive neck dissections.

The system consists of a console at which the surgeon sits and a bedside 'slave' that holds the multiple robotic arms and a high resolution endoscopic camera. The da Vinci surgical system gives the surgeon access to the hypopharyngeal area which previously was possible by only using morbid access incisions.

This robot system can perform tissue resections in deep areas along with performing flap insetting. Microvascular anastomosis is performed by the surgeon himself after withdrawl of the robot from the field. Robot-assisted surgery can enhance the ability of the surgeon to treat larger and more complex defects that are located at inaccessible areas of the head and neck region.

Reference:

1. *Garfein ES, Greaney PJ, Easterlin B et al. Transoral robotic reconstructive surgery reconstruction of a tongue base defect with a radial forearm flap. Plast Reconstr Surg 2011; 127(6): 2352–2354.*
2. *Hockstein NG, O'Malley BW Jr, Weinstein GS. Assessment of intraoperative safety in transoral robotic surgery. Laryngoscope 2006; 116: 165–168.*

50. The correct response is C

Studies have demonstrated that human adipose-derived stromal cells (ASCs) are able to repair acute calvarial defects and not chronic calvarial defects.

Human adipose-derived stromal cells (ASCs) represent a multipotent stromal cell type with a proven capacity to differentiate along an osteogenic lineage. A critical-sized calvarial defect in the mouse is a reproducible and frequently utilized model for the study of cell based skeletal repair. It has been demonstrated that ASCs from mouse or human origin heal critical sized mouse cranial defects. A critical size (4 mm, parietal bone) mouse calvarial defect shows no healing without ASC engraftment up to 16 weeks after injury. However if human ASCs are seeded onto an osteoinductive scaffold, significant bony healing occurs in as little as 4 weeks after injury. This healing is mediated by expression of various types of BMP and other factors including platelet rich plasma which are found in the acute calvarial defects.

Reference:

1. *Levi B, James AW, Nelson ER et al. Acute skeletal injury is necessary for human adipose-derived stromal cell-mediated calvarial regeneration. Plast Reconstr Surg 2011; 127(3): 1118–1129.*
2. *Cowan CM, Shi YY, Aalami OO et al. Adipose-derived adult stromal cells heal critical-size mouse calvarial defects. Nat Biotechnol 2004; 22: 560–567.*

51. The correct response is B

PlasmaBlade incisions demonstrate reduced thermal injury depth, inflammatory response, and scar width in healing skin compared with electrosurgery.

The haemostatic control and dissection capabilities of conventional electrosurgical devices is fundamental to the practice of surgery. However the underlying mechanism of action in terms of thermal ablation of tissue is associated with thermal damage to tissues, reduced surgical precision and delayed wound healing.

The PEAK PlasmaBlade is a novel electrosurgical device that uses brief (~ 40 m sec), high frequency pulses of radiofrequency energy to induce the formation of electrical plasma along the edge of a thin, flat insulated electrode. With a burst rate of less than 1kHz, a typical duty cycle that does not exceed 5 percent and a very small exposed electrode surface, the operating temperature of the PlasmaBlade remains between 40°C and 100°C. This technology has been shown to effectively dissect ophthalmologic tissues as precisely as a scalpel with the haemostatic control of conventional electrosurgery, even when completely submerged in a liquid medium.

It has been shown that PlasmaBlade reduced acute thermal injury depth by 7 to 10 fold, decreased T-lymphocyte and macrophage / monocyte inflammatory cell response and produced an approximately 2.6 fold increase in wound burst strength after 6 weeks of healing. This resulted in superior scar formation compared with conventional electrosurgery.

These findings are consistent with the PlasmBlade's favourable effects on the human skin in improving healed scar width and strength besides others and demonstrates that PlasmaBlade provides useful advantages over conventional electrosurgery during human wound healing.

Reference:

1. *Ruidiaz ME, Messmer D, Atmodjo DY et al. Comparative healing of human cutaneous surgical incisions created by the PEAK PlasmaBlade, conventional electrosurgery, and a standard scalpel. Plast Reconstr Surg 2011; 128: 104–111.*
2. *Palankar DV, Miller JM, Marmor MF et al. Pulsed electron avalanche knife (PEAK) for intraocular surgery. Invest Ophthalmol Vis Sci 2001; 42: 2673–2678.*